OXFORD MEDICAL PUBLICATIONS

Oxford Manual of Major Incident Management

Oxford Manual of Major Incident Management

Paul Hunt
Consultant and Honorary Senior Lecturer in Emergency Medicine,
James Cook University Hospital, Middlesbrough, Cleveland, UK

Ian Greaves
Consultant and Honorary Professor in Emergency Medicine,
James Cook University Hospital, Middlesbrough, Cleveland, UK

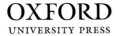

OXFORD
UNIVERSITY PRESS

Great Clarendon Street, Oxford, OX2 6DP,
United Kingdom

Oxford University Press is a department of the University of Oxford.
It furthers the University's objective of excellence in research, scholarship,
and education by publishing worldwide. Oxford is a registered trade mark of
Oxford University Press in the UK and in certain other countries

First Edition published 2017

Impression: 1

Published in the United States of America by Oxford University Press
198 Madison Avenue, New York, NY 10016, United States of America

British Library Cataloguing in Publication Data
Data available

Library of Congress Control Number: 2016960962

ISBN 978–0–19–923808–8

Printed and bound in China by
C&C Offset Printing Co., Ltd.

Foreword

A major incident is something no one wants but we are all expected and required to be prepared for. This book addresses both the preparation and practical management of major incidents in a way that is accessible to all who might be expected to respond. In an era when threats from previously unexpected sources are ever present, the potential for incidents involving novel agents and chemical, nuclear, biological, radiological, and environmental incidents must be planned for. This book caters for this. As recent events in West Africa have taught us, we must also be prepared for major or mass casualty events outside our own borders, with some of these involving real and ever-present threats to the safety of the healthcare personnel working in the environment. I commend this book to you.

Dr Bob Winter FRCP FRCA FFICM DM
National Clinical Director for Critical Care and
Emergency Preparedness, Resilience, and Response (EPRR)
Consultant in Intensive Care and Major Trauma
Medical Director East Midlands Ambulance Service

Preface

Currently, UK guidance and more generic information regarding the management of a major incident can be found scattered within a huge number of official publications and websites, as well as a relatively small number of published texts. Most of these are highly specific to certain types of incident, situations, or individual specialist groups. We believe that this book represents the first time that an attempt has been made to distil this information into a single volume and we are grateful to Oxford University Press for giving us the opportunity to do so. We accept that experts in all areas of major incident management will have a greater depth of knowledge in their own field than may be represented in this book, but we believe that there is a real need for a single source which draws together information across the whole field of Emergency Preparedness, Resilience, and Response at an appropriate level.

In many respects, this book has emerged from the large-scale review of the many materials in preparation of our previous book *Responding to Terrorism: A Medical Handbook* (Elsevier, 2011). However, it is fair to say that this volume has been far more challenging to complete and therefore has undergone a correspondingly long gestation period. Although there is no doubt that UK major incident management is highly professional and exceptionally well organized, it is also extremely complex. In some cases, the guidance provided is contradictory, in others, unclear. We have therefore in such areas of ambiguity attempted to offer logical advice which reflects the guidance available with a common-sense interpretation and in the correct context. Both authors have suffered acronym blindness on occasion—radiological incident management is especially full of often very similar and generally unhelpfully complex acronyms—and again we have tried to take a pragmatic approach.

Overall we hope that this book succeeds in bringing what will probably be familiar concepts and principles to the reader together with more useful original material and the most up-to-date guidance based on available published policies and the wider literature. Although we recognize that there will never be a 'one-size-fits-all' solution, our aim is to provide any professional who may be involved in a major incident with appropriately detailed and comprehensive directions on how to manage this as safely and effectively as possible.

Because this is the first book of its kind, we have had to take an authors' view regarding what to include. As a result, we will have included material some readers will think unnecessary and, more importantly, omitted material others may think essential. It is unfortunately inevitable that some expert readers will find errors in the coverage of their own fields, particularly those in which practices and procedures evolve quickly. A book such as this will always be something of a work in progress and we would be delighted to hear from readers with corrections or suggestions, which we will do our best to include in future editions.

PH
IG
2017

Contents

List of Abbreviations

AAIB	Air Accident Investigation Branch
ABI	Association of British Insurers
AC	ambulance commander
ACCOLC	Access Overload Control (telephone preference system, replaced by MTPAS)
ACP	access control point
ACPO	Association of Chief Police Officers
ACPOS	Association of Chief Police Officers in Scotland
AHVLA	Animal Health Veterinary Laboratories Agency
AIC	ambulance incident commander
ALARP	as low as reasonably possible
ALO	ambulance loading officer
ALP	ambulance loading point
ALSG	Advanced Life Support Group
APHA	Animal and Plant Health Agency
APO	ambulance parking officer
ARCC	Aeronautical Rescue Coordination Centre
ARS	acute radiation sickness
ATO	ammunition technical officer
ATOC	Association of Train Operating Companies
AWE	Atomic Weapons Establishment
BASICS	British Association of Immediate Care Schemes
BC	business continuity
BCM	business continuity management
BCP	business continuity plan
BHA	body holding area
BIA	business impact analysis
BIS	Department for Business Innovation and Skills
BLI	blast lung injury
BNFL	British Nuclear Fuels Ltd
Bq	becquerel (unit of radioactivity)
BRC	British Red Cross
BSE	bovine spongiform encephalopathy
BSM	bomb scene manager
BTP	British Transport Police
CAB	Citizens' Advice Bureau
CAC	community assistance centre
CAP	Central Assistance Programme
CasB	casualty bureau (also CB)
Cat 1	Category 1 responder (CCA)
Cat 2	Category 2 responder (CCA)
CB	casualty bureau
CBI	Confederation of British Industry

CBRN	chemical, biological, radiation, and nuclear
CBRNE	chemical, biological, radiation, nuclear, and explosive
CBT	cognitive behavioural therapy
CCA	Civil Contingencies Act 2004
CCC	Civil Contingencies Committee
CCDC	consultant in communicable disease control
CCG	clinical commissioning group
CCPB	Civil Contingencies Policy Branch (Northern Ireland)
CCS	casualty clearing station (sometimes CasCS) *or* Civil Contingencies Secretariat
CCTV	closed circuit television
CFOA	Chief Fire Officers' Association
CFOA – FST	Chief Fire Officers' Association Flood Support Team
CFRA	Chief Fire and Rescue Advisor
CGERT	Central Government Emergency Response Training Course
CI	critical infrastructure
CICA	Criminal Injuries Compensation Authority
CISD	critical incident stress debriefing
CLG	communities and local government
CLP	casualty landing point
CMG	crisis management group
CMO	Chief Medical Officer
CNC	Civil Nuclear Constabulary
CNI	Critical National Infrastructure
CNPA	Civil Nuclear Police Authority
COBR	Cabinet Office Briefing Room (sometimes COBRA)
COLP	City of London Police
COMAH	Control of Major Accident Hazards regulations 1999 (amended 2005)
CONCC	Cabinet Office News Coordination Centre
COSSH	Control of Substances Hazardous to Health
CP	contact premises (animal disease outbreak)
CPNI	Centre for the Protection of National Infrastructure
CPRB	Counter Pollution and Response Branch (of Maritime and Coastguard Agency)
CPS	Crown Prosecution Service
CRC	community recovery committee
CRIP	common recognized information picture
CRO	coast guard rescue officer
CRR	Community Risk Register
CRT	coastguard rescue teams
CSA	Chief Scientific Advisor
CT	counter terrorism
CTC	counter terrorism command
CTA	Chief technical advisor
CTSA	counter terrorism security advisor
CTU	Counter Terrorism Unit

CVO	Chief Veterinary Officer
CVS	Councils for Voluntary Service
DA	devolved administration
DCLG	Department for Communities and Local Government
DCLG-RED	Department for Communities and Local Government-Resilience Emergencies Division
DCMS	Department for Culture Media and Sport
DDM	designated disaster mortuary
DECC	Department for Energy and Climate Change
Defra	Department for Environment, Food and Rural Affairs
DEPZ	detailed emergency planning zone
DERC	Disease Emergency Response Committee
DfT	Department for Transport
DH	Department of Health
DipIMC	Diploma in Immediate Care
DIS	Defence Intelligence Staff
DNSR	Defence Nuclear Safety Regulator (now part of the DSA)
DPH	Director of Public Health
DRH	designated receiving hospital
DRT	disease reporting team
DSA	Defence Safety Agency (incorporates the DNSR)
Dstl	Defence Scientific and Technical Laboratories
DTI	Department for Trade and Industry
DVI	disaster victim identification
EA	Environment Agency
EC	European Commission
ECC	emergency control centre
ECS	enhanced command support
EC- RRG	Electronic Communications – Resilience and Response Group
ECSO	enhanced command support officer
EDPRT	Exotic Disease Policy Response Team (Defra)
EDW	extended direct warning
EET	emergency executive team
EFAS	Emergency Financial Assistance Scheme
EHO	environmental health officer
EMP	electromagnetic pulse
EOC	emergency operations centre
EOD	emergency ordnance disposal
EP	evacuation point
EPA	emergency planning advisor
EPC	Emergency Planning College
EPD	electronic personal dosimeter
EPIC	Emergency Procedures Information Centre managed by British Airways
EPRR	Emergency Preparedness, Resilience and Response
ERICPD	elimination, reduction, isolation, control, PPE, and discipline

EUSF	European Union Solidarity Fund
ExclZ	exclusion zone
FBP	forward briefing point
FAC	forward ambulance commander *or* family assistance centre—now humanitarian assistance centre
FBP	forward (media) briefing point
FC	fire commander
FCO	Foreign and Commonwealth Office
FCP	forward command post *or* forward control point
FFC	forward fire commander *or* flood forecasting centre
FFRC	family and friends reception centre (see FRRC)
FGS	flood guidance statement
FIC	forward incident commander
FIMC	fellowship in immediate care
FLC	family liaison coordinator
FLO	family liaison officer
FMBP	forward media briefing point
FMD	foot and mouth disease
FOB	forward operating base
FOC	freight operating company
FPC	forward police commander
FRCO	Flood Rescue Concept of Operations
FRNEP	Flood Rescue National Enhancement Programme
FRRC	families and relatives reception centre
FRS	fire and rescue service
FRSNCC	Fire and Rescue Service National Coordination Centre
FSA	Food Standards Agency
FST	flood support team
FTA	Freight Transport Association
FWD	Flood Warnings Direct
GCS	Glasgow Coma Scale
GCSA	Government Chief Scientific Advisor
GDS	Government Decontamination Service
GLO	government liaison officer
GLT	government liaison team
GO-Science	Government Office for Science
GRA	generic risk assessment
GSM	Global System for Mobile Communications
GTA	government technical advisor
GTPS	Government Telephone Preference Service
Gy	gray (unit of absorbed energy from radiation)
HA	Highways Agency
HAA	holding audit area
HAADR	holding and audit area for deceased people and human remains
HAC	humanitarian assistance centre
HACMG	Humanitarian Assistance Centre Management Group

HALO	hospital ambulance liaison officer
HART	hazardous area response team
HAT	health advisory team
HAWG	Humanitarian Assistance Working Group
HAZMAT	hazardous materials
HEMS	Helicopter Emergency Medical Service
HITS	high-integrity telecommunications system
HLS	helicopter landing site
HMCG	Her Majesty's Coastguard
HO	Home Office
HPA	Health Protection Agency (now Public Health England)
H&S	Health and Safety
HSE	Health and Safety Executive
HSWA	Health and Safety at Work Act
HTA	Human Tissue Authority
IAEA	International Atomic Energy Authority
IAH	Institute for Animal Health
ICC	incident coordination centre
ICP	incident control point or incident command post
IDB	Internal Drainage Boards
IED	improvised explosive device
IEM	integrated emergency management
IMG	Impact Management Group
INES	International Nuclear and Radiological Event Scale
IP	infected premises
IPCC	Independent Police Complaints Commission
IRMP	integrated risk management plan
IRP	incident response plan
IRR	Ionising Radiation Regulations 1999
ITU	intensive therapy unit
JARTS	Joint Aircraft Recovery and Transportation Squadron
JCC	Joint Coordination Centre
JDM	joint decision model
JESCC	Joint Emergency Services Control Centre
JESIP	Joint Emergency Services Intro-operability Programme
JSEC	Joint Services Emergency Control
JTAC	Joint Terrorism Analysis Centre
LA	local authority
LALO	local authority liaison officer
LD_{50}	[lethal dose] the dose of an agent which will cause death in 50% of those exposed to it.
LDCC	local disease control centre
LEMA	local emergency mortuary arrangement
LGA	local government association
LGD	lead government department
LHA	Local Highway Authority
LLFA	lead local flood authority

LRA	local resilience area
LRF	Local Resilience Forum
LSAM	large-scale agent model
LSI	life-saving interventions
MA	medical advisor or military assistant
MAAUG	Multi Agency Airwave User Group
MACA	Military Aid to the Civil Authority
MACC	Military Aid to the Civil Community
MACP	Military Aid to the Civil Power
MAFP	multi-agency flood plan
MAGD	Military Aid to a Government Department
MAIB	Marine Accident Investigation Branch
MBC	media briefing centre
MC	media centre
MCA	Maritime and Coastguard Agency
MCC	media communications cell
MCI	mass casualty incident
MEF	media emergency forum
MERIT	medical emergency response incident team
MERT	medical emergency response team
MFCG	mass fatality coordination group
MFP	mass fatality plan
MIA	medical incident advisor
MIC	medical incident commander
MilAAIB	Military Air Accident Investigation Branch
MIMMS	Major Incident Medical Management and Support
MIRG	Maritime Incident Response Group
MLO	media liaison officer/ military liaison officer
MLP	media liaison point
MOD	Ministry of Defence
MoU	memorandum of understanding
MPS	Metropolitan Police Service
MRC	marine response centre
MRCC	maritime rescue coordination centre
MRP	media rendezvous point
MRSC	HM Coastguard unit subordinate to a maritime rescue coordination centre (MRCC)
MTPAS	Mobile Telecommunication Privileged Access Scheme
NAIR	national arrangements for incidents involving radiation
NARU	National Ambulance Resilience Unit
National Health Service BT	NHS Blood and Transplant
National Health Service CB	NHS Commissioning Board
NATO	North Atlantic Treaty Organisation
NCAF	National Coordination and Advisory Framework
NCC	news coordination centre
NDA	Nuclear Decommissioning Authority
NDCC	National Disease Control Centre

NEAT	National Emergency Alert for Telecommunications
NEBR	Nuclear Emergency Briefing Room
NEEG	National Emergency Epidemiology Group
NEG	National Expert Group
NEMA	national emergency mortuary arrangements
NEPACC	National Emergency Planning Co-ordination Committee
NEPB	Nuclear Emergency Planning Board
NEP-C	National Emergency Plan for Communications
NEPDC	Nuclear Emergency Planning Delivery Committee
NEPLG	Nuclear Emergency Planning Liaison Group
NHS	National Health Service
NIA	Nuclear Installations Act 1965
NPIS	National Poisons Information Service
NPNG	National Police Nuclear Group
NR	Network Rail
NRA	National Risk Assessment
NRAT	National Resilience Assurance Team
NRE	National Resilience Extranet
NRL	National Reference Laboratory
NRR	National Risk Register
NSAT	National Strategic Advisory Team
NSRA	National Security Risk Assessment
NSWWS	National Severe Weather Warning Service
NTM	notice to move
NVASEC	National Voluntary Aid Society Emergency Committee
OCC	outbreak coordination centre
OIE	Office International des Epizooites
ONR	Office of Nuclear Regulation
ORR	Office of Rail Regulation
OSC	on-scene coordinator
PA	public address (system)
PAT	paediatric assessment team
PC	police commander
PDA	predetermined attendance
PFA	psychological first aid
PHE	Public Health England
PHE-CRCE	Public Health England- Centre for Radiation, Chemical and Environmental Hazards
PIM	post-incident manager
PIO	police incident officer
PLP	press liaison point
PMOC	police mortuary operations coordinator
PNICC	Police National Information Coordination Centre
POC	point of contact
PPE	personal protective equipment
PRPS	personal respiratory protection system
PSNI	Police Service of Northern Ireland (formerly Royal Ulster Constabulary)

PTE	passenger transport executive
PTSD	post-traumatic stress disorder
PWTG	Public Warning Task Group
PZ	protection zone
QC	Queen's Council
RA	risk assessment
RAF	Royal Air Force
RAG	Recovery Advisory Group
RAIB	Rail Accident Investigation Branch
RANET	IAEA's Global Response and Assurance Network
RAYNET	UK radio amateurs' emergency network
RC	rest centre
RCG	Recovery Coordinating Group
RDD	radiation dispersal device
ResCG	Response Coordinating Group
REPPIR	Radiation Emergency Preparedness and Public Information Regulations 2001
RFM	regional field manager
RIC	rail incident commander
RIO	rail incident officer
RLC	Royal Logistic Corps
RMU	radiation monitoring unit
RNLI	Royal National Lifeboat Institution
ROD	regional operations director
ROLO	rail operations liaison officer
ROTA	release other than attack
RoW	receiver of wreck
RPA	radiation protection advisor
RPS	radiation protection supervisor
RTC	road traffic collision (formerly RTA—road traffic accident)
RVP	rendezvous point (sometimes RvP)
RVS	Royal Voluntary Society (formerly WRVS—Women's Royal Voluntary Society)
RWG	recovery working group
RZ	restricted zone
SACP	scene access control point
SAG	Safety Advisory Group
SAGE	Scientific Advisory Group for Emergencies
SAR	search and rescue
SCBA	self-contained breathing apparatus
SCC	Strategic Coordination Centre
SCG	Strategic Coordination Group
SCU	salvage control unit
SECC	site emergency control centre
SEJD	Scottish Executive Justice Department
SERM	scene evidence recovery manager

SHA	strategic holding area
SIM	senior identification manager
SIO	senior investigating officer
SitRep	situation report
SMAC	Strategic Media Advisory Cell
SMC	Search and Rescue Mission Coordinator
SOP	standard operating procedure
SP	suspect premises
SPOC	single point of contact
SRC	shoreline response centre (sometimes survivor reception centre—more properly SuRC)
SRCG	Strategic Recovery Coordinating Group
SRO	senior responsible officer
SSPCA	Scottish Society for Prevention of Cruelty to Animals
STAC	Scientific Technical Advice Cell
SuRC	survivor reception centre
Sv	sievert (unit of equivalent dose of radiation)
TCG	Tactical Coordinating Group
TCZ	temporary control zone
TfL	Transport for London
TFWS	targeted flood warning service
TIC	toxic industrial chemical
TOC	train operating company
ToR	terms of reference
TSG	telecommunications sub-group
UHF	ultra-high frequency
UKAEA	UK Atomic Energy Authority
UN	United Nations
USAR	urban search and rescue
UXO	unexploded ordnance
VAS	voluntary aid societies (British Red Cross, St John and St Andrew Ambulances)
VENDU	Veterinary Exotic Notifiable Disease Unit
VHF	very high frequency or viral haemorrhagic fever
VIP	very important person (sometimes VVIP)
VSCPF	Voluntary Sector Civil Protection Forum
WIM	water incident manager
WRF	Wales Resilience Forum
WRVS	Women's Royal Voluntary Society, now the Royal Voluntary Society (RVS)

An Introduction to Major Incident Management

What is a major incident?

Emergency preparedness, resilience, and response (EPRR) principles encompass the full spectrum of prevention, amelioration, and management of significant incidents. The terminology is complex, but in general, a major incident may be defined as any incident which:

> 'requires the mobilization and use of extraordinary resources'.

The National Health Service defines a major incident as:

> 'any incident where the *location, number, severity* or *type* of *live* casualties requires *extraordinary* resources'.

Thus, in the most basic terms a major incident can be said to exist where the demand outweighs available resources. However, it should be remembered that some very significant incidents will not fall within this definition as the response, although large, will be adequate immediately an incident is declared and also, in most developed countries, it will simply be a matter of organization to ensure that an adequate response is made available in due course. This book outlines how such responses are organized as well as how resilience against such incidents can be developed.

The criteria that meet the conditions of a major incident will vary between the emergency services and an event which constitutes a major incident for one emergency responder will not necessarily constitute a major incident for another. For example, a devastating civilian aircraft crash with hundreds of fatalities will undoubtedly become a major incident for fire and rescue services, the police, and the local authorities but would not constitute a major incident for the health services. There are many ways of classifying incidents; an example is given in Box 1.1.

There are, importantly, a number of *official* definitions of a major incident; those used in the Civil Contingencies Act 2004 are shown on p. 3. This is the legislation which underpins UK civilian major incident responses.

Box 1.1 Classification system of major incidents

- Big bang: a suddenly occurring incident such as a bomb explosion or disaster caused by weather.
- Rising tide: a more slowly developing incident such as an epidemic.
- Cloud on the horizon: a serious threat developing elsewhere which might need preparatory action.
- Headline news: alarm amongst the general public or media regarding a real or perceived threat.
- Internal incidents: serious incidents within an organization such as a fire, major equipment failure, or loss of discipline or structure.
- Deliberate release of chemical, biological, or nuclear materials.
- Mass casualties: an overwhleming number and/or severity of casualties.
- Pre-planned major events that require planning and have the potential to result in a serious incident.

Part 1, Section 1 of the Civil Contingencies Act 2004

(1) In this Part "emergency" means—
   (a) an event or situation which threatens serious damage to human welfare in a place in the United Kingdom,
   (b) an event or situation which threatens serious damage to the environment of a place in the United Kingdom, or
   (c) war, or terrorism, which threatens serious damage to the security of the United Kingdom
(2) For the purposes of subsection (1)(a) an event or situation threatens damage to human welfare only if it involves, causes or may cause—
   (d) loss of human life,
   (e) human illness or injury,
   (f) homelessness,
   (g) damage to property,
   (h) disruption of a supply of money, food, water, energy or fuel,
   (i) disruption of a system of communication,
   (j) disruption of facilities for transport, or
   (k) disruption of services relating to health.
(3) For the purposes of subsection (1)(b) an event or situation threatens damage to the environment only if it involves, causes or may cause—
   (l) contamination of land, water or air with biological, chemical or radio-active matter, or
   (m) disruption or destruction of plant life or animal life
(4) A Minister of the Crown, or, in relation to Scotland, the Scottish Ministers, may by order—
   (n) provide that a specified event or situation, or class of event or situation, is to be treated as falling, or as not falling, within any of paragraphs (a) to (c) of subsection (1);
   (o) amend subsection (2) so as to provide that in so far as an event or situation involves or causes disruption of a specified supply, system, facility or service—
      i. it is to be treated as threatening damage to human welfare, or
      ii. it is no longer to be treated as threatening damage to human welfare
5) The event or situation mentioned in subsection (1) may occur or be inside or outside the United Kingdom.

Reference
http://www.legislation.gov.uk/ukpga/2004/36/section/1

Predictable special arrangements

In some cases, a major incident may result in demand for certain specialist resources which are already functioning at, or near to, full capacity. Examples may include:

- specialist adult burns centre beds
- specialist children's wards—paediatric intensive care units
- re-pressurization chambers for decompression illness treatment
- extracorporeal membrane oxygenation (ECMO) facilities.

Special arrangements could also be required for certain types of incidents, such as a radio-logical material release, where specialist teams and equipment may need to be called upon.

Mass fatalities

A very different response and set of resources will be required for situations where there are large numbers of fatalities, and relatively few injured. The events of 11 September 2001 in New York represent one example of this. While healthcare resources may not become over-stretched, the police and fire service teams will have a significant task in recovering and appropriately managing the dead. There is no specific number of casualties which is commonly used to define a mass fatality incident. The UK has special arrangements in place (see p. 162) for the handling of the mass fatalities.

Classification of major incidents

The conventional and most useful classification of major incidents uses the following system:
- Is the incident:
  - Natural versus man-made?
- Is it:
  - Simple versus compound?
- And is it:
  - Compensated versus uncompensated?

Natural versus man-made

Natural events include earthquakes, extreme weather events such as hurricanes, and severe flooding. Flooding may also be the result of seismic activity such as the Indian Ocean tsunami in 2004 and more recently the Japanese earthquake in 2011. Man-made events may include toxic industrial chemical releases (e.g. Bhopal, 1984), nuclear incidents (e.g. Chernobyl, 1986), or transportation incidents such as road, rail, or aircraft accidents.

The distinction between natural and man-made events can be difficult to distinguish, as a combination of factors may be responsible. For example, the bush fires in Australia in 2009 may have initially occurred due to human action while environmental factors, such as the local climate and weather conditions, continued to contribute to the ongoing incident.

Disaster or catastrophe?

The terms disaster and catastrophe are often used interchangeably when referring to compound uncompensated incidents where the scale of incident and the resources required often involve the organization and mobilization at a national, and in severe cases, international level.

Simple versus compound

During a simple incident, the local (or in severe cases, equally relevant to regional or national) infrastructure remains functional and effective allowing the movement of appropriate resources and transport of affected individuals. In compound incidents, the transportation, emergency services, supplies, and other infrastructure and capabilities are disrupted and ineffective.

However, what may start off as a simple incident may transform to a compound one over time as vital elements of infrastructure become overwhelmed or are additionally affected by progression of the incident or by consequences of human action, such as large-scale migration and subsequent congestion.

Compensated versus uncompensated

A compensated incident is one which can be managed by mobilizing available extra resources. For example, neighbouring emergency services are able to respond and contribute personnel or equipment to assist in the affected area. An uncompensated incident is one which cannot be managed even if every available resource is mobilized. Typical examples include natural disasters such as earthquakes or tsunamis, often requiring international assistance which will take some time to organize and deploy.

In the same way as simple versus compound definitions, an incident may transfer between compensated and uncompensated status as events unfold and the situation deteriorates, or improve as additional resources become available.

Chemical, biological, radiological, and nuclear (CBRN)

CBRN incidents are an important category of major incidents often requiring specific resources to manage effectively. These are discussed in more detail throughout Chapters 8–10. CBRN incidents may occur as a result of either deliberate or non-deliberate release.

Deliberate release

Intentional release may occur either as a component of terrorist activity or war fighting. Deliberate releases may involve the release of an agent, or agents, capable of injuring or causing disease and may arise from a variety of sources:
- Sabotage of industrial or nuclear establishments
- Acquisition of existing chemical or biological weapons
- Acquisition of radiological materials from industrial sources or medical facilities
- Novel production of chemical, biological, or biotoxin agents
- Much less likely, the detonation of an improvised or non-state-held nuclear device.

Non-deliberate release

Also referred to as 'release other than attack' (ROTA), these types of CBRN incident can occur for a number of reasons:
- Accidental causes such as incidents involving dangerous material transportation or potential sources such as failure of industrial site safety mechanisms or maintenance faults
- Collateral damage from incidents such as extreme weather, flooding, earthquake, tsunami, or transportation accidents
- Human error such as neglect, or unsafe or poor laboratory practices
- Secondary to combustion or blast causing the production of new hazardous materials or chemicals
- Unintentional detonation of a nuclear device.

Historical major incidents

Human migration to areas that provide reliable supplies of fresh water for consumption and crop irrigation, and natural areas of fertile land (often flood plains), as well as coastal regions for good access to transportation and fishing, has led to the development of many large population centres in areas at higher risk of flooding. This feature may be partly responsible for the observation that flooding, both from inland and seaborne sources such as tsunamis, is a major cause of natural disaster with subsequent loss of human life and material possessions.

History is replete with examples of natural disasters that, in modern terms, may not have actually constituted a major incident. However, despite the significant advances brought about by modern industry and technology, including an increased capacity and speed of transportation, many natural events are still responsible for major incidents due to their scale, distribution, or duration. Table 1.1 lists some examples of notable historic disasters listed by the geography and populations affected and enables basic comparisons to be drawn.

Table 1.1 Examples of notable historic disasters and major incidents

Date	Location	Incident	Dead	Injured
1556	Shaanxi, China	Earthquake	830,000[e]	
1755	Lisbon, Portugal	Earthquake	100,000[e]	
1888	Eastern Coast, USA	Blizzard	400[e]	
1913	Senghenydd coal mine	Explosion	439[c]	
1918–1920	Worldwide pandemic	Influenza	50–100 million[e]	
1931	Huang He River, China	Flooding		
1970	Huascarán, Peru	Avalanche	50,000[e]	
1977	Tenerife	Aircraft	583[c]	
1984	Bhopal, India	Chemical	11,000[e]	550,000[e]
1984	Ethiopia	Famine	1 million[e]	
1985	Mexico City, Mexico	Earthquake	10,000[e]	
1986	Chernobyl, Ukraine	Nuclear	82[e]	>2 million
1987	Zeebrugge, Belgium	Ferry	137[c]	402[c]
1988	Lockerbie, UK	Aircraft	270[c]	
1988	Piper Alpha, North Sea	Explosion	164[c]	25[c]
1989	Hillsborough, UK	Crush	96[c]	200[c]
1995	Tokyo, Japan	Chemical	12[c]	5000[e]
2001	New York, USA	Terrorist	2753[c]	6294[c]

[c] confirmed; [e] estimated.

Recent major incidents

Since 11 September 2001, terrorist atrocities have inevitably captured a large measure of the imagination of the media and public. Such events are memorable and the evil intent they demonstrate stands them in contrast to the apparently random workings of nature. However, for the majority of the human population, an environmental or transportation-related event is far more likely to be a cause of such problems. Table 1.2 lists some examples of notable disasters and major incidents that have occurred in the last decade (post '9/11').

Table 1.2 Examples of notable disasters and major incidents in the last decade

Date	Location	Incident	Dead	Injured
UK and Europe				
2003	European 'heat wave'	Climate	40,000[e]	
2005	London, UK	Bombings	52[c]	700[c]
2007	Grayrigg, Cumbria	Derailment	1[c]	88[c]
2011	Cumbria, UK	Shootings	13[c]	11[c]
2014	SW England	Flooding		
Worldwide				
2004	Indian Ocean	Tsunami	230,000[e]	
2010	Haiti	Earthquake	223,570[e]	
2011	Japanese Earthquake	Tsunami	15,188[c]	5337[c]
2014–2015	West Africa	Ebola[VHF] outbreak	11,000[e]	
2015	Nepal	Earthquake	9000[e]	23,000[e]
2015	Saudi Arabia (Hajj)	Crowd stampede	2200[e]	

[c] confirmed; [e] estimated; [VHF] viral haemorrhagic fever.

Nomenclature relating to major incidents

The first reaction to a potential major incident usually comes from a member of the public who has witnessed, or been involved in, the incident. In some cases, continuous monitoring systems may detect an event that might lead to an emergency in advance of public awareness, for example, seismic activity readings showing signs of a significant earthquake or routine radiation monitoring. However, in every case, local emergency services will be alerted and will attend the incident to assess the situation. If the incident meets the criteria for an emergency (as defined by the Civil Contingencies Act 2004) the first responder will report back through their command chain stating either '*Major incident—standby*' or, if it is clear that the emergency response will require extraordinary resources, '*Major incident—declared*'. The first responder will also provide an initial situational report after making a rapid assessment of the scene. The information required in this report is presented in a standardized format - METHANE (see below). Once declared, the immediate scene of the emergency and its surrounding area will be organized into defined zones and cordons, as described below.

Major incident scene situational report

M: Major incident 'Standby' or 'Declared'
    My call-sign/name/assignment
E: Exact location/grid reference
T: Type of incident, e.g. rail, chemical
H: Hazards encountered or potential
A: Access routes in and out, and other limiting factors
N: Number, type, and severity of casualties (usually estimated on initial notification)
E: Emergency services present, and required.

Note: the METHANE report should be sent to command as soon as possible in order for an appropriate response to be coordinated. Where information is missing or incomplete, a best estimate should be provided. Information should be regularly updated and, as the situation develops, further METHANE reports sent to command (See also: Chapter 3, p. 62).

Operational ('bronze')

The operational (bronze) zone consists of the area in the immediate vicinity of the incident and will usually include all casualties resulting directly or indirectly from the mechanism involved (see Figure 1.1). The operational (bronze) zone is bordered by the inner cordon, access across which will be restricted to emergency services personnel involved in the recovery and treatment of casualties, or control of the incident. It is not always necessary to clearly mark the inner cordon unless a specific hazard exists or in order to protect the scene of a suspected crime.

Control and safety in the operational (bronze) zone is the responsibility of the fire or police service, depending upon the circumstances and nature of an ongoing hazard.

Multiple operational (bronze) zones may exist, for example, surrounding each separate train carriage following a railway collision and de-railing incident or surrounding the immediate vicinity of each of several explosive devices that may have detonated in separate locations within a town centre.

Tactical ('silver')

The tactical (silver) zone includes the operational (bronze) zone, or multiple operational (bronze) zones, within an area the size of which is dependent on the hazard. The tactical (silver) zone includes the whole incident site. This would surround the entire site of an incident, as illustrated in Figures 1.2 and 1.3.

The tactical (silver) zone is bordered by the outer cordon. Entry and exit through the outer cordon is strictly controlled and is usually the responsibility of the police service. As with operational (bronze), more than one tactical (silver) zone may be required in order to cover a wide geographical distribution of separate incidents such as may occur due to a national disaster or from a coordinated terrorist attack.

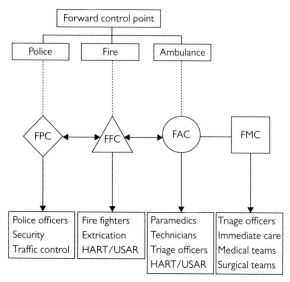

Fig. 1.1 Command structure—bronze.

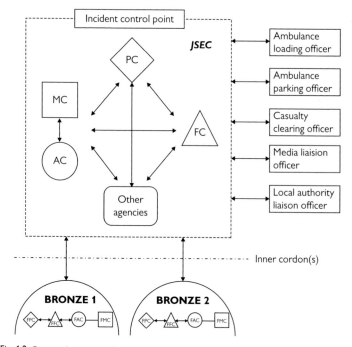

Fig. 1.2 Command structure—silver.

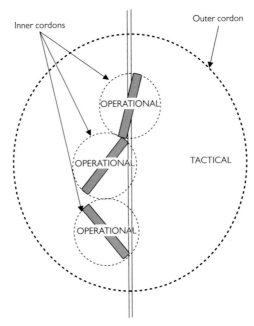

Fig. 1.3 Graphical representation of zones and cordons associated with a major incident: illustrated example of a rail crash incident with three carriages involved. Note: Conventional Joint Emergency Services Inter-operability Programme (JESIP) map marking symbols should be used in preparing site maps (see pp. 222–8).

Strategic ('gold')

The strategic (gold) 'zone' exists as a notional rather than geographical entity and represents the senior command level. It is usually located in a regional or national command centre. Senior commanders from each of the emergency services will be based in strategic (gold) in order to coordinate the response to the incident and to ensure that necessary resources are prepared and mobilized appropriately. There is normally only one strategic (gold) level for any given incident.

Grand Strategic ('platinum')

Theoretically, grand strategic (platinum) command would refer to an overarching structure or administrative level that would be in overall command of a coordinated multiagency, multiregional, or international response. In most cases, the national response is coordinated by the Cabinet Office Briefing Room. Such a high level of command might be necessary in the case of a disseminated threat or national disaster, as well as to coordinate and facilitate international assistance. However, the term is rarely used in practice.

Special cases

Where an incident may have included a 'conventional' mechanism, such as firearms or explosives use, or 'unconventional' mechanism, such as CBRN hazards, a number of special terms may be applied to zones and cordons. Zones may be referred to as 'hot', 'warm', or 'cold' depending upon the risk of exposure to any potential hazards. The number, size, and shape of these zones will depend upon multiple factors such as the type, form, and distribution of the hazard. It will also depend upon environmental factors such as weather conditions including sunlight, prevailing wind speed and direction, and the geographical layout of the surrounding ground or buildings, including drainage, elevation, and access.

Military nomenclature

In contrast to civilian terminology, the UK armed forces refer to bronze level as '*tactical*', and silver as '*operational*'. The military use 'tactics' to refer to the methodology employed to undertake missions or achieve objectives on the ground (or in air/water), and 'operations' to refer to the larger organization of forces within a defined area (i.e. the area of operations). As with civilian nomenclature, gold refers to the strategic level of command.

Hot zone (non-permissive)

The hot zone will normally comprise the area of highest risk such as the site of a toxic chemical spill or where there is an ongoing possibility of explosion. The hot zone may extend considerably beyond the immediate location of the hazard due to dispersion by wind or water (e.g. the run-off from efforts to control fire) or where the ongoing risk is mobile, such as a firearms incident. Movement into and within the hot zone will be restricted to a minimal number of necessary personnel and only those wearing appropriate personal protective equipment (PPE) such as full CBRN suits and self-contained breathing apparatus (SCBA). Treatment of casualties will not usually be undertaken within the hot zone and, if required, will be limited to life-saving interventions (LSI) only. The objective will be to remove casualties into areas of comparatively lower risk for further treatment and formal decontamination.

Warm zone (semi-permissive)

The warm zone extends to contain the area of increased risk and is bordered by the inner cordon and thus conventionally lies within the operational (bronze) area. Its size and shape are also dependent upon the threat itself and environmental conditions. For example, in the case of a CBRN incident the warm zone will usually extend in the opposite direction to the prevailing wind. Within the warm zone there may still be risk of contamination from hazardous materials although at a level that may allow initial triage and provision of life-saving treatment. Movement within the warm zone will still be restricted to authorized emergency services personnel wearing appropriate PPE. Casualties will usually be moved to the cold zone before definitive treatment and, where appropriate, will undergo decontamination when crossing the inner cordon.

Cold zone (permissive)

The cold zone will comprise those areas of the incident which are at minimal risk of contamination from the spread of, or exposure to, hazardous materials. Movement within the cold zone is not usually restricted to emergency services personnel or those wearing specific PPE. Where required, patients will have undergone decontamination before arrival in the cold zone. The threat in this zone is minimal for any given risk—anything from marauding firearms to chemical contamination.

See Figure 1.4 for a graphical representation of these zones.

Associated issues

The boundaries of the cold, warm, and hot zones are inherently mobile depending upon the extent or spread of the hazard(s) and changeable environmental conditions. For example, if the wind direction were to change, the threat from a potentially airborne chemical agent may require realignment of the hot/warm zones in order to take this into account.

Safe entry and exit to and from the hot/warm zones must be undertaken with care in order to minimize risk from exposure to downwind hazards. Figure 1.5 illustrates the best method of evacuation from downwind of the hot zone. The fastest method of evacuation is to traverse in a direction at 90 degrees to the wind direction until safely out of the 'plume' zone—a minimum distance of 400m is advised.

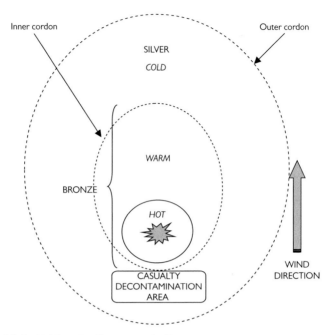

Fig. **1.4** Graphical illustration of hot, warm, and cold zones.

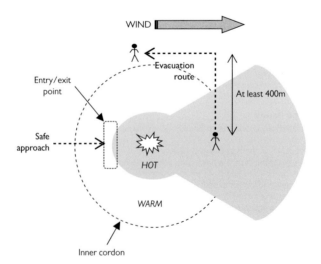

Fig. **1.5** Safe evacuation from downwind hazard (hot/warm to cold zone).

Joint Emergency Services Inter-operability Programme (JESIP)

JESIP focuses on the inter-operability of the emergency services, recognizing that the response to a major incident is a multiagency activity involving collaboration with other Category 1 and 2 responders. JESIP provides a doctrine which defines common terminology, principles, and ways of working. This approach can be applied to small-scale incidents, wider emergencies, and pre-planned operations. Commanders at every level must be able to demonstrate that they have received inter-operability training and are capable of applying the JESIP principles to both preparation and response activities.

The principles for joint working include the following:

- Co-location: allowing commanders to perform functions of command, control, and coordination, face-to-face, at a single and easily identifiable location. This will normally be known as the forward command post (FCP), located near to the scene.
- Communication: ensuring the passage of clear, unambiguous, and timely information relevant to the situation.
- Coordination: integration of priorities, resources, decision-making, and response activities of each emergency service. This avoids conflicts or duplication of efforts and minimizes risk. In order to facilitate this, one service will usually act in a 'lead' capacity, such as chairing coordination meetings. The lead service will usually be the police service.
- Joint understanding of risk: arising from threats and/or hazards which will be seen, understood, treated, or tolerated by each service differently depending upon the nature of the risk and potential control measures. Sharing this information at every level will ensure, as far as reasonably possible, that agreed aims and objectives will not be compromised.
- Shared situational awareness: common understanding of circumstances and immediate consequences of the emergency together with an appreciation of the available resources, capabilities, and priorities for the response. This can be achieved by using the Joint Decision Model (JDM) as described in the following section.

Joint Decision Model

Different organizations have a range of decision-making processes. The JDM has been developed to bring together available information, reconcile objectives, and allow the making of effective joint decisions by commanders from different organizations (see Figure 1.6.) Strict adherence to the JDM must be secondary to the need to achieve desired outcomes, especially in rapidly changing situations. The JDM is organized around three primary considerations:

- Situation
- Direction
- Action.

Situation describes what is happening, the potential risks and impacts, and what is currently being done in response. This may be described as situational awareness. *Direction* refers to the desired end-state and is made up of collective aims and objectives along with overarching values and priorities for the emergency response. *Action* refers to what needs to be done to achieve the desired end-state. Courses of action must be considered and a clear decision made and communicated to the responding organizations.

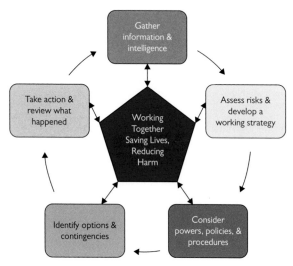

Fig. 1.6 The Joint Decision Model.

Objectives of major incident management

The effective management of major incidents relies upon successful coordination of, and liaison between, central and regional government and all emergency services and will therefore benefit from prior emergency planning. Sites at significant risk of a major incident, such as industrial complexes, nuclear installations, or airports, will present specific hazards for which major incident responses must be tailored to the available local emergency resources and environment in which they will be required to function.

Additional agencies which may be involved in the response to a major incident include local authorities, industrial and military organizations, as well as volunteer groups. A single unifying emergency response plan must therefore bring together all the relevant agencies to ensure effective management of the incident. Conducting regular 'table-top' and practical major incident exercises to test emergency plans will enable their refinement in order to ensure the most effective use of resources and to constructively highlight areas where such plans may be improved.

It is essential that each of the emergency services has well-defined responsibilities and objectives that will guide individual and combined components of the response to a major incident. The responsibilities of each of the emergency services are discussed further in Chapter 4.

The main objectives for all emergency services in the event of a major incident may be summarized as shown in Box 1.2.

Box 1.2 Objectives of an effective combined response to major incidents

Primary
- Save life and relieve suffering
- Prevent escalation of the incident
- Protect property and the environment
- Restore normality
- Deal with fatalities.

Secondary
- Facilitate enquiries from the public/media.

Phases of a major incident

There are three main phases of a major incident (see Figure 1.7).

Preparation

Prevention of incidents may be brought about by enforcement of legislation, such as transportation laws or crowd safety measures in sports stadia. Some natural incidents may be anticipated or other endemic hazards known about. Effective preparation will require appropriate planning, procurement of necessary equipment, and training (education and exercises).

Resilience is the term used to describe how well prepared an institution, organization, or population is to deal with any potential incidents.

Response

Each of the emergency services must function together and carry out their individual responsibilities within a well-coordinated system in order to provide effective scene management and to deal with multiple casualties, while preventing further escalation of the incident.

Effective scene management requires that a structured 'all-hazards' approach be followed, irrespective of the nature of the incident (see p. 20).

Recovery

Recovery following a major incident may take days, weeks, or even years although each service will experience the recovery phase differently. Healthcare resources may be able to recover within a few days while a community may take years to come to terms with a devastating local incident.

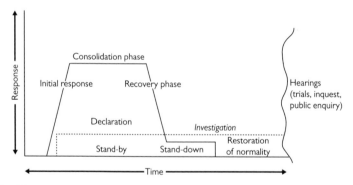

Fig. 1.7 The phases of a major incident.

Outline of casualty management

The 'all-hazard' approach is generally accepted as the most appropriate at the scene of a major incident, and can be utilized by all emergency services commanders. The generic casualty management paradigm has been developed and evaluated extensively with training provided by the Major Incident Medical Management and Support courses (MIMMS, Advanced Life Support Group (ALSG)) throughout the UK, Australia, and Europe.

The *all-hazard* approach involves seven key principles:
- Command and control
- Safety
- Communication
- Assessment
- Triage
- Treatment
- Transport.

A variation on this approach is recommended for the management of major incidents where there is suspicion, or evidence, of CBRN involvement. This is discussed further in Chapters 8–10.

Command and control

Command and control are vital to restore order to what may well be a chaotic scene at the outset of a major incident. It is vitally important that this takes place as rapidly and effectively as possible (see Figure 1.8).

Command

Each of the emergency services will have commanders working at various levels within their own hierarchy. Operational (bronze) area commanders will report up to their tactical (silver) commanders who will then report up to their strategic (gold) commanders. Command is therefore the vertical transmission of authority, within each emergency and support service.

Each service will have one individual taking the role of overall commander and will be identifiable by specific clothing or PPE. Scene commanders from each of the services will normally appoint a 'forward' commander to manage each operational (bronze) area. They will provide regular situational reports and pass on requests for further resources or personnel as required within their team.

Control

When overall responsibility falls to one service at the scene (e.g. the police at the outer cordon), this service can be said to have control of the scene. Control therefore refers to the horizontal transmission of authority, across the emergency and support services. This horizontal communication enables requests for further resources or personnel to be made between services in a coordinated and controlled manner. Each incident will have one individual in overall control of the scene.

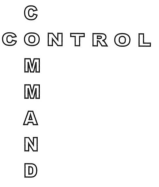

Fig. 1.8 Command and control—vertical and horizontal authority.

Safety

Safety is of vital importance and should include consideration of the individual (self), the environment (scene), and of casualties (survivors).

Self

Personal safety is of primary importance and includes the wearing of appropriate PPE, familiarity with necessary equipment (especially machinery or vehicles), and knowledge of the potential risks and hazards at the scene.

Scene

Scene safety can be achieved by establishing effective command and control, including the use of cordons. Access to the scene must be strictly limited to appropriately protected emergency service personnel.

Existing hazards, such as fire or a toxic chemical spill, will need to be managed as appropriate. Sufficient safe distances must be maintained from any hazards, including the consideration of local geography, built-up environment, and weather conditions.

Survivors

Safety of survivors will depend upon preventing escalation of the incident and providing necessary protection from scene hazards as well as the weather and climate conditions. Uninjured survivors should be guided to a place of safety and shelter as soon as possible, using appropriate evacuation routes.

Injured survivors will require recovery by emergency services, especially in the case of entrapment or immobility.

Communication

Effective and reliable methods of communication must be established early on during the response to a major incident. Modern technology should provide a number of effective methods for communication although more basic alternatives should also be considered in case these are overwhelmed or fail to function, perhaps due to the incident itself. Unfortunately, report after report continues to demonstrate that failure of communication is the commonest reason for a substandard response and incompatibility between communications systems remains unfortunately frequent. Regular person-to-person liaison is also recommended with senior commanders ideally being co-located.

Common methods of communication include:

- radio networks (e.g. VHF or UHF)
- telephone (cellular or landline)
- runners
- pager
- loud-hailer
- hand signals
- public announcement systems
- television and radio broadcasts

These are covered in more detail in Chapter 7.

Assessment

Assessment is required of both scene and casualties. (See Figure 1.9.)

Scene

An initial rapid assessment of the incident scene should be carried out by the first emergency services responder, and a report passed back to ambulance control as soon as possible—as detailed on p. 62.

Assessment should be a continuous process that enables information to be updated regularly as the incident evolves in order to ensure appropriate resources will be provided and the incident continues to be managed effectively.

Casualties

Both a global and individual casualty view will be required, with a general estimate of the number and type of casualties provided to senior commanders as well as more specific information to facilitate the work of treatment teams in the forward areas. It is essential that clinical features and patterns of injury or illness are regularly reported so that any characteristics of a CBRN incident may be detected and managed appropriately.

Assessment of casualties will require trained medical personnel to work in forward areas, which may require the use of bulky or obstructive PPE making this task much more difficult. It is important that casualties are assessed and prioritized in a simple and rapid manner to ensure timely evacuation and intervention. A process such as the triage sieve is therefore recommended.

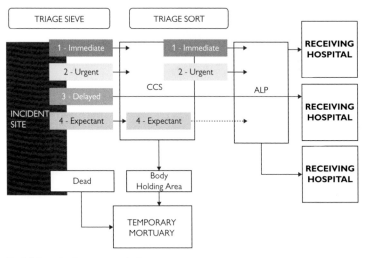

Fig. 1.9 Example of at-scene casualty flow.

Triage and categorization systems

Triage in the context of major incident management refers to the assessment and categorization of multiple casualties according to clinical need. This process requires the use of a reproducible, repeatable, rapid, and user-friendly algorithm that uses easily derived measures such as pulse rate or capillary refill time. Triage should also be repeated for individual casualties each time they are moved or a significant clinical intervention is performed.

Different triage systems may be required for different zones (zonal triage) and usually involves the use of a 'sieve' or 'sort' mechanism.

Triage sieve

The triage sieve is the most commonly used rapid triage tool and is usually the primary triage system used during major incidents. The sieve enables emergency services to identify numbers of, and to prioritise resources for, the most seriously injured casualties. The uninjured and 'walking wounded' can then be identified and assisted clear of the incident location allowing medical teams to concentrate their efforts on the remaining casualties.

An example of the triage sieve is shown in Figure 1.10.

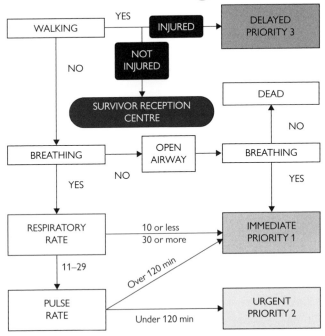

Fig. 1.10 Example of a triage sieve (MIMMS, ALSG).

Triage sort

The triage sort is intended to be a more sophisticated method of assessment and categorization. The system in Figure 1.11 is one example. As can be seen, it requires more precise physiological measurements such as the Glasgow Coma Scale (GCS), blood pressure, and respiratory rate. As a consequence, it is time-consuming and requires a significant level of clinical skill. It is inevitably poorly reproducible with significant variation between scorers. The triage sort is therefore potentially used to prioritize casualties for evacuation if sufficient resources and manpower are available. This will usually take place in the casualty clearing station. As an alternative, the sieve may be repeated or the patient may be categorized using the judgement of an appropriately skilled and experienced clinician.

The triage sort		
PHYSIOLOGICAL VARIABLE	**VALUE**	**SCORE**
Respiratory rate	10–29 >29 6–9 1–5 0	4 3 2 1 0
Systolic blood pressure	>90 76–89 50–75 1–49 0	4 3 2 1 0
Glasgow Coma Scale Score	13–15 9–12 6–8 4–5 3	4 3 2 1 0
Total score for coding (see box below)		**X**

Coded score	Priority
1–10	T1
11	T2
12	T3
0	Dead

Fig. 1.11 The triage sort. Reproduced from Greaves, Ian, and Hunt, Paul, *Oxford Handbook of Pre-Hospital Care*, 2007, with permission from Oxford University Press.

Other methods

Other methods of triage are being developed which may be more accurate and reproducible and those systems based on the shock index (heart rate/systolic blood pressure) show some promise. A number of commercial systems are also in use, although of no evident benefit compared to the conventional sieve and sort. (See Figure 1.12.)

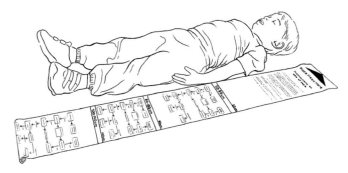

Fig. 1.12 Example of a triage system for children: The Paediatric Triage Tape. Reproduced with permission from *Emerg Med J* 2006;23:47–50 doi:10.1136/emj.2005.024893 "Validation of Paediatric Triage Tape" and from original publication "Paediatric Triage Tape" Hodgetts TJ, Hall J, Maconochie I, et al. *Pre-Hospital Immediate Care* 1998; 2:155–9.

Casualty treatment

The treatment of casualties normally takes place at three main locations:
- At point of injury (*Operational/Bronze*)
- Casualty clearing station (*Tactical/Silver*)
- Receiving hospitals.

If stable for transportation, casualties will generally be moved to the casualty treatment centre although they may receive life-saving or life-sustaining treatment at point of injury or prior to extraction from the operational (bronze) zone. This may be complicated by issues of access or entrapment, requiring the assistance of fire crews and specialist lifting or extrication equipment. Due to potential delays involved, care of casualties may need to be instituted and maintained *in situ*.

Treatment in the operational (bronze) zone is most frequently provided by paramedics although it may also be provided by fire crews, specific pre-hospital emergency response teams (e.g. MERIT), or hazardous area response teams (HART), especially in the case of CBRN incidents. Depending on the size and nature of the incident, treatment at the casualty clearing station will be provided by paramedics, doctors, and nurses. Apparently uninjured victims will be monitored at a specific location.

Introduction to roles and responsibilities

A brief summary of the roles and responsibilities of each of the emergency services is outlined in this topic. A much more detailed description of each of these is provided in Chapter 4.

Fundamentally, the priority of all emergency and health services during a major incident will be saving life, prevention of escalation of the incident, and establishment of appropriate forward control units to initiate and maintain a coordinated and timely response.

Liaison with regular and robust communication between services is essential, the organization of which is illustrated in Figure 1.13.

Fire service

The main responsibilities of the fire service include the rescue of entrapped casualties (or recovery of the dead) and saving of life, eliminating hazards, and fighting fires, as well as clearing routes in and out of any wreckage. The fire service will also provide specialist resources such as lighting and lifting equipment or shelter.

Police service

The police service will generally have overall control at the scene of a major incident although will often give control of the immediate incident zone (i.e. within the inner cordon) to the fire service in the presence of a specific hazard such as fire or chemical spill.

The police service will primarily be responsible for security and control of the scene including setting up cordons, limiting public access, and protecting the environment and property. Specific functions include evacuation and care of uninjured survivors, maintaining records of casualties, and identification of dead victims. The police service will also carry out relevant criminal investigations and assist with official enquiries, as well as liaison with the media.

Health service

The main responsibilities of health service personnel include the saving of life, prevention of further injury, and relief of suffering. Specific responsibilities include the mobilization of necessary medical resources and treatment facilities (e.g. casualty clearing station) and organization of evacuation and transport of casualties including selection of appropriate receiving hospitals.

Ambulance services may also be supplemented by additional pre-hospital care resources including the provision of triage, advanced medical procedures such as surgery to facilitate extrication (e.g. limb amputation), and prolonged field care. Medical incident advisors will have a role in coordinating the use of local and regional healthcare resources and ensuring appropriate dispersal of casualties to available treatment facilities which may include specialist centres.

Support services

Support services include both professional and voluntary services such as HM Coastguard, the military, local authorities, and various voluntary societies. All of these may have a role in the initial phase of the major incident response as well as a longer-term role in support of the recovery process.

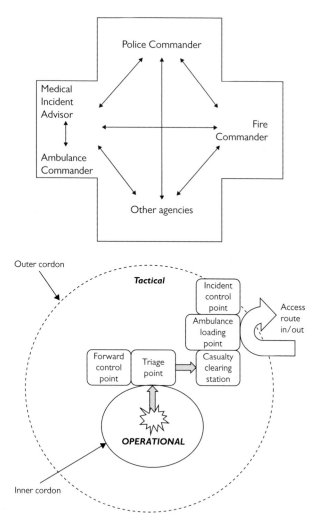

Fig. 1.13 The cross of communication.

Casualty transportation

Responsibility for casualty transport lies with the health service command and control structure. Transportation routes and access to and from the scene must be taken into consideration in order to organize evacuation safely and effectively. Ongoing triage and treatment will have direct effects upon the required order, mode, and destination of evacuation. Priority of evacuation is usually the same as priority immediately following treatment. Coordination of resources will require good communication between triage, treatment, and evacuation ('ambulance loading') officers. A designated medical incident advisor (or alternatively, an appropriately experienced ambulance officer or MERIT practitioner) will be required to ensure organization of casualties into groups by triage category for transport to each of the receiving hospitals. Again, consideration will also need to be given to those casualties in need of specialist hospital services (e.g. neurosurgery).

One or more ambulance 'circuit' is typically arranged at the level of the outer cordon in order to organize transport resources appropriately and, more importantly, to prevent bottle necks and obstructions of the available, often limited, infrastructure.

Scene movement of casualties takes place from either affected (i.e. operational/bronze) or unaffected areas of the incident site via the casualty clearing station and is prioritized by the process of triage. The flow of self-ambulant casualties (T3, delayed category) may bypass this system in order to optimize use of non-ambulance transport resources while more severely injured casualties are mobilized and stabilized for ambulance transport. (See Figure 5.3, p. 142.)

Transportation methods

Available modes of transport will also be dependent upon resources and local environment, including weather conditions.

The most common form of transport will be road ambulance provided by local ambulance services, possibly enhanced by neighbouring services if further resources are required or the site of the incident is near a border of responsibility.

In certain cases, it may be safe and a better use of limited resources for a less severely injured casualty to be allowed to transport themselves to a place where further medical care can be delivered following initial triage and assessment, and on the advice of a healthcare responder. Lists of appropriate services and relevant directions would be provided, according to local response plans.

In all cases it is vital for there to be effective communication between all transport vehicles and both sending and receiving units, in case of casualty deterioration or the need to redirect if the situation changes en route.

Examples of vehicle transport methods and their relevant strengths and limitations are listed in Table 1.3.

Table 1.3 Vehicles that may be used for casualty transport

Mode/type	Strengths	Limitations
Land		
Ambulance	Maintains ALS[a]	Limited number available
Police vans	Capacity	No ALS resources
Rail	Capacity	Limited to set routes
Buses	Capacity	No ALS resources
Air		
Helicopter	Rapid, maintains ALS[a]	HLS[b] needed, limited capacity
Fixed wing	Rapid, capacity	Runway needed
Sea		
Boat/Ferry	Capacity	Limited routes and access

[a] advanced life support; [b] helicopter landing site.

The Concept of Resilience

What is resilience?

'Resilience' is defined as the ability to detect, prevent, and, if necessary, manage disruptive challenges. In the NHS, there is an absolute requirement to ensure planning for, and effective response to, incidents and emergencies that might have an effect on health or patient care. The potential range of these incidents is exceptionally wide, from extreme weather conditions such as a severe winter to an outbreak of an infectious disease or a major accident. The Civil Contingencies Act 2004 (CCA) requires NHS organizations and providers of NHS-funded care to demonstrate that they can respond effectively to these incidents whilst maintaining a safe service. This concept can be referred to as business continuity management. This whole planning process is referred to as *emergency preparedness, resilience and response* (EPRR). The key legislation governing resilience in the UK is the CCA.

Business continuity management

This is the process of identifying key functions or components of an organization which must be maintained as a minimum during the response to a major incident. The CCA requires responders to maintain internal business continuity management (BCM) arrangements and local authorities to promote BCM to commercial and voluntary organizations in the appropriate sectors.

BCM questions worth asking (from UK Government Business Continuity Toolkit)
- What are your organization's key products and services?
- What are the critical activities and resources required to deliver these?
- What are the risks to these critical activities?
- How will you maintain these critical activities in the event of an incident (loss of access to premises, loss of utilities, etc.)?

Integrated emergency management

Integrated emergency management (IEM) is a holistic approach to preventing and managing emergencies, comprising six related activities: anticipation, assessment, prevention, preparation, response, and recovery. Emergency preparedness covers the first four of these steps whilst emergency response and recovery covers the remaining two: response and recovery. The underlying aim of IEM is to develop flexible and adaptable arrangements that will enable an effective joint response to, and recovery from, any emergency (see Box 2.1).

Emergency preparedness

Adequate preparation of all individuals and organizations that may play a part in the response and recovery effort is essential for effective major incident management. Every individual and agency will require a clear understanding of their roles and responsibilities as well as how they fit into the wider, multiagency picture.

The CCA requires those organizations likely to be at the core of an emergency response to work together to ensure that they are prepared for emergencies, as identified through the national to local processes of risk assessment.

Emergency response and recovery

This refers to the phases of managing an incident using a multiagency framework at local and regional levels.

Box 2.1 Integrated Emergency Management

Anticipation
This refers to the ongoing process of risk identification and analysis—actively 'horizon-scanning' for risks and potential emergencies. At a strategic level, the risk focus must be forwards, upwards, and outwards, with more operational risks being appropriately addressed at lower levels.

Assessment
The assessment of the anticipated risks.

Prevention
The process of eliminating, isolating, or ameliorating the anticipated risks, prioritized according to their risk assessment.

Preparation
All responders are required to be fully informed with regard to emergency plans and should regularly train and exercise to ensure an effective response.

Response
A coordinated multiagency process by which an incident is managed within a coordinated multiagency framework.

Recovery
Recovery is an active process aiming to achieve a rapid return to normality

Infrastructure and community resilience

Infrastructure resilience

The national resilience framework aims to ensure that there is an understanding by public and private sector organizations of relevant hazards and threats to infrastructure, supply, and distribution systems as set out in the National Risk Assessment. This model of resilience is intended to share best practice and advice to enable owners and operators of critical UK infrastructure to improve the security and resilience of their assets, with appropriate regulators where relevant.

Community resilience

Community resilience is about communities using local resources and knowledge to help themselves during an emergency in a way that complements the local emergency services. This includes having an awareness of potential risks such as flooding, self- and community assistance during an emergency, and how to get involved in community emergency planning. The *Civil Contingencies Secretariat* leads the development of national guidance on community and individual resilience.

It is recognized that communities are better prepared to cope during and after an emergency when everyone works together using their local knowledge. Essential community knowledge includes the anticipation of potential at-risk groups or individuals, such as frail or vulnerable adults or populations in certain geographical locations susceptible to extreme weather conditions.

Considerations for infrastructure resilience include:
- identifying and assessing risks from natural hazards
- standards of resilience
- business continuity and corporate governance
- guidance for economic regulated sectors
- information sharing
- understanding interdependencies.

The Government's community resilience programme aims to:
- increase individual, family, and community resilience against possible threats
- support and enable existing community resilience, and develop successful models of community resilience based on successful practice elsewhere
- support effective communication between the community and the practitioners supporting them
- raise awareness and understanding of risk and local emergency response capability
- provide a shared framework for cross sector, regional, and local activity that ensures sufficient flexibility to make community resilience relevant and workable in each local area/community.

The Capabilities Programme

'Capability' is a military term which includes personnel, equipment, and training and such matters as plans, doctrine, and the concept of operations.

The Capabilities Programme is the core framework through which the Government seeks to build resilience across all parts of the UK. The aim of the Capabilities Programme is to ensure that a robust infrastructure of response is in place to deal rapidly, effectively, and flexibly with the consequences of civil devastation and widespread disaster inflicted as a result of conventional or non-conventional disruptive activity and natural disasters.

The programme identifies the generic capabilities that underpin the UK's resilience to disruptive challenges, and ensures that each of these is developed. These capabilities include dealing with mass casualties and fatalities, response to CBRN incidents, provision of essential services, and warning and informing the public.

Some components of the capabilities relate to the activities of central government, such as central crisis management facilities or resilient telecommunications. Other components are delivered by regional or local responders, but developed within the framework established at the centre by the Capabilities Programme to ensure consistency and high standards.

Central Government Emergency Response Training (CGERT)

The CGERT course aims to equip appropriate personnel with the knowledge and skills required to work in crisis management at the national level. It will also familiarize those in departmental emergency organizations, devolved and regional government, and in Strategic/Gold Co-ordination Groups. (Contact cgert@cabinet-office.x.gsi.gov.uk for details.)

Emergency planning

Background

It is essential that all organizations have effective emergency plans in place which are regularly practised. This and the following sections outline the meaning of emergency planning, different types of plans, the importance of exercising them and training key staff, and the factors which planners should consider.

What is emergency planning?

Emergency planning should aim whenever possible to prevent incidents occurring. When they do occur, effective planning should reduce or mitigate the effects of the emergency. Thus, emergency planning is a systematic and continuous process which should evolve as lessons are learnt and circumstances change. Emergency planning should be viewed as part of a cycle of activities beginning with establishing a risk profile to help determine what should be the priorities for developing plans and ending with review and revision, which then re-starts the whole cycle. Plans should focus on three key groups of people: the vulnerable, victims (including survivors, family, and friends), and responders.

Vulnerable individuals

Vulnerable people may be less able to help themselves in an emergency. Those who are vulnerable will vary depending on the nature of the emergency, but plans should consider those with mobility difficulties (e.g. those with physical disabilities), those with mental health issues, and others who are dependant, such as children.

Victims

Victims of an emergency—this group includes not only those directly affected but also those who, as family and friends, suffer bereavement or the anxiety of not knowing what has happened.

Responders

Responder personnel should also be considered. Plans sometimes place unrealistic expectations on management and personnel. Organizations should ensure their plans give due consideration to the welfare of their own staff. For instance, the emergency services must have health and safety procedures which determine shift patterns and check for levels of stress and exhaustion.

Identifying and managing the vulnerable

Major incident contingency planning should ensure that, as far as is practically possible, vulnerable individuals and groups and their locations and needs are known to responding agencies. This requires detailed planning by those with statutory responsibilities in this area. It is clearly impossible to maintain accurate lists of every vulnerable person in a given area, and it is therefore recommended that planners (through the Local Resilience Forum (LRF)) ensure that lists are available of organizations which care for the vulnerable in their own homes as well as care homes, schools, and hospitals. In the event of an incident, responders can then use these contact details to ensure that appropriate care is provided for as many people as possible. Such integrated planning will also allow a reasonable estimate of the likely scale of the challenge were an incident to occur. Under the *Local Government Act 2000*, local authorities have a responsibility to ensure the economic social and environmental well-being of their community, and as a result, they have a key role to play in caring for the vulnerable in the event of an incident.

Key partners in planning care for vulnerable groups during a major incident

- Adult social services departments (local authority)
- Children's social services departments (local authority)
- Police
- Voluntary (charitable) sector including elderly care and children's charities
- NHS
- Private healthcare providers
- Education authorities and private schools and nurseries
- GP surgeries
- Job centres.

Vulnerable groups

- The elderly
- Children
- Those with impaired mobility or sensory function
- Those with mental health problems
- The acute or chronically ill (e.g. those requiring dialysis)
- Homeless
- Pregnant women
- Those whose English is limited or who do not speak it
- Tourists
- The travelling community.

Emergency planning process

There are three areas of emergency planning which must be addressed by any organization preparing an effective plan:

Prevention
Plans for preventing an emergency—in some circumstances there will be a short period before an emergency occurs when it might be avoided by prompt or decisive action following an initial warning or alert.

Mitigation
Plans for mitigating the effects of an emergency—the main bulk of planning should consider how to minimize the effects of an emergency, starting with the impact of the event (e.g. alerting procedures) and looking at remedial actions that can be taken to reduce effects. Mass evacuation may be one direct intervention which can mitigate the effects of certain emergencies.

Secondary effects
Plans for taking other actions in connection with an emergency—not all actions are directly concerned with preventing or mitigating the effect of an emergency. Emergency planning should also look beyond the immediate response and long-term recovery issues and look at secondary impacts such as extreme media attention and public response. Plans may need to consider how to handle this increased interest.

Types of emergency plans

It may be important for an organization to have more than one emergency plan. It is often the case that organizations have generic plans and specific plans.

A *generic plan* is a core plan which enables the organization to respond to, and recover from, a wide range of possible emergencies. It should, therefore, include procedures which would be used in all instances; for example, ensuring the welfare of staff and the provision of sufficient resources for responding to the emergency.

Specific plans relate either to a particular emergency or kind of emergency, or to a specific site or location. Specific plans are a detailed set of arrangements designed to go beyond the generic arrangements when they are likely to prove insufficient in a particular case. A specific plan usually relies on one or more generic plans or elements of such plans. Some organizations may have specific plans for conducting specific functions in response to an emergency. For instance, the emergency services will have plans for mass evacuation of an urban area and mass decontamination. Organizations should use their risk assessments to decide whether specific plans are necessary or desirable.

Emergency planning at the local level

Emergency planning is at the heart of the civil protection duty for Category 1 responders under the CCA (see p. 80). The Act requires Category 1 responders to maintain plans for preventing emergencies and reducing and controlling their effects. These actions should be based on relevant risk assessments and have regard for the need to warn, inform, and advise the public during an emergency.

The regulations require plans that include procedures for determining whether an emergency has occurred and provision for staff training. There is a mandatory requirement for exercising the plan to ensure it is effective. The plan must also be reviewed periodically to ensure it is up to date.

Category 1 responders should ensure that Category 2 responders, and organizations which are not subject to the Act's requirements, are involved as appropriate throughout the planning process. Category 1 responders must also be aware of the activities of local voluntary organizations when developing plans and are permitted to collaborate with these in delivering the emergency planning duty. Category 1 responders are also required to publish their emergency plans, to the extent necessary or desirable for the purpose of dealing with an emergency.

Local Resilience Forums

Regulations under the CCA require Category 1 and 2 responders in England and Wales to come together to form Local Resilience Forums (LRFs), which are based on police force areas outside London (there are six LRFs in the Metropolitan police area). These are the principal mechanisms for multiagency cooperation between local responders and help to facilitate better coordination and communication and a sense of partnership.

The purposes of the LRF (see Box 2.2) are to:

- provide a local forum for local issues
- coordinate risk assessment through the *community risk register* (CRR)
- facilitate Category 1 and 2 responders in the delivery of their CCA duties (through a nominated Category 1 lead)
- help deliver government policy in line with current guidance
- determine a procedure for the formation of a strategic coordinating group (SCG) by local responders in the event of an emergency.

The formation of the SCG is not simply a transition from the LRF and on occasion the LRF will continue to meet whilst the SCG is operating.

The LRF has no legal powers to direct its members and is not in itself a local responder. As a result, it has no specific duties under the CCA; however, during an established response the LRF will work closely with the strategic coordinating group.

Structure of the LRF

Each LRF comprises the chief officer group of the appropriate agencies, working groups, task and finish groups and subgroups (see Figure 2.1).

The LRF chief officer group should include representation at a sufficiently senior level of all responders under the CCA as appropriate (e.g. local authority at chief executive of deputy chief executive level and police at chief constable or deputy chief constable level).

The general working group is likely to be a permanent group made up of officers from the organizations represented on the chief officer group. This group takes forward business such as LRF multiagency plans and training and exercise programmes.

Subgroups of the LRF may include the general working group (executive), risk management (community risk register), capabilities (e.g. decontamination), specialist advisory (e.g. CBRN), existing standing (e.g. local search and rescue) and task and finish (project) groups. Occasionally, area groups may be established to manage smaller areas of particular risk within the LRF operating area. The secretariat to the LRF is normally provided by the Emergency Planning Unit of the local council.

Box 2.2 Specific objectives of the Local Resilience Forum

- Develop and agree policy across all responders and relevant agencies
- Identify and support lead responders
- Facilitate cooperation between responding agencies
- Inform, educate, train, and exercise local responders
- Prepare and maintain relevant Individual and Community Risk Registers
- Facilitate the development and review of multiagency plans and procedures including the voluntary agencies and the military
- Ensure awareness of, and to prepare and maintain, individual responder plans
- Be aware of the planning arrangements of voluntary sector organizations
- Prepare, review, and ensure awareness of multiagency plans
- Receive and respond to government requests for information regarding risk assessments, capabilities, and specific plans in line with the government's Capabilities Programme
- Support individual responder and multiagency training and exercises
- Prepare, maintain, and support business continuity management
- Attend multi-LRF and Devolved Administration meetings as required
- Support the response to emergencies and implement recovery plans.

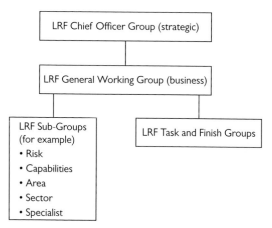

Fig. 2.1 Structure for a local resilience forum.

Reproduced under Crown Copyright from Civil Contingencies Act Enhancement Programme, revision to *Emergency Preparedness*, Chapter 2: Co-operation, March 2012, Cabinet Office. Available online at www.gov.uk/government/uploads/system/uploads/attachment_data/file/61025/Chapter-2-Co-operation-revised-March-2012.pdf

Emergency planning at the regional level

The regional level of major incident preparedness is now less formalized than the local and national tiers. In England, the Department for Communities and Local Government Resilience Emergencies Division (DCLG RED) coordinates multi-LRF planning, ensuring effective communication between local responders, relevant agencies, and central government.

As well as facilitating coordination, DCLG RED is also responsible for ensuring support to local agencies in the performance of their duties under the CCA and other legislation and guidance. DCLG RED must therefore be aware of, and fully informed of, the work and activity of LRFs of which a representative will be a standing member. This encourages cross-boundary working and sharing of good practice.

Within the devolved nations, the activities of DCLG RED fall to the deployed administrations, for example, the Welsh Government.

Emergency planning at the UK Government level

The *National Resilience Capabilities Programme* is the core framework through which the Government seeks to build resilience across all parts of the UK. The programme uses risk assessment over a 5-year period to identify the generic capabilities that underpin the UK's resilience to disruptive challenges, and ensures that each of these is developed. These capabilities include dealing with mass casualties and fatalities, response to CBRN incidents, provision of essential services, and warning and informing the public.

A national response would be expected to an incident such as an infection pandemic (e.g. the foot and mouth crisis of 2001), a significant polluting incident, or a national fuel shortage. In contrast, multi-LRF responses will be needed for more regionalized incidents such as flooding or other severe weather events including utility failures.

The Government has in place a coordinated cross-governmental exercise programme covering a comprehensive range of domestic disruptive challenges, including accidents, natural disasters, and acts of terrorism. The programme is designed to test rigorously the concept of operations from the coordinated central response through the range of lead government department (LGD) responsibilities and the involvement of the Devolved Administrations, to the regional services and local responders.

The National Risk Register (NRR)

The National Risk Register of Civil Emergencies is revised annually and forms part of the National Security Strategy which is coordinated by the Cabinet Office. It offers a brief intro-duction to the types of hazard which may occur and their management and takes account of the current *National Risk Assessment* (NRA) of which it is the unclassified version and the *National Security Risk Assessment* (NRSA). The risk assessments estimate the likelihood of different forms of civil emergency, mapping each against impact and predicted frequency. Risks are divided into three main categories: natural events, major accidents, and malicious attacks. Current guidance identifies pandemic influenza, coastal flooding, volcanic eruptions overseas, and major terrorist attacks as the highest priority risks.

Risk classification in the National Risk Register

Natural hazards
- Human diseases (e.g. pandemic influenza, Ebola)
- Animal diseases (e.g. foot and mouth, rabies)
- Flooding
- Volcanic eruption overseas
- Extreme weather (including space weather).

Major accidents
- Fires
- Contamination
- Technical failures (e.g. nuclear power plants, utilities)
- Large-scale transport incidents
- Industrial action
- Public disorder.

Malicious attacks
- Attacks on crowded places
- Infrastructure attacks
- Attacks on transport systems
- CBRN attacks
- Cyber security.

These national processes inform the devolved administrations and the regional and local levels to ensure fully integrated emergency planning at all levels throughout the UK. For any given type of emergency, a LGD will take responsibility for providing coordinated policy and other support as necessary to local responders and LRFs. As an example, LRFs would be advised regarding winter weather risks by the Department for Transport and the Department of Health as part of integrated planning for severe weather at a local level.

Official government assessments of risks to the UK from natural hazards and terrorism are held on a NRR maintained by central government.

Central government may also provide financial support for an emergency response at local level, for example, a severe weather incident or utilities failures where there is a significant threat to life and property. On rare occasions the emergency is on such a scale that the recovery process will require central government support and coordination. This is achieved through the lead departments coordinated by COBRA.

Central response
Lead department: Cabinet Office.

Regional response
Lead department: Office of the Deputy Prime Minister.

Local response
Lead department: Cabinet Office (may change).

Chemical, biological, radiological, and nuclear (CBRN) resilience
Lead department: Home Office.

Site clearance
Lead department: Office of the Deputy Prime Minister.

Infectious diseases—human
Lead department: Department of Health.

Infectious diseases—animal and plant
Lead department: Department for Environment, Food and Rural Affairs.

Mass casualties

Lead department: Department of Health associated operational framework for the NHS.

Mass evacuation

Lead department: Home Office.

Assessment of risks and consequences

Lead department: Cabinet Office.

Warning and informing the public

Lead department: Cabinet Office (Government Information and Communication Service).

Dealing with mass fatalities

Lead Department: Home Office.

Health services

Lead department: Department of Health.*

Environment

Lead department: Department for Environment, Food and Rural Affairs.*

Transport

Lead department: Department for Transport.*

Utilities

Lead department: Department of Trade and Industry.*

Financial services

Lead department: HM Treasury.*

* Much of the role of these departments is business continuity.

Critical national infrastructure

The government recognizes nine sectors of critical national infrastructure:
- Food (supply, safety, and hygiene)
- Energy (supply and network)
- Water and sanitation
- Communications
- Transport
- Health
- Emergency services
- Government
- Finance.

Central resilience planning also emphasizes the importance of potentially hazardous industrial sites, iconic (historical and cultural) sites, and those organizations of economic or strategic value to the UK. A regularly updated risk assessment by type of risk is in place and details of the potential consequences of a wide range of natural events are available if required. An unclassified version is available at the http://www.gov.uk website.

Central guidance identifies four components of resilience:
- Resistance: protection against identified risks
- Reliability: ensuring that infrastructure continues to operate in adverse conditions
- Redundancy: ensuring back-up or spare capacity
- Response and recovery: ensuring that appropriate plans are in place and sets resilience standards, for example 'as a minimum, essential services provided by Critical National Infrastructure (CNI) in the UK should not be disrupted by a flood event with an annual likelihood of 1 in 200 (0.5%)'. Regulators of commercial services such as energy, communications, and water have a key role in promoting and ensuring resilience within their sectors. In some areas of the UK, a local multiagency critical infrastructure group will have been established to coordinate resilience in those areas listed previously.

Building resilience within an organization

Building resilience has much in common with business continuity management (see p. 36 & Chapter 13). The first step is to determine which elements of the organization's function are essential and what infrastructure is needed to ensure these functions are robust. This analysis will also include dependencies on suppliers and other organizations and *their* vulnerabilities. Hazards guidance and consultation with specialist bodies such as the Met Office, Environment Agency, and British Geological Survey will then allow an informed risk assessment to be carried out.

Once the risk profile has been established, levels of resilience can be determined using national or service standards where these are available. In the light of this information, the risk profile can be adjusted and current levels of resilience determined. This allows the building of a resilience strategy which can then be embedded in the organization, regularly tested, and revised in the light of changing activity or risk.

Establishing resilience in an organization
The nine key steps for establishing resilience are summarized as follows:
Step 1. Determine critical infrastructure for essential functions.
Step 2. Identify critical links with suppliers and other organizations.
Step 3. Identify key risks.
Step 4. Understand current levels of resilience.
Step 5. Determine the risk profile.
Step 6. Review the resilience culture within the organization.
Step 7. Design the resilience strategy—what level of risk is acceptable? For example, can this risk be *terminated, treated, transferred,* or *tolerated*?
Step 8. Embed resilience in the organization.
Step 9. Engage with emergency responders.

The Framework for a Major Incident Response

Introduction

The response to a major incident consists of all the decisions and actions taken to deal with the effects of the incident in the hours immediately after it has occurred as well as those which are necessary as the incident develops. Dealing with the direct consequences of the incident may take many days or weeks, even before the recovery process is well established. Rapid implementation of necessary arrangements for appropriate multiagency collaboration, coordination, and communication is therefore vital to mounting an effective response. The major incident response will deal not only with the direct effects of the incident, such as casualty management, but also indirect effects, such as community disruption, collateral impact on other services, or media interest.

The framework of an effective major incident response should be flexible and tailored to reflect the specific situation while also following a common set of underpinning principles that will guide the process at all levels: local, subnational (previously regional), and national.

What constitutes an appropriate response to a major incident will be determined by a range of factors including:
- the type of incident and geographical extent
- duration of effects (e.g. chemical agent persistency),
- potential complexity and impacts of event
- the designated lead agency.
- local circumstances resources, and experience
- the need for regional, national, or international involvement.

Legislation: the Civil Contingencies Act 2004

The Civil Contingencies Act 2004 (CCA) relates to incidents which significantly obstruct the normal functions of the responder or demand that action be taken requiring a special deployment of resources. Such events have been known historically as '*major incidents*'. The CCA, supporting regulations, and related guidance documents use the term '*emergency*' rather than 'major incident', although this is not a legislative requirement. For the purposes of consistency and clarity, the term '*major incident*' will be used throughout this handbook: this terminology is well recognized among emergency services personnel and avoids any potential ambiguity associated with the term '*emergency*' which is context dependent and implies no sense of scale.

The well-established features which define a major incident are referenced in various provisions in the Act, and will require a major incident response from one or more of the Category 1 responders. The Act also describes an incident threshold, below which specific plans for reducing, controlling, or mitigating the effects of events or situations will not be required.

Concept of subsidiarity

The UK's approach to emergency response and recovery is founded on a 'bottom-up' approach in which operations are managed and decisions are made at the lowest appropriate level: this is the principle of *subsidiarity*. In all cases, local agencies are the key to effective response and recovery operations, with most incidents being effectively managed at the local or subnational level.

The role of central government, devolved administrations, and the subnational tier will be to support and supplement the efforts of local responders through the provision of further resources and a coordination capability.

Integrated response and recovery

Recovery is defined as the process of rebuilding, restoring, and rehabilitating the community and relevant infrastructure following an emergency. Although distinct from the response phase, recovery should be an integral part of the response from the very beginning, as actions taken during the response phase can influence the longer-term outcomes for a community.

Recovery issues should be identified at the earliest possible opportunity, thereby ensuring that the response and recovery effort is fully integrated and ensuring coherence between the two streams of activity. In some cases, resource constraints may necessitate a degree of separation, with the recovery effort gathering momentum once the initial risk to life and property has been addressed.

Use of established emergency plans

A coordinated major incident response may involve the use of established emergency plans, dependent upon the type of incident and the circumstances in which it has occurred. Emergency plans can be either generic or specific in their scope, depending on local risk or hazard assessment. Such plans may also be further defined as single-agency, or multiagency/multilevel.

Emergency responders typically use a mixture of generic and specific plans, with one or more specific plans supported by the generic 'over-arching' plan. The advantage of a generic plan over a specific plan is that it may avoid duplication and inconsistency and ensure more efficient use of resources. Generic plans may also establish a clear set of central, corporate capabilities and procedures that are transferable across emergencies and easily understood internally and by partner agencies. However, a detailed understanding in relation to particular hazards and threats could be neglected.

Generic plans are core plans which should enable a Category 1 responder to perform their functions in relation to a wide range of possible scenarios. In this section, we will discuss the organization of a generic multiagency coordinated response to a major incident as well as the relevant UK legislation relating to this. Specific features of the response to particular types of incidents are discussed further in other chapters.

Generic major incident multiagency response framework

The response and recovery effort may involve many organizations, potentially from across the public, private, and voluntary sectors, and each will have its own responsibilities, capabilities, and priorities that require coordination (see Figure 3.1).

The main stages of a generic major incident multiagency response can be summarized as follows:

- Recognize a major incident has occurred and restrict scene access.
- Report the major incident via the appropriate command chain. Consider the need to issue public warnings, information, and advice.
- Determine the type and level of response (e.g. local, regional, or national) and the initial set of capabilities and resources required.
- Delegate roles and responsibilities to responding personnel/agencies.
- Contain the incident by limiting escalation or spread of hazards and mitigating any collateral impact. Establish relevant zones/cordons.
- Coordinate multiagency capabilities and resources. Establish a robust and effective command and control structure.
- Casualty management depending on the type of incident (e.g. the CSCATTT paradigm (MIMMS), or CBRN equivalent).
- Protection and risk management for the public, responder agency personnel, local businesses, and the environment.
- Organize recovery resources and agencies including relevant investigations and enquiries (forensic or for post-incident debrief/review).

This can be remembered by the acronym **R2D2-C3PO**.

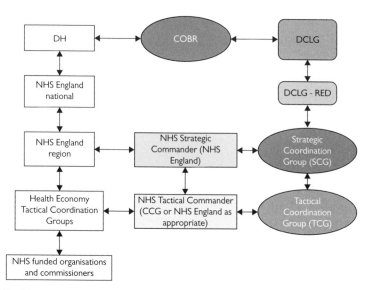

Fig. 3.1 Overview of the NHS England response framework and key partner organizations. Reproduced under Open Government Licence from NHS England National Emergency Preparedness, Resilience and Response Framework, 10 Nov 2015. https://www.england.nhs.uk/wp-content/uploads/2015/11/eprr-framework.pdf

The subnational (multi-LRF) response

Above the local level (coincident with a police area), the subnational level may consist of one or more larger geographical or functional entities able to deploy greater resources. In the deployed regions, the subnational level may be subsumed in the national response. In England, the subnational level may involve one or more local authorities, police forces, or other agencies depending on the nature of the incident. Cooperation at the subnational level will involve representatives of local responders as well as central government representatives cooperating in order to address large-scale civil protection issues. Cooperation may take place within such a multiagency setting or directly between specific responding agencies.

The generic framework and the principles and procedures underpinning it should be flexible enough to be used to manage a wide range of incidents. However, specific information and guidance regarding certain responses may be required due to the different arrangements that apply and additional agencies that are involved. As such, further guidance is provided by the supporting regulations to the Act on the considerations that may apply in relation to:

- localized incidents
- wide-area incidents
- terrorist incidents
- exotic animal disease outbreaks
- maritime incidents
- procedures and considerations for the management of mass evacuation.

Generic capabilities or procedures

Every responder agency must maintain a number of generic capabilities or procedures that ensure a predetermined response in the event of an incident, and the availability of appropriate resources and personnel. Examples of these are listed in Table 3.1. Each of these individual components can then be brought together in a coordinated manner in order to construct the framework of the overall response. This 'off-the-shelf' model will enable a bespoke framework appropriate to many different types of incident while also ensuring that each of the relevant responder agencies is adequately prepared for its own role and able to integrate effectively with others.

Specific hazards or contingencies

Similarly, a number of specific hazards may require a predetermined response which will involve certain specialist agencies, equipment, or personnel. Examples are listed in Table 3.1.

Table 3.1 Examples of generic and specific plans. Reproduced under Open Government Licence from Cabinet Office, *Civil Contingencies Act Enhancement Programme*, Chapter 5 (Emergency planning), Oct 2011 (www.gov.uk/government/uploads/system/uploads/attachment_data/file/61028/Emergency_Preparedness_chapter5_amends_21112011.pdf)

Plan category	Type of plan or planning procedure	Multilevel
Generic	Emergency or major incident	
Generic capability or procedure	Access to resources	
	Control centre operating procedures	
	Determination of an emergency	
	Disaster appeal fund	
	Emergency interpretation service	
	Emergency press and media team	
	Emergency radio and mobile communications	
	Evacuation: minor, major, mass	√
	Expenditure procedures during an emergency	
	External disasters (outside Local Resilience Forum boundary)	
	Mass fatalities	√
	Recovery	
	Rest centres	
	Secondary control centre	
	Site clearance	
	Emergency mortuary and body holding areas	
	Use of voluntary organisations by different Category 1 responders	
	Warning, informing and advising the public, including public information team	√
	Crisis support team	
Specific hazard or contingency	Aircraft accident	
	Chemical, biological, radiological or nuclear	
	Chemical hazards	
	Coastal pollution	√
	Dam or reservoir failure	√
	Downstream oil	√
	Environmental health emergencies	
	Failure of major utilities: electricity, gas, telephone, water	
	Foot-and-mouth disease	√
	Influenza pandemic	√
	Prolonged freezing weather	
	Rabies	√
	Rail crash	
	Refugees	√
	River and coastal flooding (general)	√

(Continued)

Table 3.1 (*Contd.*)

Plan category	Type of plan or planning procedure	Multilevel
	Schools emergencies	
	Severe weather	
	Smallpox	√
Specific site or location	Airport	
	City or town centre evacuation	
	City or town centre severe weather disruption	
	Methane migration	
	Multi-storey block	
	Non-COMAH industrial sites	
	Nuclear power station	
	Public event temporary venue	
	Road tunnel	
	Shopping centre	
	Specific flooding sites	
	Sports ground	

Recognition

The definition of an 'emergency' (*major incident*) in Section 1 of the CCA (see Chapter 1 for more detail regarding definitions) is concerned with the scale of consequences in terms of serious damage to human welfare, the environment, and security. Individual judgement is required to determine whether or not an event or situation falls within the definition. Box 3.1 outlines the main features that may indicate a major incident has occurred.

According to the CCA and supporting regulations, Category 1 responders are required to have emergency plans which must include a procedure for determining whether a major incident has occurred. Whilst historically this role has been undertaken by the emergency services, this is something that can be done by any Category 1 responder. The decision regarding who is best placed to determine whether a major incident has occurred will be dependent on the type of incident. For example, official review following the 2007 floods found that local authorities are best placed to trigger multiagency arrangements in relation to severe weather.

According to the Act, such a procedure must:

• enable the identification of the person who should determine whether an emergency has occurred—this will usually be a person qualified by position or training and identified as a post holder by title or role
• specify the procedure which that person should adopt in taking that decision
• specify any persons who should be consulted about the decision
• specify the persons who should be informed about the decision.

Effects of geographical scale, distribution, and onset of incidents

Recognition of a major incident will depend upon the geographical scale, distribution, and onset of the incident (see Table 3.2).

Localized

A localized incident resulting from a rapidly developing cause will usually result in a clearly identifiable scene, such as the location of a major transport incident, an explosion at an industrial site, or a building collapse. This will be quickly recognized and initiate a rapid response from local emergency services. The traditional *operational (bronze), tactical (silver), and strategic (gold) levels* of command and control are established as part of the local area response and strictly refer only to command levels within each single responder agency. In the event that a multiagency response is required, the levels of coordination are referred to as tactical and strategic (effectively tactical (silver) and strategic (gold) respectively).

Box 3.1 Main features that indicate a major incident response is required

• An event or situation which threatens serious damage to human welfare
• An event or situation which threatens serious damage to the environment
• War, or terrorism, which threatens serious damage to national security
• Threat, hazard, or incident which poses a significant challenge to a Category 1 responder agency's ability to perform its normal functions.

Table 3.2 Effects of geographical scale, distribution, and onset of incidents

	Localized	Large scale Single site	Large scale Widely distributed
Rapid onset	Building collapse Transport accident	Terrorist explosion Industrial accident	Aircraft crash Natural disaster
Slow onset	Radiation point source e.g. medical[a]	Chemical spill Radiation release	Pandemic infection Biological release

[a] Although effects may be localized, radiation casualties may travel large distances before symptoms appear.

Large scale/wide area

Large-scale or wide-area incidents can be divided into those consisting of multiple individual sites spread over a wide geographical area, such as a mid-air collision with many impact and debris sites, or where a single, large geographical area has been similarly affected, such as flooding or other natural environmental disaster.

A large-scale, widely distributed incident may be caused by a slow-onset mechanism, such as pandemic disease or flooding caused by prolonged extreme rainfall. In the event of a disease outbreak, declaration of a major incident will occur as a result of regional or centralized government surveillance systems rather than through recognition by local emergency services. In such incidents, the local (including the on-scene), response will usually be activated in conjunction with establishment of a subnational and/or national response in order to ensure higher-tier coordination.

Coordination at the strategic level is undertaken by the *Strategic Coordination Group* (SCG) which acts through the gold or strategic (gold) commanders of the individual agencies.

Restriction of scene access

In the initial stages of a major incident response, it will be necessary to restrict access to the incident scene for the following reasons:

- Safety of the public, uninjured survivors, casualties, and responders
- To ensure all responders are appropriately equipped and protected
- To maintain effective scene management, including keeping logs of anyone entering/leaving the scene
- To protect property, businesses, and the environment
- To prevent media intrusion and sensationalism, respecting the dignity and privacy of involved individuals, casualties, and the dead
- Protecting scene integrity for forensics or reasons of national security.

The outer cordon may consist of an existing physical barrier, such as geographical features or buildings, supplemented by warning tape, fencing, or other improvised barriers such as emergency service vehicles. It should also be appropriately monitored and patrolled to prevent inadvertent or intentional breaches occurring. Only those personnel with relevant identification and appropriate clothing and personal protective equipment (PPE) should normally be allowed to enter the incident scene across the outer cordon.

Control of scene access will rely upon effective control of the outer cordon and this will normally be the responsibility of the police service. At least one control point will be required at the outer cordon, across which the passage of equipment, vehicles, and personnel can be managed. A one-way circuit should be established in order to facilitate traffic movements.

Further information regarding cordons is covered on p. 84 under 'Containment'.

Reporting

Reporting of a major incident should not be delayed following its recognition and confirmation. In most cases, the first trained responder arriving at the incident scene will pass a major incident warning, or confirmation, report up to their command level by appropriate means—for example, a radio message or telephone call. By contrast, regional or central government services, such as health surveillance units or local authorities, may be the first to recognize and confirm an evolving slow-onset and widely distributed incident. In these cases, the incident will then be reported to relevant responders and other agencies and disseminated downwards.

First responders at the scene of a major incident will be expected to send an initial METHANE report (Table 3.3).

Consideration must also be given to issuing public advice, information, and any necessary warnings, such as evacuation guidance. This is discussed further later in this section (see also Box 3.2).

Involvement with media may also be required in order to effectively communicate public information and guidance. Interaction with the media is covered in more detail in Chapter 15, 'Dealing with the media'.

Table 3.3 METHANE report

M	Major incident & My callsign	Report 'standby' or 'declared'
E	Exact location	Grid reference/ transport route
T	Type of incident	E.g. explosion, transport accident
H	Hazards: present and potential	E.g. fire, chemical agent spill
A	Access	Direct of approach, routes in/out
N	Number/type/severity of casualties	Best estimate available initially
E	Emergency services	Present and required

Box 3.2 What information is needed, and when (further information is available from http://www.bbc.co.uk)

The public needs:
- Basic details of the incident: what, where, when (and who, why, and how, if possible)
- To know the implications for health and welfare
- Advice and guidance (e.g. stay indoors, symptoms, preparing for evacuation)
- Reassurance (if necessary).

The public wants to know:
- Other practical implications such as the effect on traffic, power supplies, telephones, water supplies, etc.
- A helpline number.
- What is being done to resolve the situation?

Broadcasters will require:
- Well thought-out and joined-up arrangements between the emergency services, local authority, and other organizations, capable of providing agreed information at speed
- An immediate telephone contact
- A media rendezvous point at the scene.

Public warnings, information, and advice

The CCA and supporting regulations include two specific duties for Category 1 responders in relation to communicating with the public. First, there is a duty to inform the public about civil protection matters so that the public are better prepared to deal with the consequences of a major incident if one should occur. Second, there is a duty to maintain arrangements to warn the public and provide appropriate advice if a major incident occurs. The regulations also stipulate that there is a duty to avoid alarming the public unnecessarily when making arrangements to warn, inform, and advise them. Normally, a *lead Category 1 responder* with responsibility for warning the public will be identified to save duplication of effort.

Under other existing legislation such as the COMAH Regulations (*Control of Major Accident Hazards Regulations, 1999*) and REPPIR (*Radiation Emergency Preparedness and Public Information Regulations, 2001*), there is also a duty on site operators to provide information to the public.

Under COMAH, an operator must provide information, in consultation with the local authority, to members of the public liable to be affected by a major accident at the operator's establishment. Similarly, under REPPIR, an operator or carrier must ensure that members of the public, in an area likely to be affected by a radiation emergency as a result of their operations, are supplied with appropriate information. Some Category 2 responders (e.g. utility companies) may be required under their own regulations (rather than under the CCA) to inform the public when their services are interrupted. In some specific incidents, a Category 2 responder make take the lead in informing the public.

It should also be noted that the main objectives of the major incident response must not be affected by the use of vital methods of communication to provide public advice, for example, avoiding the risk of overloading the mobile telephone networks.

Public emergency alerts

When there is a risk of a major incident, an incident is imminent, or has occurred, there is an obvious need to be able to inform the public as rapidly, easily, and effectively as possible. Methods for warning the public are listed in Box 3.3. Information should be sufficient to allow necessary actions to be taken and to reassure the public that an effective response is underway, or preparations are in place, but not so detailed as to confuse or cause concern. A lead responder for informing and warning the public is usually identified during the planning process. The lead responder will be responsible for coordinating all communications activity including emergency warning as well as managing public information in its own area of responsibility. This will require close liaison with the media (see Chapter 15). The lead responder may change as the nature of the incident changes or develops.

Box 3.3 Ways of warning or informing the public

- Landlines: for example, *Flood Warnings Direct*
- Mobile telephones
- Social media
- Conventional media: radio and television (local and national)
- Loudhailers or amplified message (from a car or helicopter or via a PA system in a shopping centre, sports facility, or workplace)
- Direct radio broadcasts to shipping
- Door knocking
- Site sirens: for example, industrial facilities, building sites
- Road side or gantry signage
- Printed materials: especially for potential risks, for example, due to a nearby nuclear complex
- Automated telephone, fax, e-mail, or text messages to communication company subscribers.

Written materials must be appropriate for their intended users and may be required, for example, in different languages, large print, or other versions.

Key features of public communications:
- *Why*: what is the event
- *Who*: who is responsible for informing the public event
- *When*: timing and urgency
- *What*: content of the message
- *How*: what means of communication will be used
- *Whom*: who needs to know—survivors, those in danger, friends and relatives, the wider public.

In general, the more people there are who require the information, the simpler it should be: complex and detailed information only being provided to those who need it. In the initial stages, the public will simply require basic details of the incident, the implications for their health and safety, and what they need to do to protect themselves: they will also require reassurance if appropriate or needed. Each message should include the location of the incident (including which areas are *not* involved), and its type, guidance regarding immediate actions (including time scales), and the source of the information.

Roles of the lead responder for warning and informing the public *after an incident has occurred* include:
- delivering urgent/emergency warnings
- provision of a media facility
- identification of spokespersons
- facilitation of interagency statements, coordinating release of information, and assisting other agencies
- ensuring all agencies are informed of action being taken
- ensuring delivery of advice within its own area of responsibility.

The public 'audience'

Six main groups (defined as groups A–F, as shown in Box 3.4) will be the main focus of attention in the first hour of an incident and beyond, each having different needs in the event of a major incident. Methods of providing this information that may be available are also summarized in Figure 3.2.

In terms of group A, those at the scene are under direct instruction from the emergency services and therefore will be kept informed and provided with advice or warnings as part of the scene management strategy. Group B will urgently need to know what they must do immediately—this may be a message to stay indoors and shut windows, to evacuate, to follow decontamination instructions, or to report somewhere for medical checks. Pre-planning should have addressed these issues. Group B may also need (and certainly will want) to know why this advice is being provided.

Group C will need to be provided with general information about the emergency, information on how the public can help, and advice on disruption in the area (e.g. traffic bulletins). Group D will usually be alerted to an emergency through the national media. The most likely

---

Box 3.4 Warning the public during the major incident response: summary of audience types
- *Group A*: survivors—those in the immediate vicinity and directly affected, possibly as wounded casualties.
- *Group B*: those close by who may need to take action to avoid further harm.
- *Group C*: those in the area who may be disrupted by the consequences of the emergency and the clear-up process.
- *Group D*: those who are not affected directly but know or are related to those who might be.
- *Group E*: those who are not affected but are concerned, or alarmed about wider implications, or simply interested.
- *Group F*: the news media.

PUBLIC AWARENESS (pre-event):
Informing and educating the public about risks and preparedness.

↓

PUBLIC WARNING (at the time of an event or when one is likely):
Alerting by all appropriate means the members of a community whose immediate safety is at risk.

↓

INFORMING AND ADVISING THE PUBLIC (immediate and long-term post-event):
Providing relevant and timely information about the nature of the unfolding event:

* Immediate actions being taken by responders to minimize the risk to human or animal health and welfare, the environment, or property.
* Actions being taken by responders to assist the recovery phase.
* Actions the public themselves can take to minimize the impact of the emergency.
* How further information can be obtained.
* The end of emergency and return to normal arrangements.

Fig. 3.2 Public communications timeline: what responders' plans need to achieve.

first response is to phone the people they know in the area, either to find out if they are safe or to get more information.

Group E are effectively 'the public at large' with their principal sources of information being news broadcasts and the Internet. The news media, Group F, can influence both the short-term handling and the long-term impact of a major incident. Category 1 responders must therefore agree what the main public messages should be and aim to provide the wider media with as much relevant material as possible, and ensure it is both accurate and consistent. As a general rule, the larger the group, the more limited the information they will require.

Responsibility for providing public information

In the earliest moments following an incident, vital operational decisions are often made by the first police officers, emergency workers, or even members of the public at the scene. Pre-planning should ensure that decisions about the nature and timing of advice to the public have a prominent place among the urgent matters to be dealt with. A responder/responder agency with lead responsibility for communicating with the public, issuing warnings and providing information should be selected in order to avoid creating duplication, contradiction, or confusion. The regulations suggest two ways in which a lead responder for warning, informing, and advising the public may be chosen—either by identification before a major incident occurs (pre-planning) or by adopting a procedure to be followed at the time of incident.

Lead responder arrangements will generally be negotiated directly or through *Local Resilience Forums* (LRFs) and should be in place before an incident occurs. In many instances, the lead Category 1 responder for warning and informing the public will be the organization which leads on the response to an emergency. In a number of instances, this role is likely to be filled by the police, although it should not be assumed that this will always be the case. The critical element in the effective delivery of information to the public will be the partnership established between the responder bodies involved (see Table 3.4).

Although not specifically covered by the Act, the Meteorological Office, the Food Standards Agency, and Defra may also provide public information or warnings in the case of certain incidents, such as severe weather warnings or from public health risk (e.g. contaminated food).

Plans for warning, informing, and advising the public will include agreement regarding:
- the identity of, and the process to identify the lead responder/agency
- joint working procedures and allocation of responsibilities to support the lead responder
- the trigger points for the handover of the lead responsibility for warning, informing, and advising from one responder body to another, and the procedures to ensure this handover occurs efficiently
- the sourcing of relevant services, facilities, or products for this role
- circumstances in which the facilities or resources of local companies and organizations (e.g. commercial premises or call centres), may be made available to the responder bodies, to help deliver advice and information to the public in the course of an emergency.

Duty to communicate with the pubic: the 10-step cycle
The 10-step cycle has been designed to assist LRFs in implementing their duty to communicate with the public as laid down in the Act.

Step1
- (a) Establish a Public Warning Task Group
- (b) Establish an audit process to log decisions taken through following the 10-step cycle.

Step 2
Use the Community Risk Register as the Task Group's starting point.

Step 3
Identify and agree the lead responders for each risk in the Community Risk Register.

Step 4
Carry out a gap analysis.

Step 5
Identify target audiences and vulnerable groups.

Step 6
Consult the public and neighbouring LRFs and seek examples of good practice.

Step 7
- (a) LRF sets standards based on steps 2–6
- (b) Implement LFR agreed measures.

Step 8
Implement training and exercise regimes in order to test the warning and informing arrangements.

Step 9
Inform stakeholder communities regularly in order to raise public awareness.

Step 10
Measure the effectiveness of the implemented control measures, review and adjusting as appropriate.

Table 3.4 Responder agencies or organizations likely to take lead responsibility in maintaining arrangements regarding public warnings, information and advice. Reproduced under Open Government Licence from Cabinet Office, *Civil Contingencies Act Enhancement Programme* Annex 7 B: Lead responsibility for warning and informing the public, March 2012 (www.gov.uk/government/uploads/system/uploads/attachment_data/file/61042/Chapter-7-Annex-7B-amends_18042012.pdf)

GENERIC HAZARD OR THREAT	1. Category 1 responders likely to have a duty to maintain arrangements to warn, inform and advise the public	2. Suggestions of Category 1 responders from whom a lead responder to maintain arrangements to warn etc. may be identified	3. Organizations, not Category 1 responders, which may also playa lead or a significant role in maintaining arrangements to warn, inform and advise the public	4. Other organizations, which may have an important role in maintaining arrangements to warn, inform and advise the public
Industrial accidents and environmental pollution	Police, Fire, Environment Agency, Maritime and Coastguard Agency, local authorities, NHS Trusts, HPA	Police, Fire, Environment Agency or Maritime and Coastguard Agency	Operators of facilities covered by the Control of Major Accident, Hazards, Radiation (Emergency Preparedness and Public Information) and Pipeline Safety Regulations	Highways Agency, utilities and Met Office
Transport accidents	Police, British Transport Police, Maritime and Coastguard Agency, local authorities, NHS Trusts	Police, British Transport Police or Maritime and Coastguard Agency	Airport or port operator, train operating companies, Highways Agency, Network Rail	Airlines, shipping companies
Severe weather	Police, Fire, Environment Agency, local authorities, HPA, NHS Trusts, Maritime and Coastguard Agency	Police, Fire or Environment Agency	Met Office, utilities, transport, including Highways Agency	
Structural hazards	Police, Fire, local authorities	Police, Fire, local authorities	Utilities, including water companies	Owners and operators of structures
Human health	Police, Health Protection Agency, NHS Trusts, Port Health Authority, local authorities	Health Protection Agency	Food Standards Agency	Utilities, Strategic Health Authority

Determining the level of response required

Within the local response framework, command authority for single agencies is undertaken at three ascending levels termed operational (bronze) (the 'lowest' tier), tactical (silver), and strategic (gold). When discussing the multiagency response, the commanders at tactical (silver) level and equivalent personnel are referred to collectively as the *Tactical Coordination Group* (TCG). At strategic level, this coordinating function is carried out by the SCG.

Construction of the framework

Where the incident has occurred rapidly within a geographically limited area, such as a transportation accident, the major incident framework is usually constructed with a 'bottom-up' approach. Escalation of the event (in severity or geographical extent) or greater awareness of the situation may require the implementation of the tactical (silver) and possibly strategic (gold) command level.

The principle of subsidiarity (as discussed on p. 53) should be applied, in other words, decisions should be taken at the lowest appropriate level while the process of coordination is carried out at the highest necessary level. It should be noted that not all tiers, single or multiagency, will necessarily be required for all incidents.

The generic response framework must be flexible and scalable to be appropriate and effective in any eventuality. The principle of subsidiarity is a key feature in allowing agencies to work within a multiagency framework that can be adapted to the response to both localized and wide-area incidents.

Localized response

The first members of the emergency services to arrive at the scene of a potential major incident will make an initial rapid assessment and report back to their control. Control will then be responsible for alerting supporting emergency services and partner agencies as required, in accordance with established plans. Each responder agency will then alert personnel or activate appropriate response procedures to the level they judge necessary.

The first priority will be to ensure that local emergency services establish control over the immediate area and coordinate individual agency responses by continuous liaison. The possible need for evacuation of the public from the immediate vicinity may also have to be considered at a very early stage.

Good communication and mutual understanding is essential, and can be improved in the preparatory stages (pre-incident) by regular training, joint exercises, and shared development of protocols. For localized incidents, responders will operate initially from a *forward command post* in the vicinity of the incident site following which an incident control (tactical) command point will be established at which the tactical (silver) commanders will work. Coordination tasks are shown in Box 3.5.

Box 3.5. Summary of roles of tactical (silver) commanders at a major incident scene assessing control measures with regard to risk (protection and risk management)

- Deciding which delegated functions will be under the control of, or shared by, each responder agency.
- Reception and engagement of Category 2 agencies (e.g. utility companies).
- Setting up appropriate scene security measures, such as cordons or barriers.
- Establishing traffic routes, direction of evacuation, etc.
- Deciding the location of key facilities such as the casualty clearing station or ambulance loading point (see Chapter 5)
- Ensure communication with, and availability of, liaison officers from local authority or other organizations such as Environment Agency, Department of Health, etc.
- Where the incident falls with its perimeter, to establish links with representatives of the relevant industrial or commercial establishment, public venue or transportation facility (e.g. airport or harbour).

Localized incidents have the potential for widespread disruption in the event of collateral consequences or interdependent impacts, for example, arising from the loss or disruption of local utilities or other essential services. Therefore, constant vigilance is required at every level to ensure an escalating incident is recognized and acted upon appropriately.

Large-scale/wide-area response

The framework for a large-scale or wide-area response will follow the same generic framework that is applicable to all major incidents. In general, many of the same challenges faced will be similar to those of single, localized incidents. In addition to the TCG at tactical (silver) level, effective interagency strategic management will require the activation of a *Strategic Coordinating Group* (SCG) bringing together commanders at strategic (gold) level. Although the SCG is often referred to as strategic (gold), strictly, this descriptor refers only to levels of command within each agency. In some instances the nature or severity of an emergency may necessitate the involvement of a subnational tier which is referred to as a multi-SCG response coordinating group (multi-SCG RES-CG). Both SCG and multi-SCG RES-CG report ultimately to COBR if it is convened.

Multiagency coordinating groups at the strategic and tactical levels will also have an especially important role in information management such as regular *situation reports* (SitReps) and building a *common recognized information picture* (CRIP).

Many challenges will be unique to large-scale or wide-area responses. These are summarized in Box 3.6. The main challenge will relate to the large number of people likely to be involved in areas with a high population density, especially in urban or built-up regions. Remaining challenges may be separated into the following domains: communication, coordination and integration. Therefore, the key role for SCGs will be to ensure an effective response is integrated and coordinated. There will also be a role for the regional tier or devolved governments in supporting or coordinating the local response, and a *lead government department* (LGD) may become involved.

Major incident responses will also need to be adaptable to slow-onset incidents, where the response is likely to be led from the top-down rather than bottom-up, due to improved situational awareness from central government.

Central government

In some instances, the scale or complexity of a major incident is such that some degree of UK central government support or coordination becomes necessary—recognized and implemented by SCGs. Examples may include multiple incidents where a number of related incidents occur close together in the same area or in different parts of the country. The central government response may also be convened before local SCGs are activated, for example, where events are driven by international developments.

Box 3.6 Challenges to management of large-scale/wide area incident responses

- Information management and inter-agency communication
- Disruption and overwhelming of local essential services such as transportation and telecommunications
- Business continuity: pressures on staff and resources
- Inter-regional and inter-agency coordination and integration ('mutual aid')
- Recognition and adaption to slow-onset incidents ('top-down response')
- International incidents: liaison and repatriation
- Effects on public confidence (e.g. fear of further attacks following a terrorist incident)
- Effects on industry/commerce (e.g. exotic animal disease outbreaks)
- Environmental effects (e.g. oil tanker spill or natural disaster)
- Specific geographical challenges (e.g. maritime incidents, see p. 196)
- Providing shelter or advice and resources for evacuation if necessary
- Managing the frail or vulnerable in a crisis (humanitarian assistance)
- Logistics: acquisition, distribution, and replenishment of essential supplies.

The strategic objectives for the UK central government response are to:
- protect human life and, as far as possible, property, and alleviate suffering
- support the continuity of everyday activity and the restoration of disrupted services at the earliest opportunity
- uphold the rule of law and the democratic process.

A designated LGD will be made responsible for the overall management of the government response. In the most serious cases, this would involve activation of COBR. The LGD's responsibilities will include ensuring that appropriate plans exist to manage relevant types of major incidents, that adequate resources are available, and to lead on public and parliamentary handling. When a major incident occurs that does not permit straightforward LGD categorization, the Cabinet Office will ensure that a lead department is identified in consultation with the Prime Minister's office and relevant departments.

Establishing an emergency call centre

As a result of lessons learned from previous incidents, an emergency call centre should be established to deal with general enquiries during a major incident and to redirect calls to other relevant organizations as appropriate. In many cases there will already be local authority, or devolved administration, contact centres who can undertake this role.

Where an emergency call centre is established, the media have an important role to play in raising awareness of its existence and the information it can provide. The telephone number should be given to the media urgently to enable them to publicize it. The role of the emergency call centre should be clearly distinguished from that of the *casualty bureau*.

Common recognized information picture (CRIP)

Information is critical to emergency response and recovery, yet maintaining the flow of information, within agencies, with partners, and to the wider public is extremely challenging under emergency conditions. Establishing systematic information management systems and embedding them within multiagency emergency management arrangements will help to ensure the correct balance is struck between accuracy and timeliness. It is important to note that voluntary and private sector organizations will typically need to be included in the multiagency response and as such they must be integrated into the information management structures and processes that are established, trained, exercised, and tested (see Figure 3.3).

The CRIP provides a predetermined template and structure to enable the effective and accurate collation, assessment, validation, and dissemination of information. Such an approach is required to support the transmission and collation of potentially high volumes of information from multiple sources.

Information will also be required for translation into appropriate information products, for example, briefing the SCG, or for release to the media for public information purposes.

Cabinet Office Briefing Room (COBR)

Collective decision-making within central government is delivered through the Cabinet committee system and decision-making during major incidents will follow the same pattern. During normal business, matters dealing with major incident responses and preparedness are managed by the *Threats, Hazards, Resilience and Contingencies* subcommittee of the National Security Council (NSC). Dedicated crisis management facilities such as COBR and supporting arrangements will normally only be activated in the event of a very large-scale or wide-area incident, or one with great political significance. Key meetings are generally chaired by the Prime Minister, Home Secretary, or another senior minister. Senior government officials from relevant departments and representatives of key external stakeholders will also be present at these meetings.

Where necessary, the senior decision-making body may also be supported by intelligence, media communication, and/or operational cells, an Impact Management Group (IMG), or a Recovery Group. If there is an intelligence cell this would be staffed by the intelligence agencies, *Joint Terrorism Analysis Centre* (JTAC), *Defence Intelligence Staff* (DIS) and others as necessary.

When COBR is activated, the early priorities will be to ensure clear lines of communication are in place and establish a common view of the issues, along with an understanding

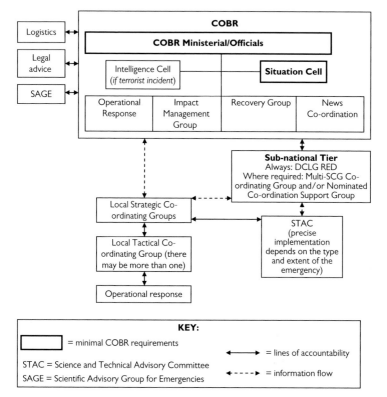

Fig. 3.3 Diagrammatic outline of the regional and central organization for major incident responses in England.

Reproduced under Open Government License from HM Government, *Emergency Response and Recovery* revised version October 2013 (www.gov.uk/government/uploads/system/uploads/attachment_data/file/253488/Emergency_ Response_and_Recovery_5th_edition_October_2013.pdf).

of immediate and emerging priorities and to identify or take any urgent decisions that are required (See Figure 3.4).

A Government Liaison Team (GLT) will act as the primary liaison channel between central government departments and local responders within the SCG, working in the local SCG (strategic (gold)).

For non-terrorist incidents, the Cabinet's *Civil Contingencies Committee* (CCC) takes responsibility for central decision-making. This body, chaired by the Secretary of State for the appropriate LGD, brings together ministers and officials from key departments and agencies involved in the response. For terrorist emergencies, the equivalent body is referred to as a *strategy group* which is chaired by the Prime Minister, Home or Foreign Secretary. This group may meet in restricted session when considering sensitive security issues.

For all level 2 or level 3 emergencies (see p. 73), a *situation cell* will be established, led by the Cabinet Office; the purpose of which is to ensure authoritative situational awareness of the evolving incident for senior decision-makers. One of the main roles of the *situation cell* is to develop and maintain a CRIP for the purposes of briefings at COBR and shared with responders at the subnational and local levels as required (see Box 3.7).

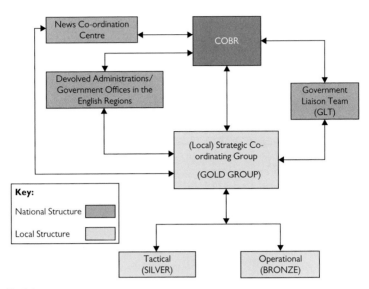

Fig. 3.4 Organization of the central response.

Box 3.7 Support to local major incident response efforts by UK central government

- Providing strategic direction based upon:
  - an agreed CRIP
  - intelligence assessments and JTAC threat levels in relation to terrorist threats, where relevant
  - advice from the local SCGs or other key stakeholders invited to attend COBR
  - advice on the wider impact and longer-term recovery
  - scientific advice provided by, or on behalf of, the LGD
- Deciding on the adequacy of existing legislation and the use of emergency powers on a UK or sub-UK basis
- Authorizing military assistance
- Mobilizing and/or releasing national assets and resources to support response and recovery efforts as appropriate
- Determining national protective security and other counter-measures
- Determining the public information strategy, and coordinating public advice in consultation with SCGs and other key stakeholders
- Managing the international/diplomatic aspects of the incident
- Determining the likely development of the incident and providing early strategic direction of preparations for the recovery phase
- Sharing information with relevant devolved administrations
- Advising on the relative priority to be attached to multi-site or multiple incidents and the allocation of national resources
- Brokering mutual aid, where necessary.

Classification of major incidents potentially requiring central government involvement

Major incidents which might require central government involvement are classified into three levels as follows:

Significant emergency (level 1)

Level 1 incidents require central government involvement or support alongside local responder agencies and the emergency services. This support is primarily from a LGD in which decision-making may require the activation of a collective central government response. Most severe weather incidents fall into this category.

Serious emergency (level 2)

Level 2 incidents require sustained central government coordination and support across several departments and agencies. The central government response will be coordinated from COBR under the leadership of the LGD. Examples include terrorist attacks, widespread urban flooding or actual or threatened severe disease outbreaks.

Catastrophic emergency (level 3)

Level 3 incidents require immediate central government direction and support due to the magnitude of their effects. Although there have been no recent UK level 3 incidents, they might include major natural disasters or nuclear industrial accidents. The response to a level 3 incident is led by the Prime Minister (see Figure 3.5).

Managing the wider consequences of an incident

Managing the wider consequences of an incident may be more complex and prolonged than the immediate management of the incident itself, which occurs in parallel. These aspects are referred to as *consequence* or *impact* management.

Elements of *impact* management include:

• preventing escalation
• preparation for stabilization and recovery
• restoration of essential services
• business continuity management
• provision of shelter to displaced persons.

The LGD for the incident response phase is responsible for consequence management, although the nature of the consequence management activity may involve other departments. In these cases, individual departments and their ministers remain accountable to the collective central government response structure for issues within their area of responsibility.

Where COBR is activated, the *strategy group* (terrorist incident) or *CCC* (non-terrorist incident) will prioritize consequence management activity. An IMG may be formally established to handle the central government component of consequence management activity. In most non-terrorist scenarios, the role of the IMG is likely to be subsumed within the CCC.

Central government responsibilities and organization in the devolved regions

Scotland

The *Scottish Executive Justice Department* (SEJD) will initiate the *Scottish Executive Emergency Action Team*, provide advice on lead allocation, and where appropriate will make a recommendation to Scottish Executive Ministers and the Permanent Secretary.

Wales

The *HR (Facilities and Emergencies) Division* of the Welsh Assembly Government (WAG) will take the immediate lead for any matters which are devolved and in which the lead role needs to be confirmed.

Northern Ireland

The *Civil Contingencies Policy Branch* (CCPB) of the *Office of the First Minister and Deputy First Minister* will provide advice on lead allocation and, where appropriate, will make a recommendation to the Head of the Northern Ireland Civil Service on this.

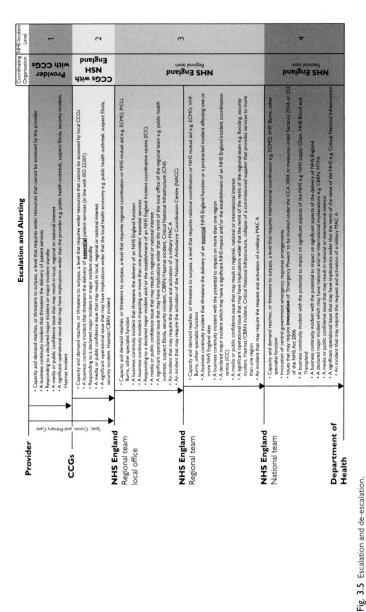

Fig. 3.5 Escalation and de-escalation.

Science and Technical Advice Committee (STAC)

In order to manage a major incident effectively, prompt access to specialist scientific and technical advice will be required. This may be public health or environmental advice or more specialist advice, for example regarding a CBRN incident. During the emergency, local responders should consider establishing a STAC to provide coordinated advice on scientific and technical issues. Scotland, like England has a STAC capability with a similar structure and function (see Box 3.8).

In Wales, public health advice for SCGs is provided by Health Advisory Teams (HATs). The National Public Health Service for Wales takes the lead in the establishment of the HAT, drawing upon scientific and technical advice as appropriate.

LRFs must ensure that plans are in place which identify a lead and core membership of the STAC. When a major incident occurs, the STAC will be activated by the SCG chair through the STAC lead or relevant duty officer. Alternatively, a senior public health professional such as the Regional Director of Public Health may recommend to the SCG chair that a STAC should be established.

Note: further information regarding STACs can be obtained from the *Provision of Scientific and Technical Advice in the Strategic Coordination Centre – Guidance to Local Responders* publication from the Cabinet Office website (http://cabinetoffice.gov.uk).

Potential membership of STAC

The core membership of the STAC should ensure provision of a sufficient level of scientific and technical advice required by the SCG. A list of potential members is given here, although this list is not exhaustive and the membership will depend on the type and location of the incident could include the following individuals/agencies:

- Emergency service technical advisers
- Site operator technical advisers
- Health Protection Agency
- Clinical Commissioning Groups (CCGs)
- Strategic Health Authority
- Environment Agency
- Food Standards Agency
- Health and Safety Executive
- Local authorities (e.g. Environmental Health Officers)
- Met Office
- Government Decontamination Service
- Defra (Welsh government in Wales).

Box 3.8 Roles of the Science and Technical Advice Committee (STAC)

- Provide a common source of science and technical advice to the SCG and Strategic Commanders
- Monitor and ensure that the responding scientific and technical community delivers the information required in order to fulfil the SCG's high-level objectives and immediate priorities
- Provide advice to inform decisions regarding deviation from previously established protocols
- Provide a consensus view on the scientific and technical merits of different courses of action
- Brief the technical lead from each agency regarding the likely ways in which the incident will develop and provide appropriate advice regarding potential interventions, and their consequences
- Identify other sources of specialist advice whose input would be valuable if invited to join STAC
- Liaise with national specialist advisors and others to ensure the best advice is available
- Ensure liaison between members of STAC and more widely
- Maintain a written record of decisions made stating the reasons why each decision was made.

Science Advisory Group for Emergencies (SAGE)

The role of SAGE is similar to that of the STAC but working at a central government level providing advice to ministers and LGDs. SAGE is activated and chaired by a representative from the LGD, *Government Office for Science* (GO Science—under the leadership of the Chief Scientific Officer) or Cabinet Office. SAGE provides scientific and technical advice to underpin the decisions made during the central government response to an incident. Depending on the complexity of the situation, this advice may be provided to the LGD minister, IMG, Civil Contingencies Committee/Strategy Group, the COBR secretariat, or to a combination of these.

The membership of SAGE is scenario specific and may change as an incident develops. The leadership of SAGE may also change as an emergency moves from the response to recovery phase.

The general responsibilities of SAGE are summarized in Box 3.9. These will be supplemented by incident specific responsibilities, which are also likely to change as the incident evolves.

Box 3.9 General responsibilities of SAGE

- Identify where scientific and technical advice is likely to be needed and prioritize and steer efforts as necessary to fill gaps or meet ministers' needs
- Provide a common source of science and technical advice for crisis managers in departments and COBR, when activated
- Provide advice regarding the likely progression of the incident and its impact and offer technical and scientific solutions to possible challenges
- Liaise with national specialist advisors from agencies represented in SAGE and, where warranted, the wider scientific and technical community to ensure the best possible advice is provided
- Provide a common view on the scientific and technical merits of different courses of action
- Monitor the scientific information being provided by individual organizations in order to identify emerging differences and consider how these might best be addressed
- Ensure consistent advice is presented nationally, and where appropriate, locally
- Ensure that scientific information is understandable by policy makers and, where appropriate, can be understood by the public.

Delegation

During the initial response to a major incident it is vital that all necessary responder agencies and individuals are briefed and directed appropriately at every level. Once the type and level of response has been determined and acted upon, relevant responders can be selected and provided with the information and instructions required to ensure a coordinated and effective response. Overarching strategic aims and supporting objectives that are agreed, understood, and sustained by all involved will ensure clarity of purpose and enable the prioritization and focus of the response effort.

The response, and recovery, will involve many organizations, from across the public, private, and voluntary sectors, each of which will have its own responsibilities, capabilities, and priorities requiring coordination.

Tactical coordinators will decide the functions to be controlled by each agency after taking account of:

• the specific circumstances (e.g. type and extent of incident)
• the professional expertise of the emergency services and other responding agencies
• relevant statutory obligations protocols
• overall scene priorities.

The individual roles and responsibilities of the main responder agencies are discussed in Chapter 4.

Responders

The CCA and supporting regulations divide responders into two categories imposing a different set of duties on each.

Category 1

Category 1 responders include all individuals or agencies involved in the core response to a major incident as listed in Part 1 of Schedule 1 to the CCA. Key Category 1 responders are listed in Box 3.10.

Category 2

Category 2 responders include all individuals or agencies not necessarily involved in the core response to a major incident, but who will cooperate and assist Category 1 responders as required. These are listed in Part 3 of Schedule 1 to the CCA. Key Category 2 responders are listed in Box 3.11.

The roles and responsibilities of the main agencies likely to become engaged in the response to a major incident are discussed in more detail in Chapter 4.

Other agencies

The following agencies may also be involved in the major incident response as part of the wider resilience community. Further details are given in Chapter 4.
- Animal and Plant Health Agency (APHA) (formerly the Animal Health Veterinary Laboratories Agency (AHVLA))
- Department of Health (via incident response centre)
- Other providers of NHS services such as Blood and Transplant, NHS 111, Supply Chain, and mental health trusts
- HM Coroner

Box 3.10 Category 1 responders
- Police services
- Fire and rescue services
- Ambulance services
- Other health bodies:
  - acute trusts including foundation trusts
  - primary care services
  - community services
  - Public Health England (and Public Health Wales)
  - NHS England
  - port health authorities
  - some independent health providers
- Maritime and Coastguard Agency
- Local authorities
- Environment Agency.

Box 3.11 Category 2 responders
- Utility companies
- Telecommunications companies
- Transport providers
- Highways Agency
- NHS Clinical Commissioning Groups
- Health and Safety Executive.

- Civil society including faith groups
- National Voluntary Aid Society Emergency Committee (NVASEC)—convened by British Red Cross
- HM Armed Forces
- Air, Rail and Marine Accidents Investigation Branches
- Private sector industrial and commercial organizations
- Association of British Insurers (ABI) and insurance providers
- Wider community.

Common responder objectives

The immediate objective of all local responders will be to save life, alleviate suffering, and contain and mitigate the impacts of the incident. Although in most cases the response phase will be relatively short, perhaps only a matter of hours, the strategic aim should look beyond the immediate demands of the response. Consideration should be given to the longer-term priorities of restoring essential services and helping to facilitate the recovery of the affected communities (see Box 3.12).

Lead responder principle

The CCA includes recommendations regarding the appointment of a lead responder agency who will take responsibility for maintaining local arrangements, such as communicating with the public, or the coordination of the activities of all responders at and around the incident scene. In most cases, the lead responder will be a Category 1 responder, often the police service although in certain types of incident, other services may lead, for example, the fire and rescue service at a major fire, or the environment agency after severe flooding (see Table 3.5).

The main aims of the lead responder will be the avoidance of duplication of effort and efficient use of resources as well as an important role in mitigating the impact of an incident on the community by ensuring consistency and accuracy of public warnings, information, and advice. Although a single agency will usually be identified at an early stage to be the lead responder, they will not have the authority to command the personnel or assets of other involved responders. The key to the success of the lead responder principle is the sustained cooperation and assistance of all non-lead responders through a process of regular consultation and sharing of information.

Ideally, LRFs will select appropriate lead responders in advance of an incident, according to established local risk assessments, saving the multiagency tactical command level valuable time.

The process of selecting lead responders will vary between LRFs and with local circumstances.

Box 3.12 Common responder objectives

- Saving life and relieving suffering
- Limiting escalation or spread of the incident and mitigating its impact
- Providing warnings, advice, and information to the public and business community
- Protecting the health and safety of responding personnel
- Safeguarding the environment and protecting property
- Maintaining or restoring critical activities
- Maintaining normal services
- Promoting and facilitating self-help in affected communities
- Facilitating investigations and inquiries (e.g. by preserving the scene and effective records management)
- Facilitating community recovery
- Evaluating the response and recovery effort and identifying and taking action to implement lessons identified.

Table 3.5 Examples of Local Risk Assessment Guidance (LRAG) hazards and likely Category 1 lead responders. Reproduced under Open Government Licence from Cabinet Office, *Civil Contingencies Act Enhancement Programme*, Emergency preparedness, March 2012 (www.gov.uk/government/uploads/system/uploads/attachment_data/file/61027/Chapter-4-Local_20Responder-Risk-assessment-duty-revised-March.pdf)

Risk categories	Outcome description	Likelihood assessment, lead department and assumptions	Variation and further information
Industrial accidents and environmental pollution			
Fire or explosion at a gas terminal as well as LPG, LNG and other has onshore feedstock pipeline and flammable gas storage sites	e.g. Up to 3km around site causing up to 500 fatalities and 1,500 hospitalisations. Gas terminal event likely to be of short duration once feed lines are isolated; event at a storage site could last for days if explosion damaged control equipment	Likelihood rating: Lead: Fire and Rescue Service (F&R)/Health and Safety Executive (HSE) Assumptions:	
Fire or explosion at a gas terminal, or involving a gas pipeline	e.g. Up to 3km around site causing up to 10 fatalities and 100 hospitalisations	Likelihood rating: Lead: HSE Assumptions:	
Transport accidents			
Rapid accidental sinking of a passenger vessel in, or close to, UK waters		Likelihood rating: Lead: Department for Transport (DfT) Assumptions:	
Severe weather			
Storms and gales		Likelihood rating: Lead: Meteorological Office (Met Office) (on behalf of EA) Assumptions:	
Structural hazards			
Building collapse		Likelihood rating: Lead: Fire/HSE Assumptions:	
Human health			
Influenza-type disease (epidemic)		Likelihood rating: Lead: Department of Health (DH) Assumptions:	
Animal health			
Non-zoonotic notifiable animal disease (e.g. FMD, Classical Swine Fever, Blue Tongue and Newcastle disease of birds)		Likelihood rating: Lead: Defra Assumptions:	

(Continued)

Table 3.5 (*Contd.*)

Risk categories	Outcome description	Likelihood assessment, lead department and assumptions	Variation and further information
Public protest			
Large scale public protest		Likelihood rating: **Lead:** Cabinet Office Civil Contingencies Secretariat (CCS) **Assumptions:**	
Industrial technical failure			
Technical failure of upstream (offshore) oil/gas network leading to a disruption in upstream oil and gas production		Likelihood rating: **Lead:** DTI **Assumptions:**	
Terrorist bombs - infrastructure			
Conventional attack on main government buildings		Likelihood rating: **Lead:** Home Office **Assumptions:**	Regions and local areas that include significant main government buildings are at greater risk.

Reproduced under Open Government Licence from Cabinet Office, Civil Contingencies Act Enhancement Programme, Emergency prepardness, March 2012 (www.gov.uk/government/uploads/system/uploads/attachment_ data/file/61027/Chapter-4-Local_20Responder-Risk-assessment-duty-revised-March.pdf)

Containment

Containment will include setting up an inner cordon to secure the immediate scene and provide a measure of protection for personnel working within the area. All those entering the inner cordon will be required to report to a designated cordon access point. This will ensure that they can be safely accounted for should there be any escalation of the incident, and affords an opportunity for relevant briefing including evacuation signals, hazards, control measures, and other issues about which they need to be aware. People entering the inner cordon must have an appropriate level of PPE, while those leaving must register their departure.

If practical, an outer cordon may have to be established around the vicinity of the wider incident management area to control access to a much wider area around the site. This will allow the emergency services and other agencies to work unhindered and in privacy. Access through the outer cordon for essential non-emergency service personnel should be by way of a scene access control point. The outer cordon may then be further supplemented by a traffic cordon if necessary (see Figure 5.3, p. 142).

The method and practical aspects of containment will depend upon the nature and extent of the incident. For instance, a large area and widely distributed incident, such as a biological agent release or pandemic, will be practically impossible to contain en masse although individual cases or groups may be isolated or quarantined for purposes of controlling spread. When organizing cordons and zones, environmental factors such as wind speed and direction will need to be taken into consideration. Chapter 7 discusses the specifics of zoning in relation to CBRN incidents in more detail.

Cordons and areas

The 'nucleus' of the incident is surrounded by the *inner cordon* and this area is defined as the *operational (bronze) area*. Command of all activity within the *operational (bronze)* area (inner cordon) is located at the *operational (bronze/forward) control* where the *operational (bronze/forward) commanders* from the appropriate agencies and services are located. By definition, the operational (bronze) area is the most hazardous area of the incident site and access to it through the inner cordon must be strictly controlled with access and egress of individuals logged and appropriate PPE worn.

The entirety of the site of an incident is termed the *tactical (silver) area* and is surrounded by the *outer cordon*. Within the outer cordon each service is under the control of a tactical (silver) commander. Other agencies will also provide commanders at this level. These commanders are usually known simply as the commanders (ambulance commander, fire commander, and others) to distinguish them from the subordinate *forward commanders*. The operational (bronze/forward) commanders report to the tactical (silver) commanders. The structural elements of the response will generally lie between the inner and outer cordons and will include the casualty clearing station, ambulance loading point, and other key functions (see pp. 144–7).

Strategic (gold) commanders will work together at a separate, usually predetermined location to coordinate the wider response to the incident and engage with the strategic coordinating group which may be termed *strategic (gold) group*.

The terms operational (bronze/forward), tactical (silver), and strategic (gold) commands should be used with caution when working with the British armed forces as they consider tactical subservient to operational and would therefore expect bronze to be tactical and silver operational.

Hazard management

At the scene of an incident, there are likely to be ongoing threats or hazards which will require control and strategies for management. Possible examples include fire, risk of explosion, building collapse, or chemical contamination. Management of such hazards will be the responsibility of the fire and rescue services although the police have overall responsibility in the case of terrorist incidents. Fire and rescue services will also deal with released chemical or other contaminants in order to restore safety of the site or will recommend evacuation and exclusion zones (see Figure 3.6, p. 85).

There will be agreement between fire and rescue and the police in terms of control of passage through cordons. Where required, fire and rescue and ambulance services will undertake decontamination of the public on behalf of the NHS. Ambulance services will also provide hazardous area response teams from strategic locations around the UK.

In England, Public Health England will be responsible for identifying and responding to health hazards from infectious diseases, hazardous chemical, poisons, or radiation. The Environment Agency is the leading public body responsible for responding to incidents affecting the natural environment which may put at risk human health or property such as floods or pollution incidents.

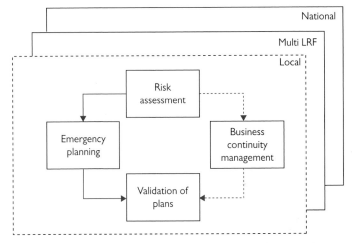

Fig. 3.6 Schematic diagram to illustrate hazard management in the context of a major incident.

Reproduced under Open Government Licence from Cabinet Office, Civil Contingencies Act Enhancement Programme, Chapter 4 Local responder risk assessment duty, March 2012 (www.gov.uk/government/uploads/system/uploads/attachment_data/file/61027/Chapter-4-Local_20Responder-Risk-assessment-duty-revised-March.pdf)

Risk

Risk is a dynamic entity during the response to a major incident. New risks emerge, previously recognized risks recede, and the balance between risks changes continuously. Active risk assessment and management should be an ongoing process. It should also enable, rather than obstruct, effective operations by providing analysis of, and solutions to, anticipated problems before they arise (see Figure 3.7 and Table 3.6).

Risk assessment

The risk assessment process can be summarized as follows:

Contextualization

Contextualization involves defining the nature and scope of the risk and agreeing how the risk management process will be undertaken.

Risk evaluation

Risk evaluation covers the identification of those threats and hazards that present significant risks, analysis of their likelihood and impacts, and the combination of these values to produce overall risk scores.

Risk treatment

Risk treatment involves deciding which risks are unacceptably high then developing strategies to mitigate these risks and evaluating what capabilities are required to achieve this.

All three phases should be cyclical and interactive as risks will vary with changes in the context, changes in the hazards and threats, and changes in available emergency response resources and capabilities.

Further reading

Please see the toolkit for communicating risk in Sections 5 and 6 of the UK Resilience *Communicating Risk* guidance at www.gov.uk/government/uploads/system/uploads/attachment_data/file/60907/communicating-risk-guidance.pdf

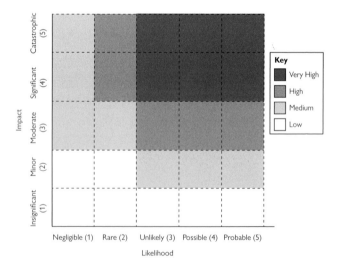

Fig. 3.7 Risk as a product of likelihood and impact.

Reproduced under Open Government Licence from Cabinet Office, *Civil Contingencies Act Enhancement Programme*, Chapter 4 Local responder risk assessment duty, March 2012 (www.gov.uk/government/uploads/system/uploads/attachment_data/file/61027/Chapter-4-Local_20Responder-Risk-assessment-duty-revised-March.pdf).

Table 3.6 Likelihood scoring scale. Reproduced under Open Government Licence from Cabinet Office, *Civil Contingencies Act Enhancement Programme*, Chapter 4 Local responder risk assessment duty, March 2012 (www.gov.uk/government/uploads/system/uploads/attachment_data/file/61027/Chapter-4-Local_20Responder-Risk-assessment-duty-revised-March.pdf)

Level	Descriptor	Likelihood over 5 years	Likelihood over 5 years
1	Negligible	>0.005%	> 1 in 20,000 chance
2	Rare	>0.05 %	> 1 in 2,000 chance
3	Unlikely	>0.5%	> 1 in 200 chance
4	Possible	>5%	> 1 in 20 chance
5	Probable	>50%	> 1 in 2 chance

Command control and coordination

The range of organizations involved in emergency response and recovery can pose difficulties for the effective management of local operations, and this underlines the importance of putting in place clearly defined structures to ensure that key agencies can:
• combine and act as a coherent multiagency group
• consult, agree, and decide on key issues
• issue instructions, policies, and guidance to which emergency response partners will conform.

This framework is based around the concepts of command, control, and coordination. To ensure consistency in nomenclature, descriptions of these terms in context of major incident management are summarized in Box 3.13.

When used, the descriptors of levels, or tiers, of the coordinating management structure as strategic, tactical, and operational (in descending order) once again does not predetermine the rank or status of the individuals involved, but acts only as a simple descriptor of their functions.

Operational (bronze) level

The operational level is the one in which the management of immediate 'hands-on' work is undertaken at the incident site(s). Individual responder agencies will usually refer to the operational level as *bronze*.

Operational commanders will concentrate their effort and resources on the specific tasks within their areas of responsibility, retaining command authority over their own resources and personnel deployed at the scene. However, each agency must also liaise and coordinate with all other agencies involved, ensuring a coherent and integrated effort. Under some circumstances, this may require the temporary transfer of one organization's personnel or assets to the control of another organization. The initial command responsibility at scene will focus on the operational (bronze) level, the first officer present being operational (bronze) commander for their own service until superseded. As the response develops, a tactical (silver) command area will be established. The initial command location is referred to as the *incident control point*, and by convention is signified by leaving the lead vehicle beacons flashing. Later, this will become a operational (bronze) or forward control point as tactical/silver command takes over the role of the incident control point (see Figure 3.8).

Operational commanders are responsible for implementing the tactical commander's plan within their area of responsibility. To do this, they need to have a clear understanding of the tactical commander's intent and plan, their tasks, and any restrictions on them.

Box 3.13 Definitions of command, control, and coordination

Command
Command is the exercise of authority that is associated with a role or rank within an organization.

Control
Control is the application of authority, combined with the capability to manage resources, in order to achieve defined objectives.

Coordination
Coordination is the integration of multiagency efforts and available capabilities, which may be interdependent, in order to achieve defined objectives.

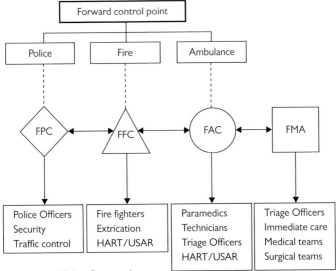

FPC: Forward Police Commander
FFC: Forward Fire Commander
FAC: Forward Ambulance Commander
FMA: Forward Medical Advisor
HART: Hazardous Area Response Teams
USAR: Urban Search and Rescue

Fig. 3.8 Operational (Bronze) tier configuration.

Tactical (silver) level

The tactical level exists to ensure that actions at the operational level are coordinated, appropriate, and integrated in order to achieve maximum effectiveness and efficiency. Individual responder agencies will usually refer to the tactical level as *silver* although from a scene management perspective, it may also be known as *Joint Services Emergency Control* (JSEC). Where formal coordination is required at the tactical level, a TCG may be convened (see Figure 3.9).

Ideally the tactical command point should be located near to the incident scene although, as the response progresses or circumstances change, it may be re-located to a point further removed from the incident site. An alternative location should always be identified.

When resources or expertise are required beyond those available at the tactical level, it will be necessary to establish a *strategic* level of command.

Tactical Coordinating Group (TCG)

A lead responder agency will usually be identified early on in the response; however, this agency, usually the police, will not have direct command authority over other emergency services or agencies. Where formal coordination is required at this level, a TCG will be convened. This will consist of the tactical (silver) commanders (or equivalents) from service or agency involved in the response.

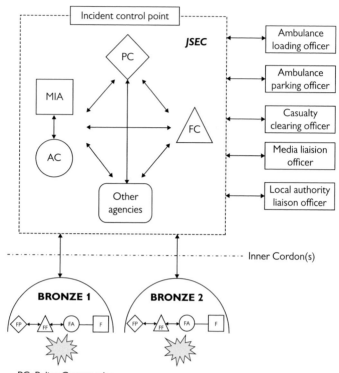

PC: Police Commander
FC: Fire Commander
AC: Ambulance Commander
MIA: Medical Incident Advisor
FIC: Forward Incident Commanders
JSEC: Joint Services Emergency Control
FPC: Forward Police Commander
FFC: Forward Fire Commander
FAC: Forward Ambulance Commander
FMC: Forward Medical Commander

Fig. 3.9 Tactical (Silver) tier configuration.

The TCG will:
• allocate available resources
• plan and coordinate the response at a tactical level
• manage resources and obtain additional resources as required
• conduct continuous risk assessments and adapt plans as appropriate.

In the event that a major incident occurs without a specific identifiable geographical location (e.g. a utility failure), a TCG may still add value in delivering an effective coordinated response.

Single agency vs multiagency command and control structures

It is important to make a distinction between single agency command and control structures (often termed strategic (gold), tactical (silver), and operational (bronze)) and the multiagency coordination structures that may be convened at strategic, tactical, and operational levels. Single agency groups have the authority to exercise a command function over their own personnel and assets. Multiagency groups are convened to coordinate the involved agencies' activities and, where appropriate, define strategy and objectives for the multiagency response as a whole. This approach can be referred to as a vertical command and horizontal coordination structure.

Strategic (gold) command

A strategic level of multiagency coordination is likely to be required when a major incident has met the following criteria:
● Significant impact (e.g. due to geographical size/spread)
● Substantial resource implications
● Involving a large number of organizations
● Lasting for an extended duration.

However, it is better to activate command at the strategic (gold) level on a precautionary basis and then stand it down, than be forced to activate it belatedly under the pressure of events (see Figure 3.10).

The strategic level of major incident management has a number of functions:
● To consider the emergency in its wider context
● To determine the long-term and wider impacts and risks arising from the incident
● To establish and communicate the overall strategy and objectives of the response
● To direct the policy for the response as it affects the lower levels of command
● To monitor progress of the response against established objectives.

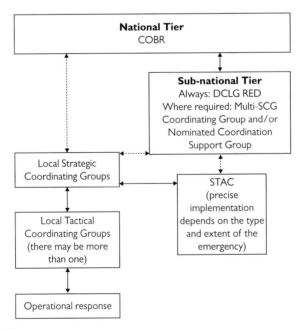

Fig. 3.10 Strategic tier configuration.

Strategic Coordinating Group (SCG)

Individual responder agencies will often refer to the strategic level as *strategic (gold) command* given that it includes their commanders at strategic (gold) level. The SCG brings together strategic (gold) commanders from all relevant organizations. It will normally, but not always, be the role of the police to coordinate all other responder agencies and therefore to chair the SCG, particularly where there is an immediate threat to human life, a possibility that the emergency was a result of criminal activity, or significant public order implications. The SCG may be referred to as *Strategic (gold) Group* (see Box 3.14).

The purpose of the SCG is to take overall responsibility for the managing the response at a multiagency level. Lower-tier command levels and the TCG will be directed by the strategic framework developed and communicated by the SCG. Unambiguous strategic aims and objectives will enable responders to focus their efforts and resources where they are most required. The SCG may establish subgroups to address specific components of the response. Examples include humanitarian assistance, forensic and legal aspects, and international or diplomatic concerns.

Multiagency major incident responder agencies are likely to be under sustained pressure and working within a complex and potentially hazardous environment. Effective communication and disciplined observance of SCG directions will therefore be fundamental to the success of the response.

SCGs must comprise representatives of appropriate seniority and authority whom should be empowered to make executive decisions in respect of their organization's resources. However, each organization represented will continue to retain its own authority, defined responsibilities, and will exercise control of its own operations via its own chain of command.

Once the initial response to the incident begins to draw to its close, it is essential that processes are established to ensure a smooth transition from the response to the recovery phase.

The SCG is the key interface with the subnational and/or central government responses to an incident. In situations where the incident is 'slow onset' or recognition is delayed (e.g. infectious disease outbreaks) and where the response is unlikely to be led by one of the emergency services, establishing the strategic aims of the response may be particularly challenging, but is all the more important. On very rare occasions, central government may itself assume an SCG-like role in setting strategic direction where coordination at the national level is required.

The location of the SCG is referred to as the strategic coordination centre (SCC) and is usually at a predetermined location such as a responder agency headquarters.

Box 3.14 Roles of the Strategic Coordinating Group

- To confirm the management framework for the overall response
- To communicate the strategic aims and objectives of the response
- To review progress and adjust plans as appropriate
- To prioritize the needs of lower-tier structures and allocate personnel and resources as they become available
- To coordinate processes for informing and warning the public
- To take appropriate planning decisions in order to facilitate the recovery process.

Subnational (multi-SCG), National or Multinational response frameworks

In some instances, an emergency may be on such a scale as to require the involvement of multiple strategic coordinating groups, distinguishing the response from that of a local strategic perspective with a single SCG. Mechanisms must also be in place to manage emergencies which straddle multiple LRF areas. An incident requiring a subnational or wide-area response will be coordinated by a multi-SCG response coordinating group (ResCG) (see Figure 3.11).

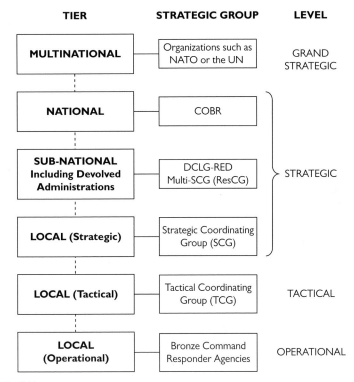

Fig. 3.11 Multi-tiered strategic perspective.

Major incident funding

The *Bellwin Scheme* (named after Lord Bellwin and introduced in 1983) is a scheme which enables central government to provide financial support to local authorities and other agencies *to assist with costs as a result of immediate actions to save life and property or to prevent suffering or severe inconvenience*. Capital expenditure is not normally covered although exceptions can be made if the work offers value for money compared to other options. Reimbursement was set at 85% of the costs incurred above the threshold. The scheme was given statutory power under the *Local Government and Housing Act (1989)*. Similar schemes operate in Wales (*Emergency Financial Assistance Scheme* (EFAS)) and in Scotland.

Bellwin funding can be activated when the costs to local government, police, fire services, or national park authorities exceed 0.2% of their *annual* budget (not the budget during the period of the incident) and is usually, although not exclusively, applied to disasters arising from extreme weather.

In 2014, following severe flooding, the Secretary of State for Communities and Local Government increased the payment to 100% of costs incurred and suspended the threshold of 0.2%. A full review of the scheme is underway. Current guidance and an application form are available at from the http://www.gov.uk website. The department must be notified of an incident likely to result in a claim within 1 month of the incident, although extensions may be granted in exceptional circumstances. The claim must be submitted in full within 3 months. Insurable costs are not covered by the scheme.

Examples of work eligible for Bellwin funding

- Hire of vehicles, plant, and machinery
- Hire and running costs of temporary premises
- Removal of obstructions from roads and public places
- Clearing watercourses and work to improve drainage
- Additional wage costs incurred as a consequence of the incident (*not wages paid to those diverted to emergency response from other duties at no additional cost*)
- Making safe dangerous structures
- Evacuation and shelter or rehousing
- Temporary mortuaries
- Emergency food and other essentials
- Maintaining communications
- Costs incurred under *Military Aid to the Civil Community* scheme
- Administrative charges including legal fees.

Handover from response to recovery phase

In order to ensure that all agencies are aware of the implications and arrangements for handover from the response to recovery phase, it is suggested a formal meeting is held within a few days of the start of the incident. Membership at this meeting should, as a minimum, include the SCG Chair and the affected local authorities. As part of the handover process, consideration needs to be given regarding how information collated as part of the response phase is effectively, efficiently, and securely handed over to those responsible for managing the recovery phase.

As part of the recovery strategy, it is recommended that various targets or milestones for the recovery are established and agreed. The community should be involved in establishing these targets which should provide a means of measuring progress with the recovery process, thereby assisting in deciding when specific recovery activities can be scaled down.

Examples of targets or milestones may include:

- demands on public services returned to normal levels (including health infrastructure and resources)
- utilities returning to fully functional state (e.g. transport infrastructure)
- local businesses return to normal trading
- tourism in the area re-established.

Recording-keeping

In order to facilitate operational debriefing and to provide evidence for inquiries (whether judicial, public, technical, inquest, or of some other form), it is essential to keep records. Single-agency and inter-agency debriefing processes should aim to capture information while memories are fresh.

A comprehensive record should be kept of all events, decisions, reasoning behind key decisions, and actions taken. Each organization should maintain its own records. It is important that a nominated information manager be responsible for overseeing the keeping and storage of the records and files created during the response, and also for assuring the retention of those that existed before the emergency occurred. All document destruction under routine housekeeping arrangements should be suspended.

Good record-keeping serves a further purpose, whether or not there is a formal inquiry. It allows lessons to be identified and made more widely available for the benefit of those who might be involved in future emergencies. Additionally, chief officers and chief executives must ensure that there is appropriate follow-up of any lessons that emerge from the debriefing process.

Debriefing and lessons learnt

Debriefing should always be honest and open, and its results disseminated widely.

Debriefing may also be 'hot' (i.e. immediately or soon after the event) to capture lessons learnt while issues are still fresh in the minds of those involved. A more structured, planned debrief may also take place at a later date during which the detail of the incident can be discussed and a more formal root-cause analysis for any aspects of management which were perceived to be ineffective or could have been improved. This more formal debrief should ideally be multidisciplinary and multiprofessional, and involve a contemporaneous examination of the events and decisions made.

Debrief is particularly important when it comes to disseminating lessons identified. These should be considered at local, regional, devolved administration, or central government level as appropriate.

Responsibilities of Relevant Agencies, Services, and Other Bodies and Individuals

Introduction

In general, the response to a major incident will probably require the involvement and coordination of all the emergency services as well as various support services and related agencies. Understanding the organization and responsibilities of each of these is vital in order to ensure an effective framework for major incident management that is flexible and appropriately prepared in order to meet the demands of the many different types of incident that may be encountered.

Central government may also have a role in the response to a major incident and therefore familiarity with various relevant legislative elements, many of which are quite recent, is also required. The organization of these elements is outlined in Chapter 2. A summary diagram appears in Figure 4.1.

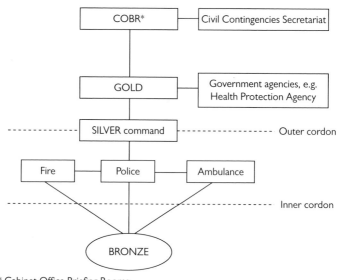

* Cabinet Office Briefing Rooms

Fig. 4.1 Basic command structure and hierarchy.
* Cabinet Office Briefing Rooms

Concept of operations

The UK government has set out eight guiding principles that highlight the key characteristics of an effective emergency response (for more detail, see Box 4.1):
- Preparedness
- Continuity
- Subsidiarity
- Direction
- Integration
- Communication
- Cooperation
- Anticipation.

Box 4.1 Guiding principles to effective emergency response

Preparedness

All individuals and organizations that might have to respond to emergencies should be properly prepared, including having clarity of roles and responsibilities, specific and generic plans, and rehearsing response arrangements periodically.

Continuity

The response to emergencies should be grounded within organizations' existing functions and their familiar ways of working—although inevitably, actions will need to be carried out at greater speed, on a larger scale, and in more testing circumstances during the response to an incident.

Subsidiarity

Decisions should be taken at the lowest appropriate level, with coordination at the highest necessary level. Local responders should be the building block of response for an emergency of any scale.

Direction

Clarity of purpose should be delivered through an awareness of the strategic aims and supporting objectives for the response. These should be agreed and understood by all involved in managing the response to an incident in order to effectively prioritize and focus the response;

Integration

Effective coordination should be exercised between and within organizations and local, regional, and national tiers of a response as well as timely access to appropriate guidance and appropriate support for the local, regional, or national level.

Communication

Good two-way communications are critical to an effective response. Reliable information must be passed correctly and without delay between those who need to know, including the public.

Cooperation

Positive engagement based on mutual trust and understanding will facilitate information sharing and deliver effective solutions to arising issues.

Anticipation

In order to anticipate and manage the consequences of all kinds of emergencies, planners need to identify risks and develop an understanding of both the direct and indirect consequences in advance where possible.

The management of an emergency occurs in three main phases:
- Preparation (pre-planning)
- Response (mitigation of immediate risks and prevention of escalation)
- Recovery (rebuilding, restoring, and rehabilitation).

Preparedness—pre-planning is covered in detail in Chapter 2 and is not discussed further here.

The police will normally take the lead in coordinating a local response where a crime has been committed, or if there is an ongoing threat to public safety. The local multi-agency response is coordinated through a Strategic Coordinating Group (SCG) located in the Strategic Coordination Centre (SCC). The chair of the group is known as the Strategic Coordinating Group Chair.

Categories of incident

UK categories of incident at a national level are described in Chapter 3. In summary, a level 1 ('serious') emergency is one that is likely to require a degree of central government involvement or support, primarily from a lead government department (LGD) or devolved administration. This occurs alongside the work of the emergency services, but without the need for a *collective* central government response. A level 2 ('significant') emergency is one which has, or threatens to have, a wide and/or prolonged impact requiring sustained central government coordination and support from a number of departments and agencies. This will usually include the regional tier in England, or devolved administration in Scotland, Wales, or Northern Ireland. A level 3 ('catastrophic') emergency is one which has an exceptionally high and potentially widespread impact and will require immediate central government direction and support.

Table 4.1 shows where each of these categories sits within the government response framework in relation to its impact and geographical extent.

Categories of responder

Part 1 of the Civil Contingencies Act 2004 (CCA) describes local arrangements for civil protection and places a legal obligation upon emergency services and local authorities to assess the risk of and plan for emergencies. These bodies are referred to as *Category 1 responders* and are also responsible for warning and informing the public as circumstances dictate. The CCA also places legal obligations for increased cooperation and information sharing between the emergency services themselves and other organizations which may have a role in responding to an incident. These other organizations are referred to as *Category 2 responders*. Examples of Category 1 and Category 2 responders are shown on p. 80.

Table 4.1 Incident levels. Reproduced under Open Government Licence from *NHS England Emergency Preparedness, Resilience and Response Framework*, 10 Nov 2015 (www.england.nhs.uk/wp-content/uploads/2015/11/eprr-framework.pdf)

Level 1 (Green)	An incident that can be responded to and managed by a local health provider organisation within their respective business as usual capabilities and business continuity plans in liaison with local commissioners.
Level 2 (Yellow)	An incident that requires the response of a number of health providers within a defined health economy and will require NHS coordination by the local commissioner(s) in liaison with the NHS England local office.
Level 3 (Orange)	An incident that requires the response of a number of health organisations across geographical areas within a NHS England region. NHS England to coordinate the NHS response in collaboration with local commissioners at the tactical level.
Level 4 (Red)	An incident that requires NHS England National Command and Control to support the NHS response. NHS England to coordinate the NHS response in collaboration with local commissioners at the tactical level.

Emergency services responsibilities

Ambulance service (Category 1)

The ambulance service NHS trusts are Category 1 responders under the CCA and will have a major role in any incident involving significant numbers of live casualties. Like all the emergency services, ambulance service personnel may be responsible for the declaration of a major incident. The actions of the first ambulance crew at the scene are to establish a control point as near to the scene of the incident as safety permits, with the senior crew member carrying out an initial scene assessment while the second crew member maintains communications with ambulance control. Routinely, the roof beacon remains on to signify that the vehicle is acting as the control point. A situation report (METHANE) is then reported to ambulance control and a major incident declared. Appropriate sites for keys areas required for command and control, treatment, and evacuation are then explored.

The generic roles of the ambulance service at or during a major incident are:

- establishing a forward control point
- saving life and prevent further injury
- relieving suffering
- liaising with other emergency services
- determining and informing the receiving hospitals
- mobilizing necessary additional medical services
- providing communications for health service resources at the scene
- provide an effective triage system
- providing a casualty clearing station
- providing an ambulance parking and loading point
- providing transport for patients, health services staff, and health resources including transport to the scene of key personnel such as medical advisors and the MERIT team
- documenting the movement of casualties
- maintaining normal levels of service cover during the incident
- acting as point of contact with the HPA, health emergency planning advisors, CBRN specialists, and others as appropriate
- providing a mobile emergency medical response team.

Like the other emergency services, the ambulance service use an organizational structure based on the following phases:

- Initial response
- Consolidation
- Recovery
- Standby
- Restoration of normality.

Provision of medical advice—MERIT

When an incident involves significant numbers of live casualties, a medical advisor may be appointed. This role was formerly referred to as the *medical incident officer*. The medical advisor will be a senior clinician with appropriate experience and training who is involved on a regular basis with the emergency services and their major incident exercises and familiar with the prehospital environment. In most areas, the medical advisor will be one of a group of individuals retained as potential advisors and available in the event of an incident occurring. Such individuals are usually part of a designated *Medical Emergency Response Incident Team* (MERIT). If such an individual is not available or there is no established pool, a medical advisor may be requested from one of the receiving hospitals which are required to provide the capability as part of their established major incident plan. Such arrangements, however, are increasingly uncommon. Responsibility for deploying a medical advisor lies with the ambulance service.

The medical advisor's role is to manage medical and nursing staff deployed to the scene, working closely with the ambulance service. The medical advisor does not usually become involved in the management of individual casualties, unless their role is as a member of the MERIT.

Fire and rescue service (Category 1)

The primary responsibilities of the fire and rescue services at the scene of a major incident are listed in Box 4.2. The fire service are normally responsible for safety at the scene of a major incident (operational / bronze areas), but in the case of incidents related to terrorism, mass gatherings, or firearms/explosives, the initial responsibility will instead pass to the police who will first ensure that there is no continuing risk such as from secondary devices, or firearms.

The fire service watch structure and rank system is available at: http://www.firesafe.org. uk/role-structure-in-the-british-fire-service. See Figure 4.2 for the rank markings of the fire and rescue service

Nationally, the role of fire and rescue services is governed by the *Fire and Rescue Service National Coordination and Advisory Framework* (NCAF) established after a number of major incidents at the beginning of the 21st century. The NCAF is designed to augment and coordinate the responses of individual services and government by providing coordinated support and advice. At the national level, the fire and rescue services will provide input through the *chief fire and rescue advisor* (CFRA) and their team who will coordinate resources through the *Fire and Rescue Service National Coordination Centre* and provide expert advice.

During the response to a major incident, the responding fire and rescue services will establish a strategic holding area (SHA) used to hold resources (vehicles, manpower, and equipment) until they are needed. Sites for these facilities have been identified by Local Resilience Forums and their locations are held on a central database; however, the nature and location of an incident may mean that other sites have to be used. Decisions regarding SHAs are usually made at strategic (gold) level. Assets are mobilized to a SHA by the FRSNCC and will act as the focus of so-called *enhanced command support* (ECS) under the command of an enhanced command support officer (ECSO) who will allocate resources on request from the incident commander through the office of the chief fire and rescue officer duty officer (*CFRA duty officer*).

The CFRA represents the fire and rescue services at the highest level during a major incident of sufficient magnitude to involve central government. They will attend COBR meetings providing advice to ministers and to strategic (gold) commanders as well as coordinating cross-government and international fire and rescue response efforts. The CFRA will be assisted by members of the *National Strategic Advisory Team* (NSAT) formed from senior officers of UK fire and rescue services. Members of the National Resilience Assurance Team (NRAT), available on a 24-hour-a-day rota will also be available for advice and support. The tasks of the fire services at a national level are shown in Box 4.3.

Box 4.2 Fire and rescue service responsibilities at the scene of a major incident

- Saving life and preventing further injury including search and rescue (SAR)
- Fighting and preventing fires
- Provision of humanitarian assistance
- Safety assessment in conjunction with the police* and safety within the inner cordon*
- Identification, monitoring, and management of hazardous materials
- Provision of expert advice regarding hazards via service scientific advisors
- Environmental protection from hazards
- Establishment of cordons in conjunction with the police
- Prevention of escalation of the incident and mitigation of damage
- Provision of specialist equipment (e.g. lifting, cutting gear)
- Decontamination (see Chapter 5).
- Ensuring health and safety of fire service responders
- Establish access to the wreckage and free dead casualties
- Liaison with other emergency services
- Maintenance of routine services during the major incident.

Role	Role collar markings	Helmet
Firefighter	N/A	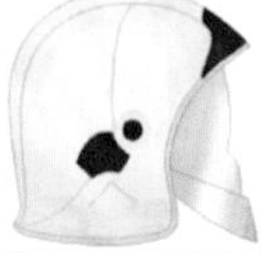
Crew manager	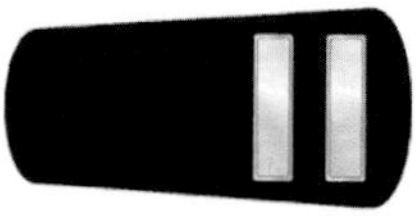	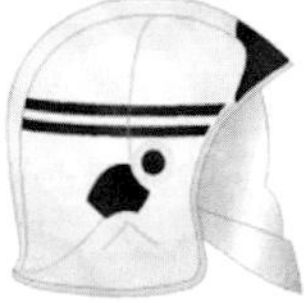
Watch manager	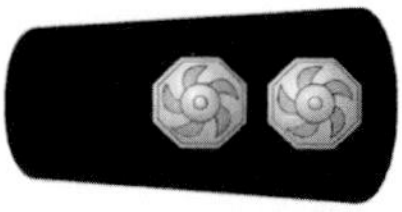	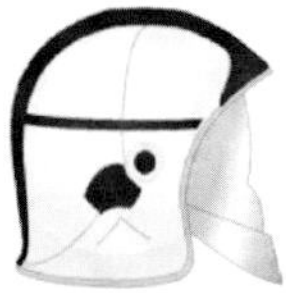
Station manager	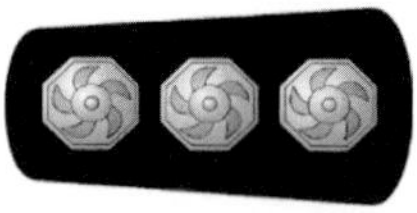	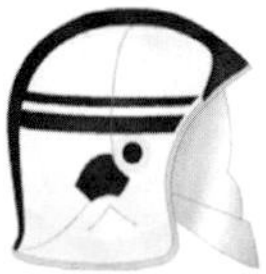
Group manager	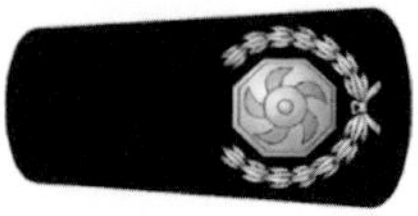	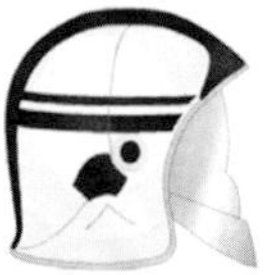
Area manager	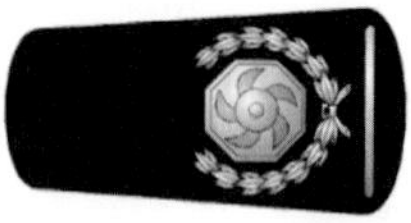	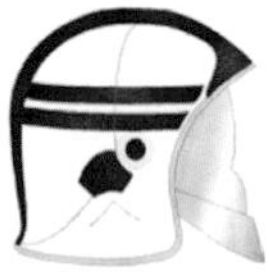
Brigade manager	Brigade manager 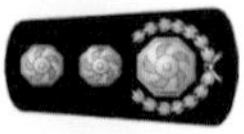 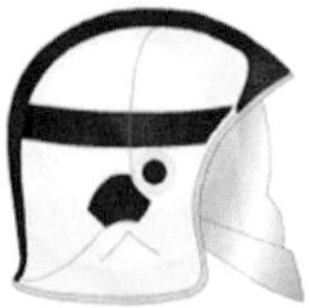	
	Deputy brigade manager	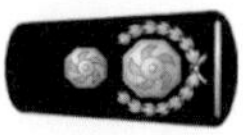
	Assistant brigade manager	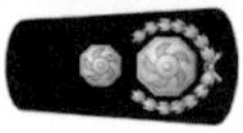

Fig. 4.2 Fire service rank markings.

Reproduced with permission from Fire Safety Advice Centre (http://www.firesafe.org.uk/role-structure-in-the-british-fire-service/) © 2015 Safelincs Ltd.

Box 4.3 Central government level fire service taskings

- Provision of expert advice to other departments and liaison with them (including the security services)
- Collection and distribution of policy information regarding fire service activity at a national level
- Provision of additional resources from within other fire services (mobilized through the NFRCC) or elsewhere (e.g. the armed forces)
- Liaison with regional resilience teams
- Coordination of cross-government and international assistance
- Provision of expert advice to, and liaison with, affected fire services and national bodies such as NFRCC
- Assistance to affected services including with business continuity
- Assistance with deployment of assets overseas if required.

Police service (Category 1)

The roles and responsibilities of the police service at a major incident include the following:
- Overall command and coordination of the incident response
- Determination of location of cordons in conjunction with the fire service
- Saving life and humanitarian actions
- Initial responsibility for safety within the inner cordon
- Regulation of access to potentially hazardous areas
- Prevention of escalation
- Evacuation of casualties
- Ensuring that all the necessary emergency services have been called
- Traffic control and maintenance of emergency vehicle routes
- Maintenance of public order and prevention of crime
- Protection of the environment and property including forensic evidence
- Maintenance of casualty records and collection and distribution of casualty information
- Identification of the dead
- Criminal investigation
- Media liaison
- Liaison with other emergency services
- Liaison with the coroner
- Deciding when military assistance is required
- Provision of security at receiving hospitals
- Determining when property may safely be returned to its owners
- Chair the multiagency SCG (*Strategic/gold Group*).

The police have initial responsibility for safety within the inner cordon at any terrorist event in order to ensure that any terrorists have been identified and disarmed and secondary devices have been identified and made safe.

See Figure 4.3 and Figure 4.4 for the rank markings of the police service.

Police responsibilities at receiving hospitals

The police have a number of key roles at each of the receiving hospitals. They will send a scene examiner to each of these hospitals which become in effect crime scenes for forensic purposes. The scene examiner will brief all staff about evidence recovery, and all patient clothing and effects will be seized and searched for ID, evidence, and debris. All injuries will be photographed if this is possible and amputated parts preserved for the coroner rather than being subject to normal disposal procedures. The scene examiner will also ensure that mortuary procedures are followed appropriately (see Chapter 5).

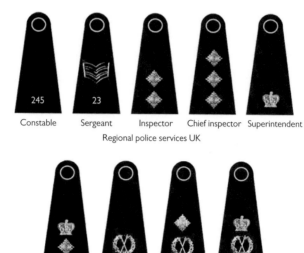

Constable · Sergeant · Inspector · Chief inspector · Superintendent

Regional police services UK

Chief superintendent · Assistant chief constable · Deputy chief constable · Chief constable

Fig. 4.3 Police service rank markings (regional).

Reprinted with permission from Greaves I et al. (2006). *Emergency Care—A Textbook for Paramedics*, 2nd edn. W.B. Saunders Ltd. Copyright Ian Greaves.

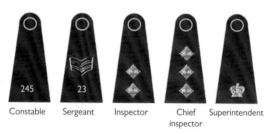

Constable · Sergeant · Inspector · Chief inspector · Superintendent

Metropolitan and City of London police

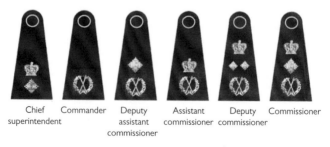

Chief superintendent · Commander · Deputy assistant commissioner · Assistant commissioner · Deputy commissioner · Commissioner

Fig. 4.4 Metropolitan Police rank markings.

Reprinted with permission from Greaves I *et al.* (2006). *Emergency Care—A Textbook for Paramedics*, 2nd edn. W.B. Saunders Ltd. Copyright Ian Greaves.

British Transport Police (Category 1)

The British Transport Police (BTP) function in the same way to local police services, although in a more specialist and limited environment. The BTP will take responsibility for the management of incidents on the rail network and at train stations.

The Security Service

The Security Service (often known as MI5) is responsible for protecting the UK against threats to national security and provides security advice to a range of other organizations, in order to reduce their vulnerability to such threats. The organization is largely based in its headquarters at Thames House in London as well as eight regional offices around the UK plus a Northern Ireland headquarters. The Service is organized into seven branches, each with specific areas of responsibility, working to counter a range of threats including terrorism, espionage, and the proliferation of weapons of mass destruction.

The role of HM Coroner

HM Coroner is required by the Coroners Act (1988) to undertake an inquest into violent or unnatural deaths and sudden deaths of unknown cause. There are other categories requiring investigation by the coroner not relevant to major incident management. The role of the coroner is to determine the identity of casualties, the cause, and the circumstances in which death occurred. The coroner does not apportion blame. A coroner is responsible for bodies lying within their district irrespective of where the death occurred. Where an incident falls across several districts, a lead coroner will be appointed.

When bodies have been recovered from the scene, the coroner will decide whether a post-mortem examination is required and if it is, will instruct a pathologist to carry it out. Only a coroner can authorize a post-mortem or specialist forensic examination of remains. Otherwise, the coroner may issue a certificate giving the cause of death. Each coroner must have in place a plan for managing multiple deaths arising from a major incident.

The coroner has the power to take and retain possession of remains until the process of establishing these facts is complete. They can also authorize removal of bodies from an incident scene to a mortuary. A number of coroners have undertaken special training in the management of incidents involving large numbers of casualties.

The inquest into a death must be carried out by the coroner in whose district the body lies. If bodies lie in more than one jurisdiction, a lead coroner may be appointed to assume responsibility for all the deaths from the incident. With deaths in or near water, jurisdiction lies with the coroner in whose area the body was brought ashore although this may be transferred if the death is known to have taken place near, or in, another jurisdiction. Again, in the event of bodies being brought ashore in a number of different areas, a single lead coroner may be appointed. An inquest may also be held regarding any body part without which an individual could not have survived and must be presumed dead. In certain circumstances, a coroner may also request permission from the Secretary of State to hold an inquest when there are no remains. The procurator fiscal in Scotland has a similar role to that of the coroner.

Use of air assets

Police helicopters

All UK police services have access to helicopters which have a number of capabilities useful at the scene of a major incident. In addition, unlike air ambulances, police helicopters fly at night. In particular, police helicopters have excellent communications facilities, visual and thermal imaging capabilities, and the ability to provide lighting at night. Helicopters carry stills cameras but can also pass video film back to control vehicles on the ground. In addition, a facility to broadcast messages from the airframe to those on the ground may be carried.

Police helicopters may thus be used to assist command and control, shoot video footage for investigational and evidential purposes, search for victims or perpetrators, identify hazards, and for traffic and access management. Police helicopters will also be used for transportation and may have a role in weather monitoring.

Military helicopters

SAR helicopters have been privatized. A contract with Bristow's began in 2015 with a phased transfer of capability from the RAF over 2 years. SAR assets can still be utilized and do not require the use of MACC regulations. Military helicopters may be called upon to assist at the scene of a major incident in a number of ways. As well as being used for transportation, military helicopters may be used in situations where access is challenging or removal of casualties is difficult and where winching may be required. Radar and infrared may be used to search for casualties. On rare occasions, military support helicopters may be used to move large numbers of casualties or personnel.

Helicopter emergency medical services

The use of helicopter emergency medical services at a major incident will be limited to the treatment and transport of single casualties. The ability to utilize more distant receiving hospitals due to greater speeds may be an advantage. The use of air ambulances will be further limited by the inability of the majority of such airframes to fly in the dark and in severe weather conditions. Air ambulances may be used to deliver highly skilled specialist teams to an incident (e.g. MERIT or specialist surgical capability). Air ambulance assets are mobilized through the ambulance commander.

Helipads

Temporary helipads must be sited to ensure maximum safety for crew and those on the ground. They should be on a level service with good all-round visibility and away from power and other cables. They should also be clear of obvious hazards, smoke, and surface debris which may be thrown up in a cloud.

> Through the Civil Aviation Authority, the police may, for the safety of those on the ground or passengers in the air, request the imposition of emergency temporary flying restrictions over the scene of an incident.

Other agencies

The Maritime and Coastguard Agency (Category 1)
The Maritime and Coastguard Agency (MCA) is responsible for the initiation and coordination of civil maritime SAR within the UK SAR region.

Animal and Plant Health Agency (APHA) (formerly the Animal Health and Veterinary Laboratories Agency (AHVLA))
The APHA is responsible for ensuring the welfare of farm animals in the UK and for controlling and eradicating notifiable animal diseases. It is the lead agency for dealing with significant outbreaks of animal disease including diseases originating abroad. In such cases, the APHA works through a National Disease Control Centre established by central government in London, Edinburgh, or Cardiff with local coordinating centres near the incident. The work of the APHA in responding to an incident will always be in close cooperation with Defra, devolved governments (where appropriate), and the Department of the Environment.

Port health authorities (Category 1)
Port health authorities are concerned with the prospect of human, animal, and crop diseases being imported into the UK at seaports and airports.

National Health Service (Category 1)
As a large and diffuse organization, the NHS will undoubtedly provide a number of key roles in the event of a major incident with significant involvement in both the pre-hospital and in-hospital settings. However, the main role of the NHS will be to provide appropriate and timely in-hospital treatment to casualties.

Specialist teams from hospital trusts may also be tasked to provide assistance in operational (bronze) areas as part of the forward medical response, such as surgical staff, or may enhance the capability of the casualty clearing station.

When the DH is acting as LGD for an incident of national or international significance, it will activate an incident response centre through its Emergency Preparedness, Resilience and Response (EPRR) team to provide a focal point for NHS and PHE activity during the response and recovery. In devolved regions, the DH will work with health bodies to ensure a coordinated response.

Other NHS bodies such as NHS Blood and Transplant, NHS Supply Chain, and mental health trusts may also have a role in responding to an incident.

Environment Agency (Category 1)
The Environment Agency has responsibilities for environmental protection in England and as such plays an important supporting role in planning for and responding to emergencies. In particular, the Environment Agency has a key role in relation to flooding, where it is the lead agency for warning those at risk and maintaining and improving flood defences (see Chapter 6). This role is fulfilled by the *Scottish Environment Agency* (SEPA) and *Natural Resources Wales* in the devolved regions.

Health and Safety Executive (Category 2)
The Health and Safety Executive (HSE) has a crucial role to play in the assessment of risk and the development of the Community Risk Register. The HSE also has a role in relation to offshore oil and gas installations. Following a major incident in circumstances for which they are the regulatory body, HSE will be responsible for determining the cause of the incident. Following the declaration of a major incident, the HSE will, if appropriate, despatch an officer to the scene who will assess the incident and inform the HSE secretariat. They will assume initial control of HSE investigation until superseded. In due course, a major incident investigation board is usually established. The HSE investigation manager will act as HSE Strategic (gold), the investigation team leader as HSE Silver. HSE is also responsible for ensuring that evidence is preserved in the event of a prosecution, determining culpability, and establishing whether broader lessons can be learnt. HSE officers may be involved in the final decision to consider an incident closed. The HSE secretariat liaises with central and devolved governments and statutory bodies.

Highways Agency (Category 2)

The Highways Agency is responsible for managing the major roads network, including both maintenance and management of traffic on those roads. In any local area, the Highways Agency is likely to be responsible for motorways and some of the A-roads. The Agency will have a particular interest in partnership with the police, responding to certain incidents and dealing with any recovery issues where appropriate on their roads, with the primary aim of getting road users moving again as quickly as possible. The Highways Agency is in charge at any incident on the road network where there are fatalities or significant numbers of injured and has a statutory responsibility to inform and warn the public.

Local authorities (Category 1)

Local authorities play a critical role in civil protection. They have a wide range of functions which are likely to be called upon in support of the emergency services during an emergency, including key statutory responsibilities such as environmental health, housing, social services, and local roads. As the response phase comes to an end, the impact on the community becomes a key issue. At this stage, the recovery phase, the local authority is likely to take the lead coordination role as part of its wider community leadership responsibility.

Local authorities will also play a key role in coordinating the voluntary effort in responding to a major incident and leading the long-term recovery process. Councils will also have responsibility for welfare and social needs through social services, psychosocial and financial support, and the provision of help lines.

Under the CCA, local authorities are required to:
- work with other responders to ensure coordination and efficiency
- ensure information sharing between responders
- perform appropriate risk assessments
- have emergency plans in place
- have plans and capability for warning the public
- establish business continuity plans and work with businesses and voluntary organizations to ensure continuity management
- provide staff and equipment for survivor reception centres
- lead the work of the voluntary agencies
- provide heavy machinery and manual labour
- provide specialist technical and engineering advice and assistance
- provide highways services and transport facilities
- Offer rehousing and accommodation
- provide environmental health and public health assistance
- facilitate access to buildings for shelter of casualties, victims, and emergency personnel
- ensure the provision of temporary mortuary facilities.

The relevant local authority will appoint a *local authority liaison officer* (LALO) who will manage requests to the local authority for assistance and will be the on-scene local authority presence at tactical (silver) level.

Other agencies and providers under the Civil Contingencies Act 2004

Although not exclusive, the following list of Category 2 responders may be called upon in the response to a major incident:
- Electricity distributors and transmitters
- Gas distributors
- Water and sewerage companies
- Telephone service providers (mobile and fixed)
- Railway operators
- Airport operators
- Ports.

Responders not included in the Civil Contingencies Act 2004

Many organizations have no requirement to contribute to resilience under the CCA, but may have a significant role in the response to an incident (see pp. 116–20). Ideally, these organizations will be built into resilience planning through the Local Resilience Forums. Some agencies will have a role in planning, but are unlikely to have a role in responding except to emergencies within their own footprint or operations, for example, airlines or oil and gas operators. Strictly speaking, the armed forces fall into this group. In view of the potential importance of their role, however, they are considered separately on pp. 124–30.

Retail organizations, including supermarkets

Large (and small) retailers may provide a useful source not only of food and clothing and other household items, but also of safe shelter and communications. Ideally, arrangements for such provision will be in place before an incident occurs.

Food Standards Agency (FSA)

The FSA is charged with maintaining public health by protecting it from risks associated with food consumption. The FSA has offices in London (head office), York, Aberdeen, Cardiff, and Belfast and will be involved in any incident which affects or may affect food safety. This rile is fulfilled in Scotland by *Food Standards Scotland*.

Transport companies

In addition to maintaining normal (or as near normal as possible) services, transport companies may be able to assist in the transport of materiel and people including emergency responders, the involved uninjured, those with minor injuries, and others providing assistance. Specialist haulage companies (and trade bodies such as the Chemical Industries Association) may provide expert advice to the emergency services. Taxi firms may assist with the discharge of patients from hospital.

Media organizations

These organizations will have an essential role in informing the general public of actions required of them as well as the progress of the incident and details of helplines (see Chapter 15).

Insurance companies

Insurance companies have a vital role to play in the recovery process following an incident and will need access to damaged properties. They will also offer advice to members of the public.

Private security firms

Staff from private security firms may be useful during a major incident, for example, in maintaining the security of a scene or preventing access to hazardous areas.

Trade and other bodies

Professional private sector bodies representing different trade groups may provide useful sources of expert advice as well as manpower and materiel.

Internal drainage boards

These organizations may, by pumping and other interventions, have an important role to play in incidents such as flooding.

Pharmacists, general medical practitioners, veterinary surgeons

Individual medical practitioners may be called upon to certify death, may deploy to the scene of an incident, for example to work in the survivor centre or casualty clearing station, or may, at their own practice, dispense advise or reassurance to the worried or those with minor injuries. Pharmacists in the community may have a similar role or be involved in the distribution of medications to affected communities. Veterinary surgeons may be involved in the response to an incident involving animals.

Providers of accommodation

Hotels, travel lodges, and other similar businesses may provide not only overnight accommodation but also conference and communication facilities.

Voluntary organizations

The *Emergency Preparedness* publication (CCA guidance) specifically identifies the following areas in which the voluntary sector can assist:
• Welfare
• Social and psychological aftercare
• Medical support
• SAR transport
• Communications
• Documentation
• Training and exercises.

A more detailed list is given on pp. 116–20, with details of each organization mapped against capability. The regulations also require Category 1 responders to have regard to the activities of certain voluntary sector responders and to include them in the planning process with regard to major incident responses and business continuity planning.

Voluntary ambulance services

The voluntary ambulance services (VAS), St. John's Ambulance, British Red Cross, and St Andrew Ambulance Service in Scotland, may be called upon to provide additional personnel and transport resources following a request by the ambulance service. Where appropriate, a properly equipped and staffed voluntary ambulance may be used to transport serious casualties to hospital. However, the main role will generally be to provide additional trained staff to support casualty treatment facilities, manning first aid posts in the survival reception centre and rest centres, and to assist as auxiliary staff and messengers ('runners'). Arrangements may be in place for the VAS to maintain business continuity by carrying out routine patient management tasks during an incident.

Other organizations

A wide range of charitable organizations will be able to offer services in the event of a major incident, some quite specialized.

Roles of the voluntary aid organizations in the event of a major incident

Welfare (supporting the local authority, social services departments, housing departments, police liaison officers, and the emergency services)
• Provision of:
  • shelter to rescuers and victims (rest centres for family, friends, victims, and personnel)
  • catering facilities
  • clothing
• Establishment of helplines and drop-in support centres
• Spiritual, emotional, and religious support
• Resettlement
• Advice regarding grants, allowances loans, and claims including insurance.

Aftercare (supporting local authorities, and health including mental health services)
• Support and counselling
• Resettlement
• Advice regarding grants, allowances, loans, and claims including insurance.

Medical support (supporting ambulance services, medical facilities at scene including the casualty clearing station)
• Medical and nursing care on scene
• Documentation
• Communications
• Assistance at receiving hospitals.

Search and rescue (supporting the emergency services)
• Mountain , cave, tunnel, industrial, cliff, moorland, mountain, flooding and urban SAR including supervision of volunteers
• Provision of specialist equipment.

Transport (supporting the emergency services and local authorities)
- Transport and escort facilities including bodies, relatives, emergency personnel
- Evacuation
- Business continuity management (ambulance services).

Communications (supporting the emergency services, local authorities, utilities, and other voluntary organizations)
- Vehicles
- Runners
- Radio and telephone communications
- Interpreters
- Translators
- Information distribution.

Documentation (supporting responders, usually the police, local authority, and NHS)
- Patient and involved uninjured tracking
- Assistance at casualty bureau
- Logging decisions and activity
- IT support.

Financial aid (supporting local authorities and other agencies)
- Fund raising appeals
- Personal advice.

Training (supporting all agencies involved in resilience)
- Instructional programmes
- Exercise planning, involvement and cooperation
- Determining good practice
- Training needs analysis.

Team Rubicon UK

Team Rubicon originated in the United States and has now been adopted in the UK. However, the numbers of volunteers in the UK are still relatively small. *Team Rubicon UK*, which is a registered charity, recruits, trains, equips, and deploys armed forces veterans to aid in disaster and major incident response operations. The philosophy is that ex-members of HM Forces have many of the skills ideally suited to coping in the austere, more challenging disaster environment as well as the ability to work effectively in a disciplined manner in adverse circumstances. Team Rubicon also aims to provide veterans with activity which generates a sense of purpose and community engagement. Team Rubicon UK volunteers have already provided assistance in Nepal following the earthquakes and in the 2015–2016 floods in the north of England.

More information is available at http://www.teamrubiconuk.org.

Voluntary organizations and capabilities

Table 4.2 shows the London Voluntary Sector Capabilities Programme. A more generic list which is not London-centric is available: www.gov.uk/government/uploads/system/uploads/attachment_data/file/61037/Chapter-14-role-of-voluntary-sector-amends-10112011.pdf

Table 4.2 Services available in London by category. Reproduced from London Voluntary Sector Capabilities Document, Fourth Revision January 2012, London Resilience (https://www.london.gov.uk/sites/default/files/gla_migrate_files_destination/archives/london-prepared-Voluntary-sector-capabilities-documentv-v4_0.pdf)

Specialist services	Available details of service	Who
Welfare services		
Staffing and/ or management of emergency centres	Providing volunteers to staff or manage various types of centres; Rest Centres, Family & Friends Reception Centres, Survivor Reception Centres, Humanitarian Assistance Centres, Emergency Mortuaries	Red Cross, The Salvation Army, WRVS, St John Ambulance, CRUSE, Faith Communities
Feeding and refreshment provision	Feeding of emergency responders and/or those affected by the emergency (taking into account cultural considerations). Continuity of services, i.e. meals on wheels	The Salvation Army, WRVS, Faith Communities
Clothing	Sourcing and distribution of appropriate emergency clothing for those in need	Red Cross, The Salvation Army
Financial & legal advice	Providing financial advice about entitlements, grants, loans, claims, etc. in relation to disaster appeals. Where direct advice is not available, signposting individuals to appropriate organisations and channels of information	Red Cross, Citizens Advice Bureau
Resettlement of affected populations such as evacuees	Providing practical & emotional support to individuals affected. May include providing such services as transport and escort, tracing & messaging, assisting individuals to access first aid services	Red Cross, The Salvation Army, St John Ambulance, Faith Communities
Support and comforting	Providing practical & emotional support through provision of telephone helplines or face-to-face meetings &/or visits. Services may include, listening, befriending, providing spiritual, religious or emotional support	Red Cross, WRVS, The Salvation Army, CRUSE, Victim Support, Samaritans, Faith Communities
Information and advice	Providing telephone helplines, drop in centres, individual visits, leaflet drops, mobile units & other single points of contact for the community. Signposting individuals to relevant specialist organisations and information	Red Cross, WRVS, The Salvation Army, Citizens Advice Bureau, CRUSE
Refugee services	Providing practical and emotional assistance to vulnerable asylum seekers & refugees, including orientation services, peer befriending, emergency support and provisions	Red Cross, The Salvation Army, Faith Communities
Home care and support services	Enabling regaining of confidence and independence through the provision of assistance with shopping, collecting prescriptions, offering companionship etc.	WRVS, Red Cross, Faith Communities
Bedding/blankets	Sourcing & distributing appropriate bedding (e.g. blankets, sleeping bags)	Red Cross, St John Ambulance
Hygiene resources & advice	Sourcing & distributing of hygiene packs (e.g. wash kits, toiletries) and/or advice	Red Cross, WRVS
Care of children	Offering support, friendship and practical assistance to families with young children	St John Ambulance, Faith Communities, The Salvation Army

(Continued)

Table 4.2 (*Contd.*)

Specialist services	Available details of service	Who
Care of pets	Sourcing temporary re-housing of pets (i.e. after a fire) providing information, advice & support or signposting to appropriate organisations	RSPCA, Blue Cross
Entertainment resources	[Where applicable & practical] Assisting with activities at centres to keep children entertained/ occupied i.e. provision of games, colouring books & pens, videos/DVDs	Faith Communities
Support at airports & other transport hubs	Meeting and greeting individuals; providing first aid, provision of clothing, spiritual, religious and emotional support etc.	Red Cross, The Salvation Army, St John Ambulance, Airport Chaplaincy, CRUSE
Support at hospitals	Spiritual, religious & emotional support	Hospital Chaplaincy
Psychosocial aftercare		
Befriending	Providing support and friendship to individuals on a one-to-one basis	Red Cross, The Salvation Army, Faith Communities, Victim Support
Providing longer term welfare & support	Giving emotional/practical support to individuals following the immediate response to & aftermath of an emergency	CRUSE, Red Cross, Samaritans, Faith Communities, Victim Support
Listening	Providing a sympathetic ear for individuals	CRUSE, Red Cross, WRVS, Samaritans, The Salvation Army, Victim Support, St John Ambulance, Faith Communities
Comforting	Providing comfort and support to individuals	Red Cross, The Salvation Army, WRVS, St John Ambulance, Faith Communities, CRUSE
Group therapy	Offering support in a group environment, incl. art therapy, workshops etc.	CRUSE
Counselling	Listening and giving support and advice to those affected	CRUSE, Faith Communities
Advice—general	Providing advice and guidance on how to deal with distress relating to incident and/or signposting to other specialist services i.e. those dealing with grief and bereavement.	Red Cross, Faith Communities, Victim Support, The Salvation Army
Advice— specialist, i.e. bereavement	Providing advice and guidance on how to deal with grief and bereavement	CRUSE, Faith Communities
Advice—spiritual & cultural	Providing appropriate pastoral care and guidance and/or multi-cultural advice, support & sign-posting	The Salvation Army, Faith Communities
Therapeutic care	Giving therapeutic massage (hand, neck & shoulders) to relieve stress and promote well-being	Red Cross
Medical support services		
Support to ambulance service	Providing crewed ambulances to support local Ambulance Services. Assisting with backfilling during major incidents	Red Cross, St John Ambulance

(Continued)

Table 4.2 (*Contd.*)

Specialist services	Available details of service	Who
First aid & medical posts	Providing first aid & medical posts at various sites including reception and rest centres, incident sites	Red Cross, St John Ambulance
Provision of field hospitals/ supplementary treatment centres	Supply and set-up of field hospitals or mobile/ supplementary treatment centres, incident sites	Red Cross, St John Ambulance
Auxiliary role in hospitals	Assisting health professionals in hospitals	Red Cross, St John Ambulance, WRVS
Assistance with vaccination	Assisting with administration, distribution of vaccines and/or public information relating to the need for vaccination	Red Cross, St John Ambulance
Assistance with medical provision	Arranging access to prescription & medication	Red Cross, St John Ambulance
Search and rescue services		
Water	Providing search & rescue teams and equipment to assist those in peril in inland waterways, coastal, sea, and flooding incidents	British Red Cross RNLI
Animal rescue & welfare	Providing people & equipment for the rescue of trapped, injured animals and/or provision of shelters and re-homing services	RSPCA, Blue Cross
Transport and escort services*		
Transport of evacuees/ displaced persons	Providing transport facilities to and from i.e. rest centres. Includes the provision of specialist transportation where applicable (i.e. disabled access)	Red Cross, St John Ambulance
Transport of injured persons	Providing transport facilities for those with minor injuries i.e. to & from hospital or medical treatment facilities	Red Cross, St John Ambulance
Transport of animals	Providing transport facilities for animals	Blue Cross, RSPCA
Communication services		
Telephone & radio operators	Provision of volunteers to man telephones and/or radios, helplines etc.	Red Cross, St John Ambulance, WRVS, The Salvation Army, CRUSE, RAYNET
Vehicle provision	Provision of specialist and/or supplementary emergency vehicles to support a response	Red Cross, St John Ambulance, The Salvation Army
Interpreters & translators	Arranging access to interpreters and/or translators for those affected (foreign language, sign language etc.), sign-posting to other organisations where appropriate	Red Cross, St John Ambulance, Faith Communities
Provision of information to the public**	Assisting Government & Category 1 responders with public information, reassurance, warnings, recommendations etc.	Red Cross, WRVS, The Salvation Army
Community participation and consultation	Training the public to respond to emergency situations i.e. public first aid training	Red Cross, St John Ambulance

(Continued)

Table 4.2 (*Contd.*)

Specialist services	Available details of service	Who
Assistance in reaching hard to reach/vulnerable individuals	Making contact with vulnerable individuals and groups either directly or sign-posting individuals to specialist organisations where appropriate	Red Cross, WRVS, Faith Communities, The Salvation Army
Assistance in reaching BME community leaders	Provide contact and assistance in reaching local BME community leaders	Faith Communities
Documentation/administration services		
Tracing & message services	Enabling restoration and maintenance of contact between families by carrying messages and helping to trace missing relatives	Red Cross, The Salvation Army
Assistance at casualty bureau & reception centres	Providing volunteers to carry out administration & reception duties, data collection & logging information from callers	Red Cross, WRVS
Logging & recording information	Documenting incident & response activities	Red Cross, WRVS
Coordination of convergent volunteers	Coordinating local convergent volunteers who respond to an emergency	Red Cross
Reception & registration duties in emergency centres	Completion of relevant local forms/police forms both manual and electronic	WRVS, Red Cross, Faith Communities, The Salvation Army
Financial services		
Disaster funds	Establishing and administering disaster fund until trustees appointed. Providing information on how to apply to disaster funds.	Red Cross
Equipment and resources available		
Bedding	Blankets, sleeping bags	Red Cross
Ambulances	Ambulance vehicles; front line, 4×4	Red Cross, St John Ambulance
Other vehicles	DPV (Disabled Passenger Vehicle), MPV (Multi-purpose Vehicle), fully-equipped major incident trucks, vans, minibuses, 4×4 off-road vehicles	Red Cross, St John Ambulance
Clothing	Emergency clothing for adults & children	Red Cross, The Salvation Army
First Aid & medical equipment	Defibrillator equipment, first aid kits, major incident first aid kits, oxygen	Red Cross, St John Ambulance
Mobility aids	Walking frames, walking sticks, wheelchairs, rolators, commodes, bedpans, bath seats	Red Cross
Catering equipment	Electric boilers/rings, gas boilers/rings, all equipment required to provide on-site hot meals	WRVS
Shelter	Tents, air shelters	Red Cross, St John Ambulance, WRVS
Hygiene packs	Wash kit, soap, shampoo, toothpaste, toothbrushes, flannels	Red Cross

(Continued)

Table 4.2 (*Contd.*)

Specialist services	Available details of service	Who
Plastic sheeting	Large units of plastic sheeting for use with provision of emergency temporary shelter	Red Cross
(Inflatable) boats	(Inflatable) boats for accessing flooded, cut-off areas	RNLI, Red Cross
Mobile first aid units	Vehicles used to provide temporary mobile communication & control (command) units	St John Ambulance, Red Cross
Satellite communications	Satellite communications equipment	Red Cross
Lighting	Portable emergency lighting (available for shelters)	WRVS, Red Cross
Generators	Portable generators	WRVS, St John Ambulance, Red Cross
Forklift trucks	All-terrain forklift truck equipment	Red Cross
Field hospital equipment	Portable shelter & equipment for use as field hospital/treatment centre	Red Cross, St John Ambulance
Stationery	Assorted emergency stationery items i.e. administration boxes	WRVS, Red Cross, St John Ambulance
PPE (personal protective equipment)	E.g. hard hats, high-visibility vests etc. (for individual volunteers)	Red Cross, St John Ambulance
Premises/ accommodation	Designated muster points and other premises which could be used for converging or for rendezvous points (either for people or vehicles)	Red Cross, St John Ambulance, Faith Communities, The Salvation Army
Radio communications	Local, regional, national radio networks together with operators for the radio systems	RAYNET

* Generally, provision of transport & escort services would be undertaken on a short-term basis and, where applicable, include the provision of specialist transportation, i.e. disabled access.

** All voluntary groups may potentially be involved in assisting in these categories.

Voluntary services response funding

As part of resilience arrangements, agreements with voluntary organizations regarding the funding and the intended nature of their activities in the event of a major incident must be in place. In general, the major agencies such as the Red Cross and St John Ambulance will not seek reimbursement of expenses although this may change in the event of a prolonged response or specific contracted or tendered services. There are exceptions: the Royal Voluntary Society 'always charges', and most smaller charities will not be in a position to provide large-scale or prolonged assistance free of charge.

The Armed Forces

The armed forces do not play a permanent role in local civil protection. They can, however, under exceptional circumstances, provide an element of the support central government can provide to Category 1 responders when responding to a disaster or emergency. They also play an important part in certain specific scenarios such as SAR (including mountain rescue) and explosive ordnance disposal (see p. 132).

The role of the armed forces in major incidents in the UK is governed by the Military Aid to the Civil Powers Regulations. These regulations divide military assistance into three main types collectively known as *Military Aid to the Civil Authorities* (MACA):

• *Military Aid to Government Departments* (MAGD) other than the Ministry of Defence (MOD), such as security at major events, or maintaining essential services

• *Military Aid to the Civil Powers* (MACP) usually to assist in maintaining law and order or public safety, for example, in terrorist incidents

• *Military Aid to the Civil Community* (MACC)—generally the provision of specialist skills such as bridge building, or of large numbers of personnel with a clear command structure to assist at the scene of an incident.

There is also a fourth category—*Training and Logistic Assistance to the Civil Police* (TLACP)— used when military personnel support civilian police activity but do not become involved in their operations.

> The armed forces have no *automatic* responsibilities under the CCA.

Requests for military aid must demonstrate:
• a clear need to act
• that other options have been discounted
• that the civil authority lacks the capability and cannot develop it in time
• or that the civil authority has the capability, but it cannot be made available in time.

See Figure 4.5 for the rank markings of the Royal Navy, Figure 4.6 for the rank markings of the Army, and Figure 4.7 for the rank markings of the RAF.

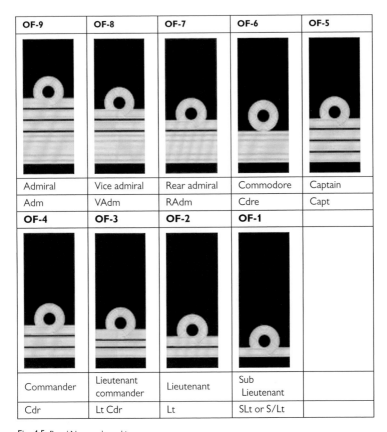

OF-9	OF-8	OF-7	OF-6	OF-5
Admiral	Vice admiral	Rear admiral	Commodore	Captain
Adm	VAdm	RAdm	Cdre	Capt

OF-4	OF-3	OF-2	OF-1	
Commander	Lieutenant commander	Lieutenant	Sub Lieutenant	
Cdr	Lt Cdr	Lt	SLt or S/Lt	

Fig. 4.5 Royal Navy rank markings.

Officer ranks

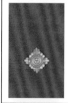	**Second Lieutenant** The first rank held on commissioning. It is normally held for up to 2 years, during which time they complete special to arms training relevant to their Corps. Afterwards they are responsible for leading up to 30 soldiers in a platoon or troop, both in training and on operations.
	Lieutenant Lieutenant is a rank typically held for up to 3 years. They normally command of a platoon or troop of around 30 soldiers, but with experience comes increased responsibilities. They also have the opportunity to gain specialised skills outside their unit.
	**Captain** Captains are normally made second-in-command of a sub-unit of up to 120 soldiers. They are key players in the planning and decision-making process, with tactical responsibility for operations on the ground as well as equipment maintenance, logistic support and manpower.
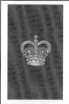	**Major** Promotion to Major follows between 8-10 years service. Typically a Major will be given command of a sub-unit of up to 120 officers and soldiers with responsibility for their training, welfare and administration both in camp and on operations, as well as the management of their equipment.
	Lieutenant Colonel Lieutenant Colonels typically command units of up to 650 soldiers, containing four or five sub-units. They are responsible for the overall operational effectiveness of their unit in terms of military capability, welfare and general discipline. Typically a two-year appointment.
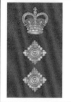	**Colonel** Colonels are not usually field commanders (except in the Royal Army Medical Corps) - typically they serve as staff officers between field commands at battalion/brigade level. It is the lowest of the staff ranks and they are the principal operational advisors to senior officers.

Fig. 4.6 Army rank markings.
Reproduced under crown copyright from British Army Website (www.army.mod.uk/structure/32321.aspx).

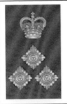

Brigadier (aka 1 star)
Brigadier is not considered to be a General Officer rank by the British Army but rather a Field officer rank. Brigadiers can command a brigade or be a director of operational capability groups such as a director of staff.

Major General (aka 2 star)
Major Generals command formations of division size and the Royal Military Academy Sandhurst, and hold senior staff appointments in the Ministry of Defence and other headquarters.

Lieutenant General (aka 3 star)
Lieutenant Generals command formations of Corps size and other commands in the UK and overseas, and hold very senior staff appointments in the Ministry of Defence and other headquarters.

General (aka 4 star)
Generals hold the most senior appointments - such as the Chief of Defence Staff, Vice Chief of Defence Staff, Chief of the General Staff, Deputy Supreme Allied Commander Europe, and Commander in Chief Land Forces.

Other ranks

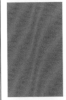

Private
On completion of Phase 1 Training, all new soldiers start as Privates although the title may be Trooper, Gunner, Signaller, Sapper, Guardsman Rifleman or even Kingsman depending on Corps/Regiment.

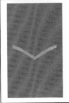

Lance Corporal
Promotion to Lance Corporal may follow after Phase 2 Training or after about 3 years as a private. Lance Corporals are required to supervise a small team of up to four soldiers called a section. They also have opportunities to specialise and undertake specialist military training.

Fig. 4.6 *(Contd.)*

	**Corporal** After 6-8 years, and depending on ability to lead, promotion to Corporal typically follows. In this rank additional trade and instructor qualifications can be gained. Corporals are given command of more soldiers and equipment such as tanks or guns.
	Sergeant Sergeant is a senior role of responsibility, promotion to which typically takes place after 12 years depending on ability. Sergeants typically are second in command of a troop or platoon of up to 35 soldiers, with the important responsibility for advising and assisting junior officers.
	**Staff/Colour Sergeant** After a few years as a Sergeant promotion to either Staff or Colour Sergeant may follow. This is a senior role combining man and resource management of around 120 soldiers, or even command of a troop or platoon.
	**Warrant Officer Class 2** (Company/Squadron Sergeant Major) This is a senior management role focussing on the training, welfare and discipline of a company, squadron or battery of up to 120 soldiers. WO2s act as senior adviser to the Major in command of the sub-unit and may also be selected for a commission as an Officer.
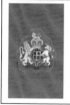	**Warrant Officer Class 1** (Regimental Sergeant Major) The most senior soldier rank in the British Army, typically reached after 18 years of outstanding service. WO1s are the senior advisors of their unit's Commanding Officer, with leadership, discipline and welfare responsibilities of up to 650 officers and soldiers and equipment.

Fig. 4.6 (*Contd.*)

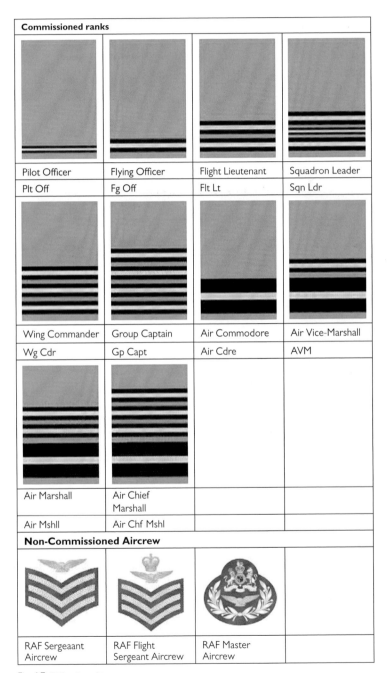

Commissioned ranks			
Pilot Officer	Flying Officer	Flight Lieutenant	Squadron Leader
Plt Off	Fg Off	Flt Lt	Sqn Ldr
Wing Commander	Group Captain	Air Commodore	Air Vice-Marshall
Wg Cdr	Gp Capt	Air Cdre	AVM
Air Marshall	Air Chief Marshall		
Air Mshll	Air Chf Mshl		

Non-Commissioned Aircrew			
RAF Sergeaant Aircrew	RAF Flight Sergeant Aircrew	RAF Master Aircrew	

Fig. 4.7 RAF rank markings.

Reproduced under crown copyright from RAF website (www.raf.mod.uk/organisation/ranks.cfm).

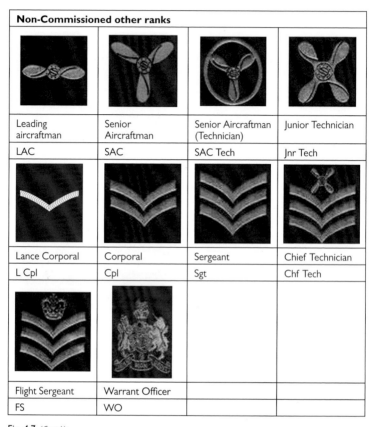

Non-Commissioned other ranks			
Leading aircraftman	Senior Aircraftman	Senior Aircraftman (Technician)	Junior Technician
LAC	SAC	SAC Tech	Jnr Tech
Lance Corporal	Corporal	Sergeant	Chief Technician
L Cpl	Cpl	Sgt	Chf Tech
Flight Sergeant	Warrant Officer		
FS	WO		

Fig. 4.7 (Contd.)

Activation and likely utilization

Use of the armed forces should only be considered where other options are unavailable, insufficient, or inappropriate and the MOD has no existing obligation to offer a specified level of assistance. Contribution of military personnel will also depend on other existing or planned commitments. Requests for military assistance should be made by Strategic (gold) Group to central government. Once armed forces are engaged, military liaison officers will be appointed at all levels.

Roles that may be undertaken by the armed forces include the following:

- Provision of:
  - large numbers of disciplined personnel
  - field facilities including tented and hard-standing structures for shelter
  - field medical facilities including accommodation, equipment, and personnel
  - Specialist equipment including generators
  - Provision of additional evacuation resources (e.g. trucks, helicopters)
- Supply of potable water and food
- Field engineering such as bridge construction
- Bomb disposal expertise
- Control of the public
- Assistance with maintaining cordons (in conjunction with the police) and control of access including prevention of looting
- Evacuation and route guidance
- Ground and incident reconnaissance
- Media handling.

Funding for military intervention

Because military aid to the civil community falls outside the stated purposes of the Ministry of Defence, the ministry is required by the Treasury to recoup the costs incurred in such intervention. Costs may be waived (i.e. no cost) if life is at risk or circumstances are exceptional for some other reason. This decision is usually a central government one, although local commanders have the authority to act immediately. In an immediate impact incident, such involvement will generally be no-cost until the recovery phase. Alternatively, the MOD may seek to recoup only those costs in excess of what would have in any event been incurred by the MOD costs (marginal). The final cost band is full costs in which every expense incurred (including pay and personnel expenses) are reclaimed.

Explosive and unexploded ordnance disposal

'Bomb disposal' may be divided into:

- explosive ordnance disposal (EOD)
- unexploded ordnance (UXO) disposal.

In the UK, all three services (Army, Royal Navy, and Royal Air Force) are involved in the disposal of explosive devices. Military 'taskings' are coordinated via a *Joint Service Cell* although the initial 'call out' in response to a suspected explosive device is the responsibility of the police.

Ammunition technicians of the Army's Royal Logistics Corps (RLC) deal with improvised explosive devices (IEDs) as well as expertise in chemical, biological, and radiation devices (including 'dirty bombs'). Ammunition technicians also liaise with, and train, the civilian emergency services as well as dealing with land service ammunition (including that of the Army Air Corps).

Bomb disposal officers of the Royal Engineers are responsible for dealing with enemy air dropped ammunition on land (e.g. World War II bombs).

The RAF is responsible for the disposal of UK service airdropped ammunition on land (apart from that used by the Army Air Corps).

The Royal Navy is responsible for ammunition found below high-tide level on Britain's coasts.

Responsibilities of first attenders on scene

The key aim of the first responder on the scene of a major incident is to make the declaration that a major incident has occurred. However, the defined response varies to some degree between services. All first attenders should avoid becoming personally involved in rescue work in order to concentrate on establishing a structured response through the tasks listed on p. 136.

Police service

The primary responsibility of the first police officer on scene is to ensure that accurate information is passed to their control room with minimum delay. The preferred mnemonic is METHANE although the alternative mnemonic CHALETS (see Box 5.1, p. 137) may occasionally be encountered. As with all the emergency services, the first officer on scene will remain in charge until a more senior officer arrives.

Fire and rescue service

The first fire officer on scene will, like the other emergency services, assume command until a designated senior officer arrives. As a consequence, he or she must carry out a careful assessment, passing information to control which will allow an appropriate and proportionate response. Initial tasks include:
- reviewing the fire-fighting measures (if any) already underway
- determining what additional resources are required
- assessing the hazards which are present or may develop (information may be available from the brigade Operational Risks Register available through a mobile data terminal)
- developing an initial plan for the use of fire service resources
- liaising with other services to ensure recognition of threats and coordination of efforts
- providing a safety briefing based on, where possible, joint services assessment
- providing a safety briefing and determine levels of PPE
- preparing to brief the designated ambulance commander.

Ambulance service

The first ambulance crew on scene, like the fire service or police, declare a major incident where necessary. The senior crew member will assume the role of ambulance commander until replaced by a designated senior officer. The acronym METHANE should be used to pass information to control. An incident log should be established and maintained; ensuring accurate recording of all decision-making and communications in a contemporaneous fashion.

Chapter 5

Casualty and Scene Medical Management

Declaration of a major incident

Rapid-onset 'big bang' incidents are generally obvious events that result in potentially large numbers of dead or injured casualties, as well as a significant number of uninjured bystanders and potential witnesses. Such incidents are recognized and responded to by emergency services personnel, usually following 999 calls from the public, leading to a major incident standby or declaration being made as appropriate by the first member of the emergency services to arrive at the scene. This will result in a 'bottom-up' response and escalation as necessary according to the evolving situation.

In the case of a chemical or radiation release incident, public or emergency services alarm may not be raised until suspicion is aroused by clusters of casualties with similar and/or unexpected symptoms coming forwards. There may be considerable delay until the nature, or causation, of the incident can be confirmed. For biological agent release or disease pandemic incidents, the delay will often be even greater and relies upon detection by regional or national health surveillance organizations. In such cases, the response to these so-called slow-onset 'rising tide' incidents is often initiated and managed from regional or central government institutions downwards.

This chapter is concerned with the management of a rapid-onset 'big bang' incident occurring at a defined location. The management of slowly developing incidents such as flooding is considered elsewhere in this book. The wider roles and responsibilities of the emergency services are covered in Chapter 4. This chapter brings together the elements of the medical response at scene.

Generic actions for the first emergency service personnel on scene are to:
- issue a major incident warning or major incident standby as appropriate
- control the scene to prevent unnecessary access and spread of contamination
- assess the scene for access and location of key elements of the response
- complete and send a METHANE report (see p. 137)
- commence a log of decisions and briefing with timings
- act as focus for the development of the response from one's own service (incident commander until relieved).

Initial information from the scene

It is vital that key information is passed from the scene to the emergency services control as soon as possible. In order to prevent confusion and ensure that important information is not missed, a standard formula should be used; conventionally this is by use the mnemonic METHANE (see Box 5.1).

Box 5.1 The **METHANE** and **CHALETS** formats

METHANE
My call sign/major incident alert
Exact location
Type of incident
Hazards at the scene
Access
Number of casualties and severity
Emergency services present and required

CHALETS (generally no longer used)
Casualties, number and severity
Hazards, present and potential
Access and egress
Location—exact
Emergency services—present and required
Type of incident
Safety

Summary of the medical response to a major incident

Medical responders at the scene of a major incident must be prepared to integrate fully within a multiprofessional multiagency team with shared understanding and objectives, following the systematic CSCATTT approach as shown in box 5.2.

Command and control

There are seven strands to the medical management of the on-scene response to a major incident. However, these strands provide an effective structure for the discussion of all aspects of scene management. *Command* is a vertical process, and *control* is horizontal. On-scene command and control meet at the *incident command centre* (tactical / silver command). Unless an effective command structure is established at the earliest opportunity, the management of the incident is likely to be significantly compromised.

Safety

Appropriate personal protective equipment (PPE) must be worn at all times and personnel who are to use it must be comfortable and confident to do so. High levels of PPE will only be used by the fire service, armed services, and specialist teams (such as HART teams). Those unfamiliar with the use of PPE or with the pre-hospital environment should be allocated to working in the casualty clearing station or other safe area. A safety officer will be appointed by the ambulance service (*ambulance safety officer*) to oversee health, safety, and welfare at the scene.

Communications

An effective communications system must mirror the command structure. The ambulance service will provide a *communications officer* at the tactical (silver) command who will coordinate arrangements. Communications will also be established and maintained with *strategic (gold) command* and with receiving hospitals. A hospital liaison officer will be appointed by the ambulance service. Communications are covered in more detail in Chapter 7.

Assessment

Commanders at both tactical (silver) and operational (bronze) levels must ensure that regular accurate reassessments of the scene are carried out. Information must be passed from operational (bronze) to tactical (silver) to *strategic (gold)* command (and vice versa) and shared across agencies at each command level.

Triage

Triage is the process by which priorities for treatment or transport from the scene are assigned to patients on the basis of their clinical condition. The aim is that patients who are more seriously injured or most likely to benefit from more rapid treatment will be allocated a higher category. Each casualty is likely to be triaged more than once at different stages of their rescue and evacuation.

Treatment

In general, treatment at the scene should be restricted to the minimum necessary to save life or limb. More complex treatment may be necessary if the patient is trapped. Wherever possible, casualties should be removed to the safety of the *casualty clearing station* where treatment can be performed more easily and safely.

Box 5.2 The CSCATTT paradigm (MIMMS)

Command and control
Safety
Communication
Assessment
Triage
Treatment
Transport

Transport

Transport of patients to hospital is an ambulance service responsibility. Careful records must be kept of patient destination. The tactical (silver) ambulance commander will appoint *ambulance loading* and *parking officers*.

Command structure

The key to the emergency services response at the scene of an incident is the *Joint Emergency Services Control Centre* (JESCC) (see Figure 5.1). The control centre is a tactical (silver) level command comprising the *tactical (silver) commanders* of each emergency service and the medical incident advisor as well as others depending on the nature of the incident such as environmental, railway, or scientific authorities. The fire, police, and ambulance commanders will be recognizable by their identifying tabards and headgear. Each service will also have at least one *forward commander* who reports to their commander at tactical (silver) level.

Forward commanders

In order to establish command and control in the operational (bronze) area, the fire, police, and ambulance services will each appoint a *operational (bronze/forward) commander* responsible for its operations within the inner cordon. In very significant incidents, a *forward medical incident advisor* operational (bronze) may be appointed to assist the *medical incident advisor* in the forward areas. The term *forward incident officer* may occasionally be encountered, although it has been replaced with the term *commander or advisor (medical)*. Overall control in the operational (bronze) area lies with the fire service with the specific exception of a terrorist incident when it falls to specialist police.

Commanders tactical (silver)

The emergency services responses at the scene are controlled by the individual service *commanders*, who together make up the JESCC or *tactical (silver) command*. The tactical (silver) commanders will report to *strategic (gold) command*. Although the ambulance, police, and fire services will usually appoint commanders, a *medical incident advisor* (MIA, or equivalent appointment) is likely to be requested only in incidents involving significant numbers of live casualties where direction may be required to distribute the load most appropriately to several hospitals or other medical facilities, especially where specialist services may be required (e.g. burns or children). Overall control at tactical (silver) level normally remains a police responsibility.

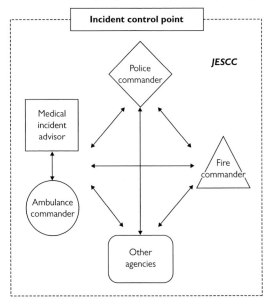

Fig. 5.1 Schematic representation of JESCC.

Organization of the on-scene medical response to a major incident

Figure 5.2 is a schematic diagram of the layout of the response at the scene of an incident involving significant numbers of live casualties. The early establishment of this framework is the key to an effective emergency services response. Figure 5.3 is a schematic layout of the organization of the casualty clearing station (or equivalent facility).

Casualty clearing station

The casualty clearing station (CCS) will be established by the ambulance service and initially staffed by ambulance service personnel. In due course, doctors and nurses may be allocated to work there as they become available. The CCS is the main location for treatment at the scene of an incident. Ideally, where possible, pre-existing buildings should be used although temporary accommodation, often tentage, is an alternative. Whatever location is used, lighting, heating, communications, and sufficient space are essential (see Box 5.3). The CCS may be extended in size if necessary, depending upon casualty numbers, their severity, and the existing capacity to effectively manage the casualty load.

The ambulance service will appoint a *casualty clearing station officer* who will ensure its effective operation. The casualty clearing station officer is also responsible for managing patient flow through the CCS including transfer to hospital in conjunction with the *ambulance loading officer* and hospital liaison officers. Medical and nursing staff who are not familiar with pre-hospital practice but who are sent to or turn up at the scene are best utilized at the CCS.

Ambulance circuit

In order to avoid congestion, an ambulance circuit must be established. Empty vehicles are parked at an *ambulance parking point* and called forwards as required to the *ambulance loading point* next to the CCS. Once loaded, the ambulance follows this predetermined circuit from the site. Patients will be transferred to appropriate receiving hospitals according to the clinical severity and nature of their injuries. Liaison officers at each receiving hospital in consultation with personnel on scene are responsible for matching patients with clinical facilities taking into account the clinical needs of the patient and the location and capacity of available hospital services including appropriate specialist centres. A medical incident advisor may be appointed to *strategic (gold)* to act in an area hospital liaison role.

Body holding area

There are only two reasons for moving the dead bodies of victims: to allow access to living casualties or if there is a risk that they might be destroyed or damaged. A body holding area should be identified in incidents where there are large numbers of dead and must provide appropriate shelter and protection from the elements as well as being away from any possible media intrusion. A police officer must be present at the body holding area at all times to ensure maintenance of the chain of evidence.

Temporary mortuary

A temporary mortuary is not to be confused with the body holding area. Temporary mortuary facilities - local emergency mortuary arrangements (LEMAs) - may be established *away from the scene* for the accommodation of large numbers of bodies. Local major incident plans will normally have pre-identified potential sites for temporary mortuaries such as aircraft hangers or industrial units. LEMAs require a licence from the Human Tissue Authority (HTA) under the Human Tissue Act 2004.

Box 5.3 Key features of a casualty clearing station
- Access from the incident site operational (bronze) area(s)
- Easy access and egress for emergency vehicles from outer cordon to ICP
- Shelter/covered area
- Heating
- Lighting
- Water supply
- Appropriate storage for medical equipment—both electrical and consumables.

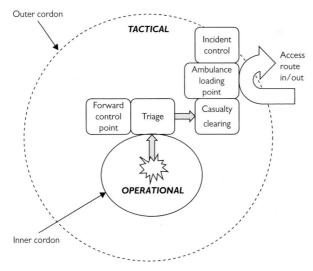

Fig. 5.2 Schematic layout of the organization of medical response facilities at the incident scene.

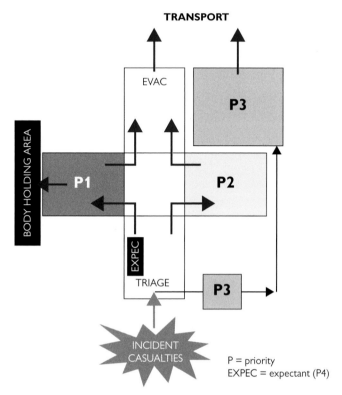

Fig. 5.3 Example of casualty clearing station layout.

Survivor reception centre (SRC)

Uninjured survivors should be moved to a SRC and not transferred to the CCS. However, the CCS should be close enough to the reception centre for survivors to be transferred if they show signs of becoming unwell or unrecognized injuries become apparent. The reception centre should offer shelter, warmth, and lighting and provides a location for the police to collect required information before people are dispersed from the scene. Where possible, existing buildings such as school halls, leisure centres, and supermarkets should be used in order to reduce the need to improvise the required facilities. Key requirements are shown in Box 5.4.

Rest centre/reception centre

The rest centre is an interim place of safety for those evacuated as a result of an incident. The local authority will usually coordinate this provision which will be provided until more suitable longer-term arrangements can be made.

Friends and relatives reception centre ((FFRC)

The FFRC provides a location at which survivors can be reunited with their loved ones, information can be disseminated to friends and relatives, and there is a quiet and private area for friends, family, and victims to meet and communicate. Emotional support should also be made available.

Box 5.4 Key requirements of a survivor reception centre

- Privacy and security (the public and the press must be excluded)
- Provision of food and water
- Toilet/sanitation facilities
- Dry clothing
- Facilities for basic first aid, recognizing and initial management of acute medical illness
- Facilities for documentation and communication
- Social and welfare support.

Key medical roles and responsibilities at scene

Medical incident advisor (Strategic and Tactical)

In general, a medical incident advisor (previous designations include medical incident officer and medical incident commander) will be utilized to assist in the management of large numbers of live casualties at the scene of an incident. The medical advisor will usually be chosen from a pool of suitable experienced and trained individuals maintained by the ambulance service. Resilience planning must ensure that arrangements are in place for the provision of a medical advisor and that MERITs are available (see p. 102) when required (in conjunction with acute hospitals within the region).

It is the role of the medical incident advisor to work closely with the ambulance incident commander as part of the tactical (silver) command. Both commanders will also work closely with the tactical (silver) commanders of the fire and police services (and other equivalents) in addition to the other key players at tactical (silver) level.

Enhanced Care Team Doctors (Operational)

The Enhanced Care Team Doctors will be responsible for the provision of specialist medical care in the operational (bronze) area, working closely with the ambulance forward commander and other service forward commanders as part of operational (bronze) command. Such individuals will normally be members of skilled pre-hospital care teams such as HART and extensively experienced in working in challenging circumstances.

Casualty clearing station medical lead

An appropriate clinician may be appointed to head the medical treatment teams within the CCS. This is not the same as the casualty clearing station officer who bears managerial responsibility for the facility.

Further information can be found within National Ambulance Resilience Unit guidelines (www.naru.org.uk).

Responsibilities of medical incident advisors

- Provision of strategic medical advice and direct clinical support to the emergency services
- Supervisory clinical responsibility for the medical care of all casualties at the scene
- Working with liaison officers to ensure the evacuation and transport of patients to the most appropriate receiving hospital according to their priority and specific clinical needs
- Provision of a doctor for the confirmation of death in conjunction with the police service (via the police incident commander)
- Liaison with receiving hospitals regarding:
  - emergency department capacity
  - bed availability
  - intensive therapy unit (ITU) bed availability
  - Theatre capacity
- Liaison with public health agencies, the Health Protection Agency, and other healthcare bodies
- Cooperation with media requests for information in conjunction with the emergency services
- Maintenance of a log of timings and decisions.

Other healthcare roles and responsibilities

Casualty clearing station officer
The responsibilities of the casualty clearing station officer include:
- establishing and monitoring triage and treatment at the CCS
- overseeing and allocating medical and nursing staff
- ensuring adequate equipment supply
- liaison with the ambulance loading officer
- liaison with the ambulance commander
- ensuring appropriate medical records are made at the CCS.

The site of the CCS is determined by the ambulance tactical (silver) commander.

Ambulance loading officer
The responsibilities of the ambulance loading officer are:
- establishment of an ambulance circuit (in conjunction with the police)
- coordination of evacuation by clinical priority, availability and location of beds, and availability of vehicles (in conjunction with the medical advisor and ambulance commanders)
- liaison with the ambulance parking officer, calling forward vehicles as required
- supervision of packaging of patients
- determination of appropriate evacuation methods
- collection and return of equipment when the incident is closed.

Ambulance parking officer
The tasks of the ambulance parking officer include:
- logging staff and ambulance service vehicles as they enter and leave the site
- ensuring best use of ambulance service and other evacuation vehicles
- sending vehicles forward for loading and coordinating waiting vehicles.

Equipment officer
In the largest and most prolonged incidents, an equipment officer will be appointed by the ambulance service to take responsibility for the provision and resupply of medical equipment at the scene.

Communications officer
The communications officer is also appointed by the ambulance service and will take responsibility for:
- communications between the site and ambulance control
- communications between different emergency services command vehicles
- communications between the site and receiving hospitals
- assessment of the most appropriate communications modalities
- keeping an appropriate record.

Ambulance safety officer
The ambulance safety officer is responsible for:
- ensuring that all health services personnel are wearing appropriate PPE
- identification of hazards at the scene (working with fire service personnel) and appropriate action to deal with them
- welfare of health services personnel
- liaison with other emergency services on health and safety matters
- obtaining appropriate advice on health and safety matters (including decontamination) in conjunction with the relevant statutory authorities.

Triage officers
The ambulance service will appoint individuals to carry out triage in the operational (bronze) area (*primary triage officers*) and at the CCS (*secondary triage officers*) See pp. 148–53.

Key initial actions for the ambulance service

- Declare a major incident/major incident standby
- Inform receiving hospitals
- Appoint and send a hospital ambulance liaison officer (HALO) to each hospital to ensure crew welfare and collate patient numbers
- Appoint and send (where possible) a hospital ambulance liaison control officer (HALCO) to each hospital to liaise with the hospital coordination team
- Commence an incident log
- Alert other agencies such as the National Blood Service, bed location services, etc.
- Determine whether medical incident advisor(s) or MERIT teams are necessary and if so arrange for them to be collected and transported to the scene
- Deploy sufficient heavy equipment to the site
- Establish communications between the incident scene and the wider NHS
- Establish the ambulance circuit
- Establish a full incident command structure
- Ensure that PPE and identifying tabards are available at scene
- Establish triage.

Triage

Principles of triage

Triage is the active process of sorting casualties into priority for treatment, evacuation, or transport and is the key to optimizing the management of large numbers of patients where available medical personnel and resources are limited. *Primary triage* is carried out in the operational (bronze) area and patients are usually re-triaged (*secondary triage*), at the CCS. *Triage for transport* will be carried out before patients leave the site in order to ensure the most appropriate distribution of casualties to receiving units. In the majority of incidents, triage is used to determine the order in which patients are treated, although in overwhelming incidents triage could be used to determine who is treated and who is not.

Triage categories

Casualties are triage into one or other of the categories listed in Table 5.1.

Immediate category
Casualties in this category require immediate life-saving treatment.

Urgent category
These casualties require significant intervention as soon as it can be given.

Delayed category
These patients will require medical intervention, but not urgently.

Expectant category

Some patients will be so severely injured (or so seriously ill) that any attempt to treat them would have very little chance of a successful outcome and, in doing so, would divert limited resources from other casualties who may have a greater chance of survival. When the available resources are inadequate to provide everyone with the treatment they need, such patients may be assigned to the *expectant* category. The decision to invoke this category should be taken at tactical (silver) level and only after discussion with strategic (gold) command. To date, the expectant triage category has never been invoked in a UK major incident.

If the expectant category is to be used, a recognized patient triage and labelling system must be agreed. The most widely recognized are:

- blue card (rarely available)
- P3 card overwritten *expectant*
- P3 card with the green corners turned back to reveal red underneath.

Triage sieve

The triage sieve is intended to be a rapid, simple, and reproducible triage system for use at first contact with the casualty (see Figure 5.4). It may also be used at secondary triage in place of the more conventional *triage sort*, depending on the casualty flow. Because it is physiologically based, different values must be used for children. Triage sieves for children are found on pp. 151–3.

Table 5.1 Triage descriptions

Triage (T)	Priority (P)	Description	Colour code
1	1	Immediate	Red
2	2	Urgent	Yellow
3	3	Delayed	Green
4	1 (hold)	Expectant	Blue
Dead	Dead	Dead	White or black

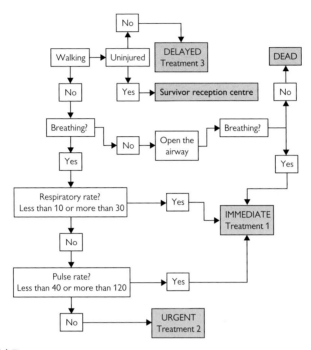

Fig. 5.4 Triage sieve.

Reproduced from Greaves, and Porter, *Oxford Handbook of Pre-Hospital Care*, 2007, with permission from Oxford University Press.

Triage sort

The triage sort is a more complex technique than the sieve and consequently takes longer to perform (see Figure 5.5). It is therefore intended as a tool for secondary triage at the CCS. The triage sort may require measure such as respiratory rate, blood pressure or an assessment of the Glasgow Coma Scale (GCS) score. As a result, lack of staff or pressure of patient flow may mean that the sieve rather than the sort is used for secondary as well as primary triage.

Triage in children

The triage sieve is based on normal *adult* physiological values. If it is used on children, significant over triage will result. Substitute values are necessary. Sieves are available for children based either on length (top of head to feet) or weight (see Figures 5.6, 5.7 and 5.8).

The approximate weight of a child can be worked out from their age using the following formulae (*APLS*):

Weight:	1–12 months	$= \dfrac{\text{months} + 4}{2}$
	1–5 years	$= (\text{years} \times 2) + 8$
	6–12 years	$= (\text{years} \times 3) + 7$

As an alternative, paediatric triage tapes can be used to identify the appropriate algorithm estimated by weight according to a child's size (e.g. the Broselow system).

The triage sort		
PHYSIOLOGICAL VARIABLE	**VALUE**	**SCORE**
Respiratory rate	10–29	4
	>29	3
	6–9	2
	1–5	1
	0	0
Systolic blood pressure	>90	4
	76–89	3
	50–75	2
	1–49	1
	0	0
Glasgow Coma Scale Score	13–15	4
	9–12	3
	6–8	2
	4–5	1
	3	0
Total score for coding (see box below)		**X**

Coded score	Priority
1–10	T1
11	T2
12	T3
0	Dead

Fig. 5.5 Triage sort.
Reproduced from Greaves, Ian, and Porter, Keith, *Oxford Handbook of Pre-Hospital Care*, 2007, with permission from Oxford University Press.

The need for evacuation

In some circumstances it may be necessary to advise the public on whether they should evacuate a given area or remain and shelter indoors. This may take place rapidly (e.g. if there is a risk of fire spreading or explosion), or more slowly during flooding or other extreme weather, when phased evacuation may be possible. Circumstances which might justify evacuation include:
- acts of terrorism
- release or threatened release of radioactive materials or other hazardous substances
- spread of fire
- risk of explosion
- damage caused by severe weather
- risk from serious flooding
- risk of environmental contamination
- transport failures.

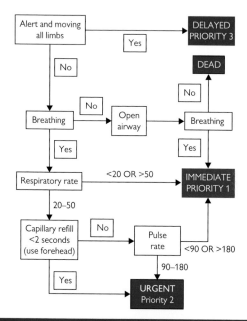

Fig. 5.6 Triage sieve: child 50–80cm or 3–10kg.
Reproduced from Greaves, and Porter, *Oxford Handbook of Pre-Hospital Care*, 2007, with permission from Oxford University Press.

Planning will mitigate the effects of evacuation on the individuals concerned but the evacuation will be both emotionally charged and require rapid mobilization of facilities including transport and safe shelter. Ideally, the LRF will have determined which organizations can initiate the decision to evacuate and identified triggers for evacuation (such as flood water levels), but if time allows, this is a decision best made at *Strategic Coordination Group* (SCG) level usually on the advice of the police in consultation with other agencies. The police will also define the area to be evacuated. (See Figure 5.9.)

The decision to carry out a mass evacuation would normally involve central government. The police can only recommend evacuation and have no power (except within the inner cordon in response to a terrorist incident) to require responsible adults to leave their homes.

Plans for evacuation and shelter should take into account:

• Transportation of people and traffic management
• Shelter and rest centre accommodation
• Supporting people sheltering *in situ*
• Assisting groups with specific needs
• Developing multiagency crime prevention strategy
• Arrangements for pets and livestock
• Arrangements for business continuity management
• Protecting items of cultural interest and high value
• Special considerations for flooding, CBRN, hazardous materials, and pandemic flu
• Return and recovery
• Communications.

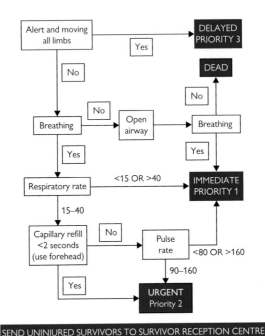

Fig. 5.7 Triage sieve: child 80–100cm or 11–18kg.
Reproduced from Greaves, and Porter, *Oxford Handbook of Pre-Hospital Care*, 2007, with permission from Oxford University Press.

LRFs should develop a generic evacuation plan and consider how best to structure their evacuation planning activities, for example, by establishing a sub-group to focus specifically on evacuation and shelter issues.

Once the decision to evacuate is taken, the public and other responding organizations should be informed as soon as is practical. Effective safe evacuation will require identification and management (including policing) of safe egress routes which do not obstruct emergency services access to the incident. Plans should include means of acquiring transport facilities, especially for those with particular needs, bearing in mind that the ambulance service may be busy with emergency evacuation of casualties. Plans for all areas must include the contact details of those who are especially vulnerable such as the elderly, children and those with disabilities and planners must be aware of the likely scale and type of needs these groups will present. (See Figures 5.10 and 5.11, and Tables 5.2 and 5.3.)

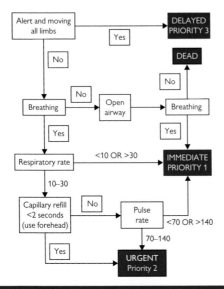

Fig. 5.8 Triage sieve: child 100–140cm or 19–32kg.

Reproduced from Greaves, and Porter, *Oxford Handbook of Pre-Hospital Care*, 2007, with permission from Oxford University Press.

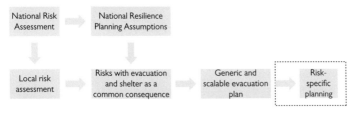

Fig. 5.9 Risk and planning process for emergency evacuation and shelter.

Reproduced under Crown Copyright from HM Government, *Evacuation and shelter guidance*, January 2014 (www.gov.uk/government/uploads/system/uploads/attachment_data/file/274615/Evacuation_and_Shelter_Guidance_2014.pdf).

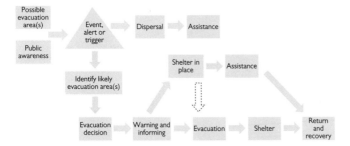

Fig. 5.10 Stages of evacuation.

Reproduced under Crown Copyright from HM Government, *Evacuation and shelter guidance*, January 2014 (www.gov.uk/government/uploads/system/uploads/attachment_data/file/274615/Evacuation_and_Shelter_Guidance_2014.pdf).

Table 5.2 Scales of evacuation

Definition	Decision to trigger taken by	Resources likely to be required for this magnitude	Example
Small-scale/local evacuation	Incident controller or SCG	Local responders	One or two streets evacuated. E.g. gas leak
Medium-scale evacuation	SCG	Local responders, possibly with mutual aid or national support	Evacuation or dispersal of parts of a city or large industrial site
Large-scale evacuation	SCG	Local responders, with mutual aid or national support	Evacuation in response to a major chemical release
Mass evacuation	SCG coordination with central government	Local responders, mutual aid, and national support	Evacuation in response to significant flooding

Reproduced under Crown Copyright from HM Government,

Evacuation and shelter guidance, January 2014 (www.gov.uk/government/uploads/system/uploads/attachment_data/file/274615/Evacuation_and_Shelter_Guidance_2014.pdf)

Table 5.3 Roles and responsibilities. Reproduced under Crown Copyright from HM Government, *Evacuation and shelter guidance*, January 2014 (www.gov.uk/government/uploads/system/uploads/attachment_data/file/274615/Evacuation_and_Shelter_Guidance_2014.pdf)

Role/responsibility	Organization
Evacuation	
Decision to evacuate	SCG, relevant emergency service, and other agencies, as determined by the LRF
Evacuation route planning	Highways authorities
Use of publicly owned transport	Local authority
Use of railways and stations	Train operation companies and Network Rail
Specialist medical vehicles	NHS, commissioned service providers, voluntary sector
Hospitals	NHS
Care homes	Provider
Home care	Local authority, in coordination with NHS and commissioned service providers
Schools	School
Children's homes	Service provider
Prisons	Prison service and NOMS
Immigration detention and removal centres	Prison Service, in coordination with Home Office
Shelter	
Provision of short-term shelter	Local authority
Registration of evacuees	Local authority

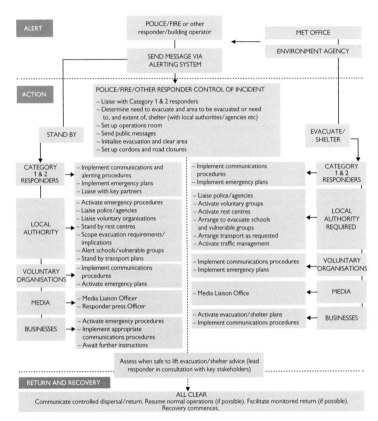

Fig. 5.11 Overview of emergency evacuation and shelter processes.

Reproduced under Crown Copyright from HM Government, *Evacuation and shelter guidance*, January 2014 (www.gov.uk/government/uploads/system/uploads/attachment_data/file/274615/Evacuation_and_Shelter_Guidance_2014.pdf).

Decontamination

General principles

If deemed necessary due to an identified or suspected hazard, decontamination of all casualties and uninjured survivors should take place at the scene. However, it is likely that a significant number of casualties, or individuals who suspect they have been exposed, will also self-present to local hospitals and other medical facilities. Some of these may potentially be contaminated therefore plans must also be in place to deal with them. A balance must be achieved between mitigating risk to, and protecting, emergency responders and healthcare facilities, as well as providing timely care to self-presenters.

A dynamic risk-based approach should be utilized to take into account the rapidly evolving nature of any CBRN incident (see Figure 5.12). Three areas should be considered:
1. The need for, and type of PPE
2. Medical interventions that may be necessary
3. Decontamination procedures (dry vs wet).

Dry decontamination

Dry decontamination should be considered the default process for non-caustic chemical incidents. This involves the use of dry absorbent material (e.g. blue paper roll) to blot exposed skin following full disrobing, unless casualties are showing any signs of caustic or irritant substance exposure. All waste materials should be double-bagged into clinical waste (or equivalent).

At the scene, casualties (and the uninjured if necessary) should be removed from the area of maximum contamination into the open air, upwind of the incident and should be fully disrobed. Patients who can do so should undress themselves under supervision. Casualties should have their glasses or hearing aids removed. Additional support may be necessary for these patients. Glasses needed for reasonable function may be returned after they have been decontaminated. If there is reason to believe that a release is ongoing, removal of casualties to a closed area may be safer.

Key principles should focus on the person being disrobed and decontamination, rather than the process itself. These must include:
• good communication at every stage of the process
• clear and accessible instructions and information
• safety and protection from hypothermia
• modesty: culture and gender.

Careful removal of clothing will remove around 90% of contamination, with a further 9% removed by dry decontamination—as expressed in the 'rule of tens'(see Figure 5.13). Details of all discarded clothing and personal articles should be documented and linked to an individual.

Wet decontamination

Wet decontamination should only normally be used with signs of caustic chemical substance (acids and alkalis) exposure (e.g. redness, itching, blistering, or burning of the skin or eyes). Wet decontamination should also follow confirmed biological or radiological contamination. There is no national standard for the method of wet decontamination. Any available water source may be considered such as showers, taps, and hose reels or sprinklers. Duration of wet decontamination should be no more than 45–90 seconds.

Facilities

Clinical decontamination using purpose-designed decontamination equipment may be involve collapsible temporary mobile decontamination units at the hospital reception, static decontamination units which are semi-permanent structures usually situated outside emergency departments, or permanent decontamination rooms within the hospital infrastructure. NHS organizations should consider fixed decontamination facilities when designing new buildings.

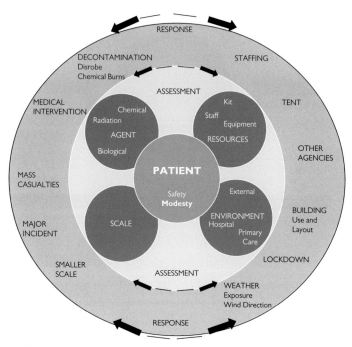

Fig. 5.12 Main elements of dynamic risk assessment for emergency decontamination (NHS England London Region, 2014).

Reproduced under Open Government Licence from NHS England *Emergency Preparedness, Resilience and Response (EPRR), Chemical incidents: Planning for the management of self-presenting patients in healthcare settings*, 1 April 2016 (www.england.nhs.uk/wp-content/uploads/2015/04/eprr-chemical-incidents.pdf).

The pathway for patients self-presenting with suspicion or evidence of hazardous substance contamination is outlined below (with acknowledgement to Pennine Acute Hospitals NHS Trust):
1. *Isolate*: limit movement of, and contact with, patient.
2. *Disrobe*: instruct patient to remove all clothing and place in bags provided.
3. *Contain*: switch air conditioning off and consider unit compartmentalization or lockdown.
4. *Assess*: approach based upon knowledge of substance involved, specialist team required, pre-hospital information or central guidance.
5. *Decontamination*: wet for caustic substance skin/eye contamination, dry for all others. Consider secondary sources (e.g. relatives or others).

On reception of suspected or confirmed contaminated persons, local response plans should be followed if these have not already been activated. Further considerations include the following:
• Possibility of further self-presenters
• PPE (resilience stocks)
• Observation for secondary contamination exposure
• Inform Public Health England (or other devolved administration)
• Liaise with specialist sources of advice
• Need for countermeasures (resilience stocks)
• Need for mass decontamination facilities (fire service)
• Early business continuity and recovery arrangements.

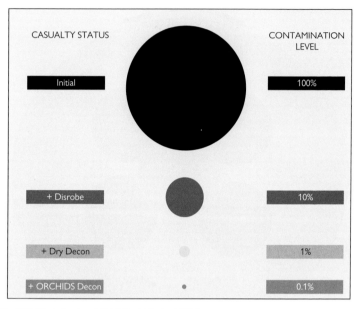

Fig. 5.13 The 'rule of tens' (Public Health England, 2014).

*ORCHIDS: Optimisation through Research of Chemical Incident Decontamination Systems.

Reproduced under Open Government Licence from Department for Environment, Food, and Rural Affairs, *Contingency Plan for Exotic Notifiable Diseases of Animals in England*, March 2016 (www.gov.uk/government/uploads/system/uploads/attachment_data/file/508753/exotic-notifiable-disease-contingency-plan-2016.pdf)

Responsibilities for decontamination.
- Decontamination of the sick and injured is the responsibility of the ambulance service but may be carried out by the fire service in some areas by local arrangement.
- The ambulance service is responsible for ensuring that appropriate advice is available regarding necessary decontamination.
- The fire service is responsible for mass decontamination.

General principles for mass decontamination
- Focus must be maintained on the person being disrobed and decontaminated
- Good command, control, and communication are vital
- Considerations include safety (risk of hypothermia) and modesty
- Is normally undertaken at the inner cordon
- Should be sited taking into account the wind direction and typography.

The response at medical facilities other than hospitals, such as urgent care centres or general practice, should follow the same basic principles and must be appropriate and proportionate to the setting and scale of the incident. Specific guidance is available from the NHS England website under EPRR.

Decontamination run-off

Water used for decontamination should ideally be contained in order to reduce environ-mental damage. If the fire and rescue service are likely to be unable to contain the run off, the Environment Agency, or SEPA in Scotland, and the local water and sewerage companies should be alerted in order to mitigate the potential adverse effects. The police may take samples of run-off water for forensic analysis.

Decontamination of the dead

Decisions regarding the decontamination of dead bodies are the responsibility of HM Coroner and police senior investigating officer.

Personal protective equipment

All scene responders must have access to a basic standard of PPE. It is the *personal responsibility* of anyone who regularly provides pre-hospital care, or is likely to be called upon to do so, to have this level of protection immediately available.

By the nature of terrorist incidents, it is possible that responders are placed in situations of some personal hazard. Although, in general, medical care in such situations should only be provided by those with special training, it is essential that anyone who enters such an area is appropriately protected. It is the responsibility of the police and other emergency services to ensure that such protection is available and that healthcare staff are not exposed to any unnecessary risk.

NHS issue personal protective equipment

All NHS receiving hospitals are issued with suits offering respiratory protection. It is essential that all staff are familiar with wearing, and working in, this clothing. Putting on the standard NHS PPE takes time and is best achieved with assistance from a colleague. The length of time medical staff can safely operate in the suit is limited and should not exceed 1 hour (see Figure 5.14).

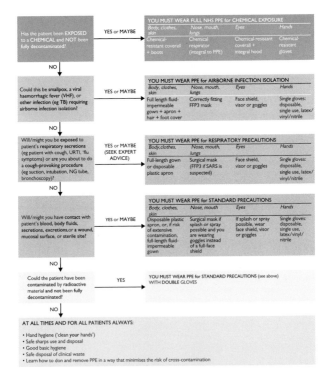

Fig. 5.14 HPA guidance regarding requirement for NHS personal protective equipment.

Reproduced under Open Government License from Heptonstall J, Gent N, *CRBN incidents: clinical management & health protection*, Health Protection Agency, London, November 2006 (Revisions v4.0 September 2008), www.gov.uk/government/uploads/system/uploads/attachment_data/file/340709/Chemical_biological_radiological_and_nuclear_incidents_management.pdf

Dealing with the dead and human remains

The following simple guidelines should be followed when dealing with the dead once they have arrived at the mortuary. Mass fatality incidents are covered on p. 162 and forensic and legal aspects on p. 164. Whilst at the scene, bodies must remain under police supervision to ensure continuity of evidence. The police will appoint a *police mortuary operations coordinator* (PMOC) at any mortuary used during a major incident. Some police forces have a specially trained *victim recovery team* expert in the safe and forensically appropriate removal of remains.

Mortuary procedures (police)

- If there is more than one incident scene, a separate mortuary should be used for the casualties from each.
- Bodies identified as belonging to terrorists or suspects, should be sent to a separate mortuary.
- Scene examiners will be appointed solely to deal with each mortuary in order to avoid cross contamination.
- Bodies will be X-rayed on arrival wherever possible for the identification of debris.
- Bodies will be traced swabbed for explosive residue where appropriate.
- A scene examiner will attend each post-mortem examination.
- All clothing and effects will be collected, searched and recorded as exhibits.

The PMOC will ensure evidence is collected and handled appropriately and that continuity is demonstrated as well as that all relevant documentation is correctly completed. In addition, the PMOC is responsible for health and safety within facility, security, liaison with funeral directors and forensic specialists, implementing investigation and identification strategies, and working with specialist mortuary staff.

Staff at a temporary mortuary

- Police mortuary operations coordinator (PMOC)
- Mortuary facilities manager/emergency mortuary coordinator:
  - Manages facility, liaises with HTA, ensures health and safety
  - Ensures staff and equipment available, works closely with PMOC and supervising forensic pathologist
  - Ensures proper disposal or storage of waste.
  - Supervises decommissioning of facility
- Police mortuary officers: search and strip bodies and ensure that all evidence is bagged labelled, and preserved
- Mortuary documentation officer: is responsible for all documentation of victims and evidential samples
- Mortuary exhibits officer: records and labels all non-tissue evidential items
- Supervising forensic pathologist (appointed by the coroner)
- Mortuary technicians
- Forensic specialists.

Mass fatalities

Most major incidents will not involve mass fatalities. Unfortunately, those that do will be associated with the highest degree of scrutiny and the greatest levels of anxiety and distress. An effective mechanism for managing mass fatalities is therefore essential. A mass fatality incident is sometimes described as an incident *where the number of fatalities exceeds* what normal local mortuary facilities can handle, although each coroner's area must identify designated disaster mortuaries. In managing large numbers of bodies, forensic aspects including preservation of evidence, chain of evidence and avoidance of contamination, issues relating to possible or actual contamination, and equally importantly the cultural or religious sensitivities of the deceased and their relatives must all be taken into account.

Information regarding mortuary capacity must be continually updated during an incident and the information passed to Strategic (gold) Group. Some UK coroners have been specially trained to deal with mass fatality incidents.

In some cases, a *Mass Fatality Coordination Group* (MFCG) may be established which will report to and work in close cooperation with Strategic (gold). Potential membership is shown below.

The stages of the process of dealing with disaster victims are:
• recovery
• identification
• reconciliation (forensic matching)
• repatriation (if required).

MFCG membership
• HM Coroner
• Senior identification manager (SIM)
• Senior investigating officer (SIO)
• Casualty bureau manager
• Senior evidence recovery manager (SERM)
• Supervising pathologist
• Policy mortuary operations coordinator (PMOC)
• Family liaison coordinator (FLC)
• Survivors reception centre manager
• Family and friends reception centre manager
• Hospital investigation team coordinator
• Planning, intelligence, and logistics manager
• Finance manager
• Local authority representative
• Human Tissue Authority (HTA) representative.

The chair is usually the coroner or senior identification manager.

Senior investigating officer (SIO): the senior police officer in charge of the criminal investigation into an incident.

Senior identification manager (SIM): appointed by Strategic (gold), the SIM is a senior specially trained police officer responsible for the recovery and identification of the deceased. Other responsibilities include collection and storage of forensic evidence and personal property from the deceased, management of appropriate passage of information to the media regarding the dead and missing, and welfare of staff involved in managing the dead. The SIM is also required to ensure that the families of the deceased are kept informed at all stage of the investigation.

Identification of the deceased
This is dealt with in Chapter 13 (p. 394).

National emergency mortuary arrangements

Central government currently has a contract with a logistical company to provide emergency mortuary arrangements for very large numbers of victims when local mortuary facilities are overwhelmed. This facility will be activated by central government though the *Central Assistance Programme* (managed by the Home Office Emergency Preparedness fatality Team) and at the request of the Mass Fatality Coordination Group, but the costs will generally fall to the local authority.

The Central Assistance programme includes:

- temporary structures capable of housing up to 600 casualties
- mortuary equipment which may be used in the temporary accommodation or made available to designated disaster mortuaries
- post-mortem X-ray equipment (as above)
- temporary storage areas used to enhance NEMA or designated mortuaries.

Potential sites for NEMA should have been identified in advance and built into resilience planning. NEMA is stored in Oxfordshire with stockpiles of general mortuary equipment stored in London, Yorkshire and Humberside, the North West, and South West.

Management of contaminated fatalities

Ideally, contaminated casualties will be decontaminated on scene. Where this is not possible, they will be removed from the scene on the authority of the SIM and coroner. Full PPE will be required by all attending personnel and suitable dedicated vehicles will be required. Examinations will generally be carried out at the temporary mortuary where storage will usually occur, although refrigerated vehicles can also be used which may require destruction after the incident. Bodies may be disposed of by cremation in a special body bag or burial, often deep and avoiding ground water and other hazards, in an airtight metal coffin containing charcoal.

Role of the police senior investigation manager (SIM)

The SIM will work closely with the commanders at tactical (silver) and strategic (gold) and with the SIO to establish an appropriate plan which does not interfere with the management or rescue of live casualties as well as agreeing terms of reference with the coroner (or equivalent). In the event of a terrorist incident either Counter Terrorism Command (CTC) or the relevant *Counter Terrorism Unit* (CTU—outside London) will be informed. The SIM will explain the evidence retrieval strategy at tactical (silver) level and ensure the presence of evidence recovery personnel under a *scene evidence recovery manager* (SERM). Victim recovery teams of specially trained police officers will also be used.

The SIM must ensure that family liaison officers have been tasked by a *family liaison coordinator* (FLC) and that police personnel are present at the *survivor's reception centre, CCS*, and *family and friends' reception centre*. They should also ensure that hospital documentation teams and a casualty bureau are in place and that appropriate information is being collected. The SIM is responsible for ensuring that appropriate management of the dead and human remains is in place including compliance with the Human Tissue Act 2004. The decision to establish a mass fatality group will be jointly taken with the coroner as will decisions regarding identification of the dead and management of the bereaved. All decisions taken by the SIM should be logged for evidential purposes.

Circumstances may arise, for example, following a natural disaster, when there is a SIM but no SIO. Following a terrorist incident, an explosive ordnance officer may manage the scene until it is made safe before handing over to a *bomb scene manager* (BSM) from the counter terrorism unit or command.

Evidence

There are five categories of evidence at the scene of a major incident: bodies, body parts and human remains, personal property, evidential property (anything not personal to the victims but required for the investigation), and technical property required for any technical enquiry, for example, by any of the accident investigation boards. Body parts collected at the scene may be held at a holding audit area (HAA) before being removed from the scene. A chain of evidence must be maintained at all times. The Maritime and Coastguard Agency is responsible for the recovery of human remains from an incident at sea.

Special Incidents

Animal health

Mass outbreaks of animal disease are unfortunately relatively common and their impact on the wider population is likely to vary. At their worst - for example the foot and mouth disease (FMD) outbreak of 2001 - the impact on farmers, the rural community, and Britain as a whole, as well as the political fallout from allegations of mishandling can be immense. This section will not consider the management of diseases transmitted from animals to humans (*zoonoses*), or threats of such transmission, as these are managed through well-established disease surveillance processes, nor will it consider longstanding animal health risks to humans such as the management of tuberculosis in badgers and commercial cattle.

Government policy
Management and policy for animal disease outbreaks in England is the responsibility of the *Department for Environment Food and Rural Affairs* (Defra). In the devolved regions, responsi-bility lies with the Scottish and Welsh governments. However, planning guidelines stress the importance of a coordinated response to outbreaks which are likely to cross administrative borders. Defra maintains contingency plans for notifiable diseases such as FMD as well as for exotic diseases, defined as those not normally present in the UK. The main agency for the response to such an incident is the *Animal and Plant Health Agency* (APHA).

Animal and Plant Health Agency (APHA; formerly the Animal Health and Veterinary Laboratories Agency)
The APHA is an agency which works on behalf of Defra, the Department of the Environment, and the Scottish and Welsh governments. The agency is responsible for pre-venting and controlling animal diseases and for providing specialist laboratory services as well as providing policy advice on animal health-related issues. The Agency acts as a global refer-ence laboratory for some exotic and zoonotic diseases and regulates control in endangered species as well as overseeing import regulations and controls designed to protect the UK's food supplies. APHA offers a wide range of services including serological testing from its UK-wide offices and laboratories. APHA offers a 24-hour helpline to report potential suspicious disease outbreaks in animals (03000 200 301).

Aims of animal disease control
Like all plans for the management of a major incident, the most important component of dealing with a major outbreak of animal disease is containment. Similarly, rapid recognition will be a key factor in restricting the impact of any outbreak. The central government frame-work recognizes the following requirements for an effective response:
• Prevention of incursion of an exotic disease into the UK
• Rapid recognition through effective surveillance
• Minimization of the cost to and impact on the taxpayer and wider society
• Minimization of the cost to and impact on individual farmers and agriculture
• Minimization of the number of animals which require culling and the effects on animal welfare.

Wherever possible, therefore, disease will be isolated and contained where it is first dis-covered. Further spread will be reduced or prevented through selective culling of affected animals and contacts and mandatory restrictions on movement of animals. Further meas-ures will include vaccination (if appropriate and available), enhanced national imposition of biosecurity measures, and risk assessment before interventions are lifted.

Preparedness
As in all types of major incident, preparedness is crucial in reducing the likelihood of an event and moderating its impact. Defra is the lead agency for preparedness in matters regarding animal health; it is not a statutory responder under the CCA. Defra's Exotic Disease Policy Response Team (EDPRT) is responsible for the development of policy, while the APHA leads the operational aspects of preparing for an outbreak. Each APHA office has a *regional operations director* responsible for ensuring that plans are in place and that training occurs to optimize the response to an incident. Each APHA region also appoints *resilience and*

operations and *readiness and resilience managers* with specific responsibility for prepared-ness. All planning is done in close cooperation with the agencies described in Chapter 2 and the APHA will be actively engaged in LRF arrangements. In the event of an outbreak, the regional resilience manager supports the regional operations director in establishing and managing the *local disease control centre*.

UK disease alert status

White alert

The disease is not present or suspected in the UK. This is the 'normal' alert state for exotic diseases.

Black alert

This indicates a higher than normal risk, for example, due to disease in a nearby EU member state. The decision to raise the alert state is made by the chief veterinary officer.

Amber alert

There is a strong suspicion of the presence of the disease on a specified premises based on clinical evidence after assessment by a vet. By this time, samples will have been submitted for analysis.

Red alert

The disease has been confirmed or an operational response commenced.

Definitions

An *exotic* disease is one that does not normally occur in the UK.

Zoonotic diseases are those transmitted to man through an animal reservoir: they may or may not be exotic.

Notification

When the owner of an animal, usually but not invariably a farmer, suspects that one of their animals has a notifiable disease (see p. 168), they must immediately inform the duty veteri-nary surgeon from the APHA. By far the most significant of these diseases is FMD. Other notifiable animal diseases are listed in Box 6.1. Further information is available on the http://www.gov.uk website. It should be remembered that some of these conditions present with sporadic low numbers of cases and are unlikely to be the cause of a typical major incident: in major incident terms, the most important of these conditions are *FMD, anthrax*, and *rabies*.

Defra maintains a permanent standing *National Expert Group* (NEG) on exotic disease which includes representatives of the APHA and *Pirbright Institute* as well as epidemiologists, virologists, meteorologists, and other experts as appropriate. In the event of an outbreak of disease, it will provide advice to responding agencies.

Foot and mouth disease

FMD is a notifiable disease of ruminants, including cows, sheep, and pigs, and other cloven-footed farm animals as well as similar wild species, such as deer. The last UK outbreak was in 2007. Animals have a high fever and painful vesicles or blisters on the feet and in the mouth and sometimes the teats, making suckling and milking difficult. They do not eat, becoming subdued and separating themselves from other animals. Movement is painful and the animals will generally lie down. Laboratory testing is required to confirm the diagnosis. The national reference laboratory is the *Pirbright Institute* (formerly the *Institute for Animal Health*) in Pirbright, Surrey. There are seven strains, some of which cause high levels of death in young animals. In adult animals, the disease is not usually fatal although lameness and reduced productivity may result. Current 'on farm' tests are effective at confirming the diagnosis when the clinical picture is clear in cattle, but less so in sheep (in which the disease may occur as a subclinical infection and which, like pigs, generally present with lameness) and may produce false negatives if sufficient viral material is not present.

Box 6.1 Notifiable animal diseases
- African horse sickness[a,b]
- Classical[a] and African swine[a,b] fevers
- Anthrax
- Aujeszky's disease[a,b] (pseudorabies)
- Avian influenza
- Bluetongue[a]
- Bovine spongiform encephalopathy (BSE and similar diseases)
- Bovine tuberculosis[c]
- Brucellosis
- Chronic wasting disease[a,b] (of deer)
- Contagious agalactia[a,b] (in sheep and goats)
- Contagious bovine pleuro-pneumonia[a,b]
- Contagious epididymitis[a,b] (in sheep and goats)
- Contagious equine metritis[a]
- Dourine[a,b] (affects horses, donkeys, etc.)
- Enzootic bovine leucosis[a]
- Epizootic haemorrhagic disease[a,b] (deer and cattle)
- Epizootic lymphangitis[a]
- Equine infectious anaemia[a] (swamp fever in horses)
- Equine viral arteritis[a]
- Foot and mouth disease[a]
- Glanders and farcy
- Goat plague[a,b]
- Lumpy skin disease[a,b] (cattle)
- Newcastle disease (chickens and other birds)
- Paramyxovirus infection[a,c] (pigeons)
- Porcine epidemic diarrhoea[a]
- Rabies
- Rift Valley fever[b] (sheep goats, cattle humans)
- Rinderpest[a] (cattle)
- Scrapie (sheep and goats)
- Sheep and goat pox[a]
- Sheep scab[a,c]
- Swine influenza[c]
- Swine vesicular disease
- Teschen disease[a]
- Vesicular stomatitis[a,b] (cattle, pigs, horses, goats)
- Warble fly[a] (horses and deer)
- West Nile fever (horses birds humans).

[a] Does not affect humans. [b] Not yet recorded in UK. [c] Currently present in UK.

The virus is present in the vesicular fluid as well as in saliva, milk, and faeces, all of which may spread the disease. It may also be spread through the medium of infected food, equipment, vehicles, or footwear. Animals which do not suffer from FMD may nonetheless transmit it to animals that do. Airborne spread is also possible and may occur over several miles. The virus is killed by heating or disinfectant.

Imported diseases
Defra is responsible for monitoring outbreaks of animal disease abroad and ensuring that appropriate plans are in place to deal with them including the imposition of appropriate restrictions *before* the disease is confirmed in the UK. Generic and disease specific guidance is available on the Defra website: http://www.gov.uk/Defra.

In the case of FMD, imports of animals from outside the EU are only allowed from countries which meet appropriate EU standards for control. Imports from all countries must be certified not to be from an area under FMD or other disease restrictions and must enter at designated *Border Inspection Posts* where they will be subject to veterinary inspection. Live animals and genetic material may not be imported from a country outside the EU with FMD. However, meat and dairy products from certain countries may be imported if they comply with EU legislation and have been treated to eliminate FMD.

Dealing with an exotic disease outbreak

Local disease coordination centre

At the operational level, the APHA will establish one or more *local disease control centres* (LDCC), each headed by a *regional operations director*. LDCCs report to the OCC in London (see Figure 6.1). The LDCC coordinates and implements the control of the disease, following higher direction from a *field operations team* (part of the OCC) and established guidelines. Delivery of disease eradication measures at the level of individual premises will be under the control of a *regional field manager*. Forward operating bases (FOBs) may be established close to the site of outbreak. Once an outbreak is confirmed, the regional operations director will brief the other agencies involved in local resilience including the chair of the LRF. Local authorities (particularly highways, health, and emergency planning departments) will have a very significant role during a disease outbreak.

Higher-level arrangements

The higher-level response in the UK is coordinated through a National Disease Control Centre (NDCC) which has both operations and policy functions and is headed by the *outbreak operations director* who reports to the chief veterinary officer through the chief executive of the APHA. The chief executive of the APHA bears responsibility for the delivery of the operational response and has the authority to activate the NDCC. The operational component of the NDCC is the *Outbreak Coordination Centre* (OCC) under a *head OCC*. As part of the NDCC, the *exotic disease policy response team* heads the policy response. The NDCC coordinates the response at a local and national level and against the international background and plays an essential role in business continuity and returning to normality. VENDU, the Veterinary Exotic Notifiable Disease Unit, provides veterinary advice to policymakers on control of disease. A National Emergency Epidemiology Group will be established to provide advice to the chief veterinary officer and relevant management groups and Defra's strategic decisions will be made under the authority of its Emergency Executive Team (EET). Defra will also convene the core expert group for the disease in question. The impact of a disease control measures on human health will be assessed by Public Health England, the DH providing expert advice regarding the potential impact of the disease on humans.

Where the geography of the outbreak makes it necessary, representatives of the deployed administrations will be based at the OCC. Defra will also provide advice and information for those affected via the website http://www.gov.uk.

Role of central government

The decision to activate COBR in the form of the *National Security Council Sub-Committee on Threats, Hazards, Resilience and Contingencies* in response to an exotic disease outbreak will depend on the scale of the incident and will be taken by the Cabinet Office (Civil Contingencies Secretariat). The decision to establish SAGE (Scientific Advisory Group for Emergencies) will be taken by Defra and the chief scientific and chief veterinary officers. The secretary of state at Defra (the LGD) is likely to be involved in a large-scale incident, especially one which may affect human health.

International arrangements

Under the 2004 *International Animal Health Emergency Reserve* agreement, the USA, Canada, Australia, and New Zealand undertake to provide veterinary and technical staff in the event of an outbreak of an animal disease. EU member states may also assist following communication between chief veterinary officers.

The *Office International des Epizooites* (OIE) is the international standard-setting body which establishes and maintains the sanitary safety of international trade in land animals and their products. It is responsible for setting out the requirements a country must meet to be declared free of a particular disease. Not all countries are members. The UK representative is the chief veterinary officer.

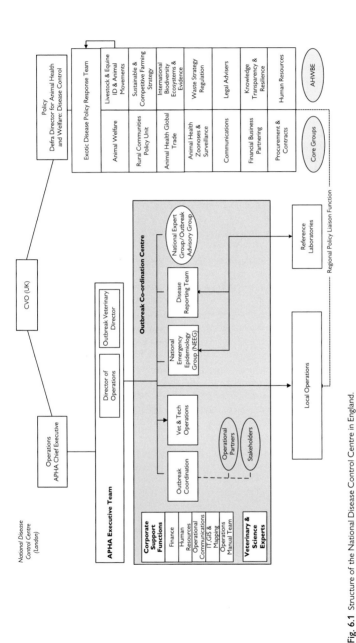

Fig. 6.1 Structure of the National Disease Control Centre in England.

Reproduced under Crown Copyright from Department for Environment, Food, and Rural Affairs, Contingency Plan for Exotic Notifiable Diseases of Animals in England, March 2016 (https://www.gov.uk/government/uploads/system/uploads/attachment_data/file/508753/exotic-notifiable-disease-contingency-plan-2016.pdf).

Disposal of animals

Many animal-borne diseases are controlled, at least in part, by rapid implementation of culling, in some cases on a very large scale. There is extensive EU and UK legislation concerning the welfare of animals during the culling process. Culling must be carried out by or under the supervision of an APHA veterinary surgeon. Culling of livestock and pet animals will be by lethal injection, electrical stunning, captive bolt, or free bullet, each with or without sedation. Different methods, including gassing and neck wringing, are available for poultry. Rare breeds *may* be exempted from culling programmes.

The preferred method of disposal of carcases is commercial fixed plant incineration followed by rendering and landfill. On farms, burning and burial may be considered in very remote areas.

Debriefing

Following any disease outbreak, appropriate debriefings will be held to ensure that effective practice occurred and to identify lessons for the future.

Stages of a foot and mouth disease incident

Suspicion stage

Once the duty veterinary officer has been informed, they will discuss the presentation with the individual reporting it. Based on this information, they may be able to rule out infection. If this is not possible, a vet will be sent to the premises, now referred to as the *suspect premises* (SP). This is the *suspicion phase* of the response. Once a vet has assessed the situation at the premises, if disease cannot be ruled out, a number of steps will be taken:

• Warning signs are erected at the entrance to the premises prohibiting unauthorized access
• A record of all animals on the premises together with other transition risks is established
• Movements on and off the premises are halted unless there is a pressing welfare need in which case exception may be made
• Disinfection equipment is placed at all entrances to the premises
• Movement of vehicles, equipment, people, and other materials such as food or waste onto or off the premises are banned.
• Rodent control measures are put in place.

In addition, information gathering begins in order to facilitate investigation of the potential outbreak. This will include details of previous animal movements (including those from the premises which might have spread the disease further) and how long the features of the disease have been present.

If laboratory tests are needed to rule out the presence of the disease, a temporary control zone (TCZ) will be established with a default radius of 10km, although it may be larger. Movement of animals within this zone is not permitted without a licence. Similar arrangements exist for circumstances in which a disease is suspected in animals at a slaughterhouse.

Advice to a farmer suspecting FMD

• Isolate the animal (if it is in a field, leave it there as long as fences are secure).
• Do not allow anyone who has been in contact with it to come into contact with other stock.
• Never ask a neighbouring stockman to look at a suspected animal.
• Do not move the animal across a public road.
• Do not move animal, milk, animal feed, or vehicles from the premises.
• Where possible, do not allow people to leave the premises—those who do must clean and disinfect boots, wash hands, and ideally change clothes.
• Shut in or tie up dogs, cats, and poultry.

Restrictions within the temporary control zone (TCZ)

Movements of susceptible animals are banned except for movements through the zone without stopping and to complete a journey started before the zone was enforced. Stray or feral susceptible animals may be destroyed.

Confirmation stage

Once the presence of the disease has been confirmed by laboratory testing, the *confirmation stage* has begun and the SP becomes an *infected premises* (IP). The chief veterinary officer will formally confirm the outbreak and notify the European Commission and the World Organization for Animal Health. Exports to the EU of live animals, meat, and dairy products from the restricted zone will be prohibited as will export of meat, genetic material, milk, and by-products produced in the restricted zone for at least 21 days before the outbreak. The APHA regional resilience manager will support the regional operations director in establishing and managing the *local disease control centre*. Defra will contract private vets to support its own staff once an outbreak is confirmed.

Some specific exports may be allowed following treatment to kill any potential virus and are subject to strict handling and documentation requirements. Arrangements outside the EU will vary from country to country.

Three zones will now be put in place:
- *Protection zone*: with a minimum radius of 3km around the site (different rules apply for slaughterhouses; see Defra guidance for further details)
- *Surveillance zone*: a minimum of 10km around the site
- *Restricted zone*: to establish a national movement ban across the UK (may extend from England into a devolved nation).

Public access to IPs is banned, access to other areas usually remains open with intensified biosecurity arrangements (see Boxes 6.2, 6.3, and 6.4,). Culling of animals will then begin for disease purposes and the premises are then disinfected.

Animal welfare advice is available during a disease outbreak from Defra, RSPCA, and SSPCA (Scottish Society for Prevention of Cruelty to Animals).

Box 6.2 Banned and restricted activities during a FMD outbreak: restricted zone (RZ)

Banned
- Susceptible animals in or out of the RZ
- Animal gatherings
- Stalking and shooting except under licence
- Sheering and dipping sheep except under licence
- Ultrasound scanning or other livestock services to susceptible animals except under licence.

Restricted/controlled
- Slaughter of susceptible animals
- Products from slaughterhouses
- Vehicle movement and associated biosecurity
- Feral susceptible animals may be destroyed.

Box 6.3 Banned and restricted activities during a FMD outbreak: protection zone (PZ)

Banned
- Movement of susceptible animals except for:
  - slaughter under licence
  - between connecting parts of the same premises using a public highway (licence needed)
  - movement in or out of the zone remains banned with the exceptions of transfers across the zone without stopping and transport from outside the zone for immediate slaughter
- Movement of non-susceptible animals to and from premises with susceptible animals (except pets, and horses under licence). Movement within the same premises using a public highway is permitted under licence
- Animal gatherings
- Hunting and stalking including similar gatherings
- Movement of vehicles used in the transport of animals from premises with susceptible animals (except under licence)
- Shearing, dipping, and other livestock services except under licence or where there are specific exemptions.

Restricted/controlled
- Collection of milk and milk products
- Dogs and poultry movements.

> **Box 6.4 Banned and restricted activities during a FMD outbreak: surveillance zone (SZ)**
>
> *Banned*
> - Movements of susceptible animals from premises except :
>   - to slaughter (following clinical examination, and under licence)
>   - movement to pasture within SZ following clinical and serological testing and more than 15 days after last case in PZ
> - Shearing, dipping, and other livestock services except under licence or where there are specific exemptions
> - Sale of hides and skins of susceptible animals (exemptions apply)
> - Animal gatherings
> - Gatherings of people including appropriate sports.
>
> *Controlled*
> - Dogs and poultry must be under control
> - Drivers of vehicle used to carry susceptible animals must adhere to required biosecurity measures
> - Collection transport and processing of raw milk.

The government has the authority to exclude certain animals or groups of animals (e.g. in wildlife parks) subject to an individual risk assessment. Although a lasting image from the 2001 outbreak is of huge pyres of burning animals or mass burial pits, it is intended in the future that disposal should be by commercial incineration, rendering, or licensed landfill (see 'Disposal of animals', p. 172). Compensation is paid to owners for slaughtered animals.

Exit phase

Restrictions will remain in place until the occupier of an IP has undertaken cleaning under the direction of the AHVLA and 'test animals' placed on the premises show no sign of the disease clinically or on laboratory testing. For FMD, restocking may begin under licence at least 21 days after the AHVLA is satisfied that cleaning is to a sufficient standard. Alternatively, a prolonged period may be allowed to pass to ensure that the virus has decayed naturally. This is usually 1 year. Restrictions in the wider protection and surveillance zones will be lifted once an epidemiological survey demonstrates negative results on all premises with susceptible livestock.

Exports from the UK will resume once disease control measures have eradicated the disease and control zones have been lifted and when any extra measures imposed by the EU have been complied with. Arrangements for other countries will vary. The World Organisation for Animal Health will restore the UK's disease-free status once the disease has been eradicated, usually 3 or 6 months after the end of the outbreak depending on the methods used to eradicate the disease.

Vaccination for foot and mouth disease

Routine preventive vaccination is illegal under EU law. In the event of an outbreak, the government may consider its use and the authority of the Secretary of State will be required, following advice from the National Expert Group. The decision to use vaccination is complex and the vaccine available in EU stocks must be effective against the strain causing the outbreak. If used, it is intended to reduce the number of animals requiring slaughter. Effective immunity in cattle takes 4 days, reaching a peak after a week. Specific movement and other restrictions apply to areas in which animals have been vaccinated.

Major incidents on the rail network

Major incidents on the UK rail network are exceptionally rare. However, when they do occur, there is the potential for very significant loss of life, not to mention massive disruption of the transport and business infrastructure. As a consequence they tend to be very high profile. Some selected recent and historical incidents are given in Table 6.1.

Resilience

The railway system in the UK is complex, including national and international passenger and freight services, commuter services, tram and metro systems, industrial railways, underground services, and heritage lines. Management is usually divided into three groups: infrastructure managers (Network Rail in England, Wales, and Scotland), train operating companies, and freight companies. There may be considerable overlap between operating companies, both in terms of role and geographically. By its very nature, an incident on the railway network is likely to have a significant impact. In addition, the rail system provides a conduit for National Grid cabling and other communications and utilities. As a result, pre-planning for the response to a rail incident is not only complex, but vital.

National level

The *National Emergency Planning and Co-ordination Committee* is a national body with membership including representatives of the *Association of Chief Police Officers* (ACPO), *British Transport Police* (BTP), *Chief Fire Officers' Association* (CFOA), *Network Rail and London Underground*, as well as HM Inspector of Railways (from the *Office of Rail Regulation* (ORR)).

Railway tracks are traditionally described as main or freight, up or down (see Box 6.5, 'Glossary', p. 179) although all combinations are possible on the same line at different times. In general, trains run on the left (like roads in the UK); however, some tracks are both way and some may be reversed for operational reasons.

Local level

Similar meetings will occur between the emergency services and rail bodies (operating and infrastructure) as part of LRFs.

Important information

Agencies which will be responsible for responding to a rail emergency must be aware of the following information:
- Operations within their operational area, including the number of companies involved and frequency of services
- Geographical areas of different operating bodies and boundaries of responsibility for managers
- Number and location of control/signal facilities under the authority of each manager
- Types of traction power used
- Established emergency procedures
- Specific local hazards due to materials carried
- Generic emergency services' intervention plans.

Sources of information

A number of official bodies and industry associations will provide information useful in planning the response to a rail incident, these include:
- Department for Transport Rail Group
- Passenger Transport Executive (PTE)
- Network Rail
- Association of Train Operating Companies (ATOC)
- Freight Transport Association (FTA)
- British Transport Police (BTP)
- operators of local tram, metro, and underground services.

Table 6.1 Historical examples of significant rail incidents

Date	Incident	Cause	Casualties
Recent			
2007	Grayrigg	Points failure	1 killed 88 injured
2004	Ufton level crossing	Suicide by road vehicle driver	7 killed 37 injured
2004	Tebay	Faulty brakes, runaway trailer	4 killed 3 injured
2002	Potters Bar	Points failure	7 killed 71 injured
2001	Great Heck	Driver of road vehicle fell asleep and ran vehicle onto track	10 killed 80 plus injured
2000	Hatfield	Track failure	4 killed 70 injured
1999	Ladbroke Grove	Driver error passed signal at danger	31 killed 400 plus injured
1997	Southall	Driver error passed signal at danger	6 killed 150 injured
Historical			
1991	Cannon Street	Train hit buffer stop	22 killed 240 injured
1988	Clapham Junction	Signal failure due to wiring error	35 killed 1000 plus injured
1975	Moorgate (tube station)	Driver error	43 killed 74 injured
1967	Hither Green	Rail failure	49 killed 78 injured
1957	Lewisham	Missed signals in fog	90 killed173 injured
1952	Harrow and Weald stone	Missed signal at danger	112 killed340 injured

Box 6.5 Railway glossary

Railway terminology is complex and extensive. Some of the more common terms are defined as follows:

Authorized walking route
Designated route providing safe access.

Ballast
Crushed stone used to support sleepers and track.

Bogies
Multi-wheeled platforms on which a train runs.

Catenary
Overhead electric power line system.

(Continued)

Box 6.5 (Contd.)

Cess
Area immediately outside railway tracks beginning at the edge of the ballast shoulder.

Detonator (fog signal)
Small explosive device placed on a rail to warn the driver of a hazard ahead.

Down (and up) lines
The down line is traditionally that away from London, or alternatively the left line facing in the down direction (railways usually follow the same patterns as road carriageways) or away from the headquarters. Although all lines are named, the terms are best avoided and the direction of travel on a particular line established.

Fastening
Method of attaching rail to sleeper.

Four foot
The space between the rails of one line (not four feet!).

Level crossing
Unprotected: no warning is given of an approaching train. Protected: warning is given through gate closure, lights, or audible alarms.

Lineside
Within the railway boundary fence to a distance no closer than 3m to the nearest line.

Pantograph
Mechanism for picking up electric power from an overhead line.

Refuge
Designated safe place to stand when a train is passing.

Rolling stock
Railway vehicles other than locomotives.

Running rail
The metal rail on which the train runs.

Signal passed at danger
When a train fails to stop at a stop signal.

Six foot
Space in between two adjacent sets of track (even if not six feet!).

SPT
Direct telephone link to a signal-box, positioned on or near a signal.

Ten foot
A wider space between two pairs of track or similar when there are multiple lines (not ten feet!).

Trackbed
The base on which the rail tracks lie.

Trainset
Rolling stock permanently or semi-permanently coupled together.

Trains stopped
No train movement on a section of track.

Other specialized sources of information during an incident include:
- premises information boxes
- infrastructure managers
- station control rooms
- train and freight operating company representatives
- Rail Accident Investigations Branch
- HM Inspector of Railways from ORR
- rail industry engineers
- manufacturers of rail vehicles.

Developing generic operational plans

The challenges at a rail incident are particularly great for the fire and rescue services. Under the *Fire and Rescue Service Act 2004*, fire and rescue services must ensure that plans consider:
- access including stations (above and below ground), tunnels, rendezvous points, cuttings, bridges, level crossings, and sidings
- potential rendezvous and intervention points including hard standing for appliances, water supply, and communications. Inter-tunnel evacuation passages should be identified
- location of rail network control rooms
- information box location
- traction power supply systems (electric, steam, diesel, or battery)
- line speeds
- hazardous materials transport
- complex locations involving multiple managers with different areas of responsibility
- communications
- fixed installations such as fire detection systems, sprinklers, inert gas systems, electricity supplies for fire service use, and hydrants
- ventilation systems—some tunnels and underground lines have ventilation systems which may assist in control of fires or other hazards.

Types of rail incident

The possible types of rail incident include derailment, bridge strike, terrorist incidents, flooding, hazardous materials incidents, fire (on trackway or on train), persons trapped on the trackway, and collision with other vehicles, for example, at a level crossing.

Responding to a railway incident: specific issues

Many of the details of the response to a major incident will depend on the specifics of the accident or its location. However, there are certain elements which will be common to all plans and constitute the generic response.

Following the receiving of a call to the emergency services, the first emergency service on scene will assess the situation, passing back information to augment that already available. Each service will then dispatch emergency personnel and vehicles. In the case of the fire and rescue services, this will be in accordance with a *predetermined attendance* (PDA), although this may be increased if reports suggest a very significant incident. Further information is likely to become available en route. Relevant agencies will be notified including infrastructure and services managers, although in most cases, these individuals will already be aware of the incident. Utility company managers are also likely to need to be informed.

The emergency service incident commanders at the scene (tactical / silver level) should have access to pre-planning information. Identification of the precise location of an incident is the key to an optimal response. Access routes must be identified, usually by the fire and rescue services, as must areas of specific risk such as tunnels, viaducts, utilities such as power cabling, embankments and cuttings, and standing water. Information will also be needed regarding the motive power system. As soon as possible, details of the train set involved should be gathered including the estimated number of passengers, type and number of carriages, carriage of passengers or freight, nature of the evacuation underway, whether there are any passengers with special evacuation needs and if any hazardous materials are being carried.

Determining the location of a rail incident

In addition to details such as grid references, the following may be used:
- Signal gantry and box numbers
- Bridge numbers
- Overhead line support numbers
- Track side mile posts
- Electrical substation name plate
- Nearby features such as level crossings, geographical features, road intersections, or buildings
- Point numbers
- Track side telephones.

Black and white hatching on a trackside phone indicates that it is a signal post to signal box telephone. A red telephone symbol indicates a telephone connecting with the electrical control room. Other telephones are marked with a black cross and can be used to communicate widely within the Network Rail system.

Command and control at the incident scene follows the structures described in Chapter 5. Interagency cooperation is especially important because of the complexity and lack of familiarity with the operating environment. As long as safety is not compromised, appropriate efforts should be made to keep disruption to normal services to a minimum. Indirect results of an incident are likely to include passengers stranded at stations, passengers stranded on trains stopped outside stations (who may put themselves at further risk by leaving the carriages), overcrowding on other trains or on platforms, and widespread service disruption. Passengers on stranded trains are likely to suffer from heat, thirst, hunger, and anxiety due to their inability to contact loved ones. The key priority is to establish as safe an environment as possible for rescuers and victims.

Cordons at a rail incident will follow the structures described in Chapter 5. There may be the need for more than one operational (bronze) area if the incident can only be accessed at certain specific points such as the ends of a tunnel or embankment, or if wreckage is distributed over more than one location.

Staff from infrastructure and train operating companies will act as important sources of information regarding the operating environment as well as carriage types and methods of access. The rail infrastructure company will provide to the scene a *responsible person at tactical (silver)* or *rail incident officer* who will provide experience, knowledge, and appropriate authority to assist rescuers. This individual will advise regarding the suitability of control measures and on the most appropriate control actions, as well as assessing and advising with regard to the impact on the wider network and how it might be minimized. They will also arrange for specialist personnel and equipment and coordinate the return to normal service. The train operating companies are represented on site by *rail operations liaison officers* (ROLOs).

Establishing control over the railway following an incident

The key component in establishing as safe a working environment as possible is gaining control over the railway. The following escalating levels of control over rail activity are possible:
- The rail infrastructure manager is informed of a minor incident on or near the tracks. Such incidents might include a small fire, or a vehicle stuck under what appears to be an intact bridge.
- Rail vehicles are requested to '*run at caution*'. This is usually implemented to protect emergency workers near the track and ensures that the train can stop safely and in time due to a reduced speed.
- The infrastructure manager is requested to stop all vehicles. This will protect individuals from injury or death, but may take some time to come into effect as moving trains must reach or receive a stop sign before halting
- '*Power off*' is requested. This procedure will protect individuals at risk of coming into contact with live rails or wires. It will not stop diesel vehicles, and trains travelling at high speed will take some time and distance to come to a halt. Stoppage of power is likely to have very widespread effects, but may also be requested to specific sections of track.

Different levels of control are likely to apply to different areas following a single incident.

Maintaining safety at a rail incident

Safety is a key concern at a rail incident for obvious reasons, and especially in the early stages of the response. The emergency services will appoint safety officers responsible for reducing risk throughout the response; however, when it is unclear whether train movements have been halted, it may also be necessary to place individuals to warn of rail movements. Stopping times will depend on, amongst other factors, whether power has been switched off, train speed, weather conditions, and the motive power system. Safety is likely to be compromised by the noise and the confusion of the scene, factors reducing visibility, track with trains running in both directions, and geographical considerations. Responders to an incident must be aware of established danger or warning signals and the actions to be taken when one occurs.

When it is necessary, a train may be stopped by raising both arms above the head in a clearly visible position, or in darkness waving a light. When crossing track, it is important not to stand on either sleepers or running rails. Points should be avoided as they can trap feet even if the power has been turned off and feet should never be placed between a running rail and a conductor rail.

Overhead cables and powered rails

Where power is provided by overhead lines, there is a risk to responders working within 1 metre of such cables; in such cases, rail managers will be requested to isolate or earth overhead cables after power is off. 'Power off' alone rather than with earthing may be requested to facilitate removal of casualties in contact with live cabling who are at risk of death as earthing will be slower.

When power is supplied by a third or fourth rail, the highest control levels should be implemented. If rescue is attempted before *power off* is confirmed, full PPE and dry gloves should be worn and rescuers must stand on non-conducting material and use dry on-conducting material for the rescue. The same applies to overhead cable rescues after power has been switched off.

Underground railway incidents

A number of UK cities have railways systems which run underground for some or most of their length. Inevitably a major incident on such a system will present special challenges. Particular concerns include access routes, ventilation systems, and passenger welfare as a result of overcrowding, heat, dehydration, and anxiety if trains are stopped for prolonged periods in tunnels. Underground transport providers will inevitably have complex and site-specific plans in place in conjunction with the emergency services.

Types of electricity supply

Third rail

These are DC current systems at 750V often used on underground railways where charge is picked up by a pick-up shoe.

Fourth rail

These systems are less common, but are used on the London Underground, where there is a third rail beside the track, energized at +420V DC, and a fourth rail is located centrally between the running rails at −210V DC, combining to provide a traction voltage of 630V DC. Sections of track on both third and fourth rail systems can be electrically isolated by rail personnel.

Overhead line equipment (railways)

Used on main lines usually (in the UK) at up to 25kV alternating current, the current is fed from a feeder or sub-feeder station. The overhead power cable is connected to the running rail by a *bond*.

Overhead cabling (trams)

In modern systems, this is usually a 550–750V direct current system

Rail Accident Investigation Branch (RAIB)

The RAIB was established in 2005 after recommendations in Lord Cullen's report into the Ladbroke Grove incident. The RAIB must by law investigate all rail incidents in which there has been a derailment or collision or which have resulted in, or could result in death, serious injury to five or more people, or extensive damage to stock, infrastructure, or the environment. They may also investigate *near miss* incidents. Following an incident, RAIB investigators will be appointed who have the power to enter railway property, seize any material relating to the accident, demand access to and disclosure of records, and require people to answer questions about matters relevant to the inquiry. The RAIB is charged with determining the cause of an accident, it does not apportion blame.

British Transport Police (BTP)

The BTP are effectively the railways' own police service. At an incident they will assist with cordons and lead the investigation into whether a crime has been committed. BTP will be informed of an incident by Network Rail.

Railway hazards

Responsibility for scene safety
The fire service will appoint one or more safety officers at the scene of an incident.

Stopping distances
A conventional intercity train travelling at 125 mph may take up to 1 mile (1.6km) to stop and an international service at 186mph up to 2.8 miles (4.5km). The location and weather conditions may prolong these times.

Air turbulence
High-speed trains produce air turbulence which may suck individuals towards the train.

Power
See p. 183.

Diesel trains
For obvious reasons, diesel locomotives will not stop when motive power is turned off by Rail Track.

Steam trains
Risks include high-pressure steam and fire.

Utilities
Gas pipes and electricity supply cables may be routed along railway tracks.

Track components
Bridges, tunnels, viaducts, embankments cuttings, and points are all potentially hazardous.

Office of Rail Regulation

The Office of Rail Regulation (ORR) is both the economic *and* safety regulator for UK rail operations. As such, it is tasked with ensuring that not only are the railways operating safely, but efficiently and effectively and offer value for money to customers. In the event of a major incident, ORR will mirror the strategic (gold), tactical (silver), and operational (bronze) structure of the emergency services, providing expert advice and information. In large-scale incidents, a designated individual at strategic (gold) will be termed the *rail incident commander* (RIC). At least two inspectors will be sent to the site to work at tactical (silver) and operational (bronze) who will work closely with all other agencies and services, the representative at tactical (silver) being the ORR *rail incident officer* (RIO). In particular, the ORR representatives will work closely with staff from the RAIB.

The main roles of the ORR following an incident are to investigate potential breaches of health and safety legislation, collect evidence for future enforcement, monitor the safety of recovery operations, ensure immediate actions arising from the incident are being undertaken by the rail industry, and producing an initial so-called fast stream report. The ORR will ensure that the central government is informed where appropriate.

Flooding

Flooding appears to be occurring increasingly frequently, although the causes, which are undoubtedly complex, are subject to often heated debate. The most significant incidents in recent years are shown in Table 6.2. Such incidents are increasingly likely as climate change increases and planning permissions for housing developments do not always avoid flood plains. According to government figures, one in six homes is at risk of flooding, and a total of 2.5 million properties are at risk of flooding from rivers or the sea, half a million at significant risk. One million of these are also at risk from surface water flooding. A further 2.8 million homes are at risk from surface water flooding alone.

The Royal Institute of British Architects (RIBA) has estimated that 1.5% of the UK is at risk from direct flooding from the sea and around 7% of the country is likely to flood at least once a century from rivers. Flooding is estimated to cost the UK economy around £2.2bn a year.

Government guidance for England is given in the *National Flood Emergency Framework for England* developed following the significant floods of 2007. Responsibilities for those responding to a flood are laid down in the CCA, *Flood and Water Management Act 2010* and *Reservoirs Act 1975* as well as the *Flood Risk Regulations 2009*. The key legislation in Scotland is *The Flood Risk Management (Scotland) Act 2009: Delivering Sustainable Flood Risk Management* published by the Scottish government. The Environment Agency (EA) (*Scottish Environment Protection Agency* (SEPA) in Scotland) maintains a strategic overview of flood defences and response and the LGD is Defra. The devolved government are responsible for planning in their respective areas of responsibility.

Sources of flood water

The main sources of flood water are:

- sea
- rivers and canals
- surface water
- groundwater
- reservoirs and lakes.

Groundwater flooding is likely to occur following saturation of land by heavy rain or flooding from another source, which will therefore be exacerbated. Building on flood plains and prevention of effective drainage by building over areas which might otherwise absorb water will further worsen flood damage.

Table 6.2 Recent UK flooding incidents

Date	Location	Consequences
2015	Cumbria, Dumfries and Galloway, Lancashire, and North Yorkshire	One estimate suggested these floods will reduce GDP by 0.2%
2014	Somerset levels	
2012	Various locations 11 major floods, 6000 flood warnings	7950 properties flooded (May–June) Estimated cost £320 million
2010	Cornwall	400 properties flooded
2009	Cumbria	1800 properties flooded 1 death
2008	Morpeth	1000 homes and businesses affected
2007	Various locations	55,000 properties flooded 500,000 people without water or mains drainage 13 deaths

Resilience

The EA (and its equivalents) maintains a strategic overview of flood resilience in England. *Lead local flood authorities* (see p. 188) are responsible for assessing, mapping, and planning local flood risk and work with water companies to manage surface water flooding. Surface water flood maps are available to lead local flood authorities, LRFs, and local planning authorities. Flood resilience planning is likely to be a key priority in those areas where there is a significant longstanding flood risk.

Defra has issued detailed guidance for LRFs on developing a *multi-agency flood plan* (MAFP): depending on the area, such a plan may not be relevant for all LRFs. In general, it is recommended that a MAFP is prepared for any area with more than 250 properties in significant or moderate flood risk areas. The guidance also recommends the formation of tactical and strategic flood plans corresponding with tactical (silver) and strategic (gold) levels of command at an established incident and covering larger areas at risk.

Involvement of infrastructure companies, including the utilities will be important in both planning for and responding to significant flooding.

Guidance for flood resilience identifies the priorities as outlined in Box 6.6.

The role of central government

Defra

Defra is the LGD for flood resilience and response and will act as the focal point for communication between central government and agencies responding to an incident, taking the central decisions necessary for such agencies to respond optimally, ensuring that Parliament is informed and coordinating requirements such as funding for large scale interventions.

Flooding incidents graded *Level 1—serious* (see p. 189 for an explanation of this categorization) are usually handled within Defra. *Level 2—significant* incidents are coordinated by Defra but also through COBR and *Level 3—catastrophic* by the Civil Contingencies Secretariat through COBR with Defra support. Defra maintains a 24-hour duty rota for reports of possible or actual flooding and an *Emergency Operations Centre* (EOC) located in London. Defra is also responsible for assessing and managing the impact of flooding on its other areas of responsibility.

Action in response to a significant risk of serious flooding will usually be taken after a *National Flood Advisory Service* teleconference between Defra, the EA, the Met Office, and the *Flood Forecasting Centre* (p. 189).

Box 6.6 Key elements of flood resilience

- Communications (including with the public, the media, and between responding organizations and pre-prepared announcements)
- Provision of advice to the public (see p. 192)
- Public warnings including loudhailers and sirens
- Structures to be established in the event of an incident and contact details
- Detailed allocation of roles to responding agencies (reflecting conventional task assignments)
- Arrangements for mutual aid (between CCA responders and others) and cooperation
- Care of vulnerable groups or individuals[a]
- Managing and reducing disruption to infrastructure and business continuity[b]
- Evacuation and shelter for affected or at-risk groups or individuals
- Engagement with the voluntary sector
- Establishing community resilience.

[a] Providing adequate warning to vulnerable people is a key priority and plans should include maps identifying vulnerable groups, institutions for such groups, and individuals. Information should also include access details including keyholders, carers, and community leaders.

[b] The UK critical infrastructure is divided into nine sectors: water, energy, transport, telecommunications, health, food, financial services, emergency services, and government. Arrangements must be in place to gain access to relevant premises.

Organizations involved in flood prevention and management

The impact of flooding on communities is usually profound, complex, and prolonged. Inevitably, therefore, a significant number of organizations are involved. These are listed below. See also Table 6.3.

Lead local flood authorities (LLFAs)
Lead local flood authorities are county councils and unitary authorities which are required to prepare and maintain local flood risk strategies, lead emergency planning and post-flood recovery, investigate flooding incidents, develop sustainable drainage systems, and review planning applications which affect relevant structural or water features.

Water and sewerage companies
These privatized utilities must ensure that they have appropriate levels of flood resilience and continue to provide essential services during an emergency. They must also manage water and sewerage in order to reduce the risk of flooding, manage its impact, and work with developers, landowners, and LLFAs to understand and manage risk. Water and sewerage companies also provide advice to LLFAs and work with other bodies including the EA (SEPA in Scotland) and local authorities to coordinate their normal business with risk management strategies.

Department for Communities and Local Government (DCLG)
During a major flood, the DCLG will provide a government liaison officer and support team who will attend the SCG on behalf of Defra and other central government departments. They are responsible for ministerial and VIP visits and ensuring effective interdepartmental working, especially in consequence management. DCLG, through the *chief fire and rescue advisor* (CFRA), coordinates fire and rescue service (FRS) assets at a national level using the fire and rescue service *National Coordination and Advisory Framework* (NCAF).

During the recovery phase of a flooding incident, DCLG will act as the liaison point between local agencies and central government ensuring clear aims and an effective recovery process by coordinating capabilities and taking executive decisions where necessary. The DCLG is also responsible for the dissemination of information to parliament and the public.

District and borough councils
Local councils are actively involved in flood risk management in partnership with LLFAs

Internal Drainage Boards (IDBs)
IDBs are public bodies responsible for managing water levels in low-lying areas. They are responsible for supervising land drainage and flood defence works on ordinary watercourses as well as managing groundwater. IDBs will use drainage channels, management of watercourses and pumping facilities to optimize water management.

Table 6.3 Flood warnings: agencies providing flood warning advice and information

Type of advice	Agency	Type of flooding
Daily flood guidance statements	Flood Forecasting Centre	All types of flood
Public flood warnings	Environment Agency	River, coastal, and groundwater flooding
Rivers and sea levels (Internet)	Environment Agency	River and coastal flooding
National Severe Weather Warning Service (NSWWS)	Met Office	All types of flooding
Targeted flood warnings	Resellers using Met Office data	River and coastal flooding
Road and rail disruption	Highways Agency and National Rail Enquiries	All types of flooding

Highways authorities

Highways authorities (Highways Agency (HA) and unitary authorities) have the lead responsibility for managing drainage from roads and managing road ditches. The HA must identify high-risk flood areas on the strategic road network, provide mitigation, and ensure that plans are in place should disruption due to flooding occur. Contingency plans for flooding on local roads are the responsibility of the LRFs and local highways agencies, working with DCLG during the response to an incident.

Flood Forecasting Centre (FFC)

The FFC is a partnership between the EA and the *Met Office* and responsible for forecasting river, surface and ground water, and coastal flood risk. The FFC delivers flood warnings to Category 1 and 2 responders and is part of the National Flood Advisory Service teleconference (see p. 187). The *Flood Guidance Statement* (FGS) issued by the FFC is a daily flood risk assessment for CCA responders by county across England and Wales for the following 5 days. It combines information from the FFC, EA, and *Natural Resources Wales*, and covers all types of flooding.

Environment Agency (EA)

The EA maintains a strategic overview of all sources of flooding. It is responsible for flood risk management on main rivers and the coast, regulating reservoir safety and working with the Met Office to provide flood warnings. As part of its responsibility, it develops flood management plans including water capture schemes in conjunction with local bodies. The EA does not take the lead for surface water, groundwater (except in certain designated areas) or ordinary watercourses, although it does support the relevant responsible bodies. The EA is responsible for communicating the risk of flooding to those potentially affected and alerting LRF partners to actual flooding and engaging in tactical (silver) and strategic (gold) levels of flood response. The EA is responsible for the provision of flood data and flood mapping.

Department of Health

The DH is responsible for the health aspects of flooding, providing advice and information to local responders, government departments, and ministers. The DH will work with *NHS England* to ensure capacity and continuity, *Public Health England* (PHE) regarding public health including infectious disease, and the social care sector in conjunction with the DCLG.

Met Office

The Met Office (this is now its official title) will provide advice to central government and to regional responders via *civil contingencies advisors*. The Met Office also provides *Hazard Manager*, an Internet-based information service for the response community.

Department for Transport (DfT)

The DfT has responsibility for resilience planning with regard to transport infrastructure in conjunction with owners and operators. Train operating companies, Network Rail, airport operators, and port owners are responsible for managing the impact of flooding on their operations in conjunction with official bodies. Network Rail has primary responsibility for flood resilience on the rail network.

Armed forces

Requests may be made under the *Military Aid* regulations (see p. 124–32) for assistance with specialist tasks, logistics, or manpower in the event of a large-scale flooding incident.

Categorization of flood risk

The Flood Forecasting Centre classifies potential flooding into *minimal impact, minor impact, significant impact*, and *severe impact*. The disruption due to minimal impact flooding will be limited to potentially difficult driving conditions, minor flooding in remote areas, and heavy wave activity. Minor impact flooding will affect individuals with localized disruption. Significant and severe impact floods have the potential to endanger life and cause structural damage; in severe incidents, building collapse and disruption of whole communities and infrastructure may occur.

FLOOD ALERT
FLOODING IS POSSIBLE. BE PREPARED.

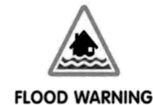

FLOOD WARNING
FLOODING IS EXPECTED. IMMEDIATE ACTION REQUIRED.

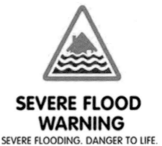

SEVERE FLOOD WARNING
SEVERE FLOODING. DANGER TO LIFE.

Fig. 6.2 Flood warning signs.

Sign images reproduced under Crown Copyright.

Flood warnings

Alerts and warnings

A *flood alert* means that flooding may occur. Simple actions including monitoring flood warnings and weather forecasts and ensuring communications should be undertaken. A *flood warning* means that flooding is imminent. Individuals should be ready and equipped to evacuate if necessary and possessions should be moved to a safe area if possible. Gas and electricity should be turned off and local flood plans complied with. Alerts are generally issued more than 24 hours ahead, warnings up to 24 hours ahead. The warning signs are shown in Figure 6.2.

Severe flood warnings

A severe flood warning will be issued if there is significant risk to life from deep, fast flowing water, rapidly moving debris, possible collapse of buildings, or if particular groups or areas are at additional risk due to their location. Such a warning may also be issued if there is a risk of significant disruption to a community due, for example, to individuals being trapped by rising water in remote areas, loss of critical infrastructure, or large numbers of individuals requiring evacuation.

Flood Warnings Direct

Flood Warnings Direct (FWD) is a scheme run by the EA operating in flood-prone areas giving access to flood warnings via the Internet or via a dedicated telephone number (*Floodline*: 0845 988 1188). Members of the public are required to register for FWD. *Extended Direct Warning* (EDW) is a facility which allows the EA to contact properties at risk by means of recorded telephone messages sent to a landline. *Floodline* also provides a 24-hour helpline service for members of the general public requiring information regarding flood risk in their area.

Advice to those who are at risk of flooding

Government agencies have effective and well-practised systems in place for using social media to disseminate flood warnings and associated information. The EA issues clear guidance for those at risk of flooding or who have been flooded (see also p. 192):

Before flooding happens
- Find out what the local risk of flooding is
- Sign up for free flood warning messages
- Know what the levels of warning and alert are and mean
- Have a personal plan for if a flood occurs
- Prepare your home using simple measures
- Ensure the property is insured.

If a flood is forecast
- Listen to local media and monitor the flood warning services
- Prepare a flood kit including phone numbers, insurance documentation, money, bank cards, medicines, medical devices (and batteries), clothing and personal items, and baby items if relevant.
- Know how to turn off the gas, water, and electricity supplies.

Effects of flooding

The adverse effects of flooding are considerable, some obvious, others less so. Flood water may be fast flowing, of unknown depth, and contaminated with sewage chemical or other toxins. Fallen trees, collapsed buildings, and downed power lines may all increase the hazard level. Ironically, lack of safe drinking water may also present risks. Businesses will be disrupted and homes and livelihoods lost. The effects on health include:
- drowning and near drowning
- trauma from concealed objects or landscape features
- water shortage or contamination
- infectious diseases from water contaminants and other agents such as rodents
- carbon monoxide poisoning from pumping equipment
- mental health issues (acute and long term) such as depression and anxiety.

In addition, displaced populations may find access to routine healthcare challenging, a problem which may be further exacerbated by damage to healthcare systems and buildings. As is reflected in the resilience priorities, these issues may disproportionately affect the vulnerable.

Advice to those affected by flooding

During the flood
- Do not walk or drive in flood water.
- Stay safe and listen to broadcast information.
- Do not touch electric appliances if standing in water.
- Follow the instructions of the emergency services and evacuate if told to do so.
- Where possible and safe, assist the vulnerable.
- Move to a high place with means of escape.
- Avoid contact with flood water and wash hands regularly.
- Inform your GP if you develop gastrointestinal symptoms after swallowing flood water.

After a flood
- Take care in flood water (risks include displaced manhole covers and water of unknown depth).
- Ensure good ventilation if using heating appliances to dry out indoor areas (due to the risk of carbon monoxide poisoning).
- Do not turn gas or electricity back on until they have been checked by a qualified technician.
- Seek advice from the water company regarding whether your water is safe to drink.
- Do not eat fresh food that has been in contact with flood water or food from switched off refrigerators or freezers.
- Maintain good personal hygiene with regular hand washing.
- Ensure regular medications are taken and health appointments attended where possible.
- Stay with friends or family or seek alternative accommodation through the local authority.
- Contact your insurance company and take photographs before and after cleaning up. Do not throw property away until authorized to do so.

Cleaning up
- Rubber boots, gloves, and masks should be worn during the cleaning up process.
- Soft items should be washed on a 60-degree cycle with detergent and clothes used for cleaning should be washed separately.
- Hard surfaces cleaned with hot water and detergent.
- Dead rodents/other animals should be disposed of in plastic bags ensuring appropriate PPE is worn while this is being carried out.
- Rubbish should be placed in hard bins away from accommodation.

Prevention of flooding effects on health

Prevention of the effects of flooding on health can be considered under three headings:

Primary prevention
These measures should be in place before a flood occurs and include flood defences and watercourse management, building control, landscape and architectural design, and emergency planning.

Secondary prevention
Secondary preventative measures will be taken just before a flood is expected or during a flood in order to reduce its impact. Such measures will include protection of the vulnerable and dissemination of information.

Tertiary prevention
Tertiary prevention measures are taken during or after a flood to minimize risks to human health such as moving at-risk individuals, ensuring safe drinking water, and health surveillance.

Flood rescue

The *Flood Rescue National Enhancement Programme* (FRNEP) led by Defra is a national coordinated programme designed to improve flood rescue across England and Wales. As part of the FRNEP, a national register of all flood rescue resources including personnel is maintained and available in the event of an incident. Rescue itself is covered by the *Flood Rescue Concept of Operations* (FRCO) developed as part of FRNEP. The FRCO covers all aspects of flood response involving a wide variety of agencies such as RNLI and the RSPCA who have the capability to rescue animals from flooding. A *water incident manager* (WIM) will be appointed at each level of the response to coordinate water rescue.

The response to localized flooding is usually managed at a local level and coordinated by the police. Specialist flood rescue teams may be deployed. Larger-scale flooding will require mutual aid from agencies outside a single LRF. In these circumstances, rescue capability is requested through the Fire and Rescue Service National Coordination Centre (FRSNCC) in London who will initiate a *Chief Fire Officers' Association* (CFOA) *Flood Support Team* (FST). The FST in conjunction with the Flood Forecasting Centre will determine the most appropriate response and request the necessary assets. Air assets for flood response are requested and coordinated through the *Aeronautical Air Rescue Centre* (ARCC). (See Table 6.4.)

Table 6.4 Levels of flood rescue response capability

Category	Team type[a]	Capability
A	Advanced water rescue boat team	Not currently used
B	Water rescue boat team	Technical water rescue, water-based searches, power boat rescue, in-water operations, flood response
C	Water rescue technician team	Technical water rescue, water-based searches, in-water operations, non-powered boat operations, flood response
D	Water first responder team	Support operations, limited in-water operations, bank-based safety, flood response
E	Water awareness team	Support operations, bank-based safety, logistical support, pumping operations

[a] Team leaders wear white helmets; rescue boat operators and water rescue technicians, red helmets; and water first responders, yellow helmets. Standard training packages are available for each of the levels of response in the table.

Air incidents

Regrettably, many incidents involving aircraft will result in few, if any, survivors. However, some, most notably from a UK perspective the Kegworth incident of 1989, may result in large numbers of injured survivors. The response to such an incident will vary greatly from Lockerbie in 1988 (259 fatalities), where the emphasis was on body recovery and forensic investigation, to Kegworth, where almost 80 passengers survived and the immediate need was to extricate survivors and transfer them to hospital. In every incident involving an aircraft, a detailed and often highly technical inquiry will inevitably be held, as well as the usual coronial proceedings. In the event of such an incident, advice regarding potential hazards may be obtained from the *Air Accident Investigation Branch* (AAIB) and the Ministry of Defence (MOD).

Investigation

AAIB

The AAIB investigates all civilian aircraft incidents in the UK and will assist at military incidents if requested to do so by the MOD, just as the military may assist with civilian incidents. Following a major incident, the police will contact the AAIB. In smaller incidents this responsibility will fall to the pilot or operator.

The AAIB maintain a dedicated 24-hour accident reporting line (01252 510 300), together with a separate number for press enquiries (0207 944 3118). The RAF *Joint Aircraft Recovery and Transportation Squadron* (JARTS) based at RAF Boscombe Down may be requested to assist with the removal of wreckage.

The AAIB has six teams of inspectors and is headed by a *Chief Inspector* and *Deputy Chief Inspector of Air Accidents*. Inspectors fall into the categories of operations, engineering, and flight recorder inspectors and have both technical knowledge and extensive experience of the aviation industry. The role of the AAIB is to determine the circumstances and cause of the accident as well as identifying lessons which may allow the avoidance of accidents in the future. It does not apportion blame or liability.

JARTS

The RAF JARTS is part of the MOD. It includes the *Military Air Accident Investigation Branch* (MilAAIB) with similar responsibilities for military aviation to the AAIB for civilian incidents.

River and maritime incidents

These incidents are fortunately rare, but when they do occur, present special challenges to responders. A list of recent significant UK maritime and river incidents is shown in Table 6.5.

Agencies and responsibilities

The *Maritime and Coastguard Agency* will coordinate search and rescue efforts, and may appoint an *on-scene coordinator* (OSC) on a suitable vessel. Some major rivers and ports have dedicated fire and police vessels which are able to assist other assets such as the RNLI. Harbour masters have authority to control river traffic during an emergency and will be involved in the establishment of exclusion zones. Just as in a land-based incident, vessels entering the area of a major incident must be logged. Cordon positions and access points may have to be moved during an incident with changes in tides. There is a statutory duty on the masters of vessels to go to the assistance of ships or persons in distress. Rendezvous points should be identified, ideally on both banks in a river incident.

Casualty management

Predetermined safe *casualty landing points* (CLPs) should be identified in areas where there is a risk of a significant marine incident. An ambulance officer should be present at each CLP to coordinate casualty landing and ensure that information is passed centrally regarding numbers and type of casualties.

Marine Accident Investigation Branch (MAIB)

The MAIB, based in Southampton, and established after the *Herald of Free Enterprise* disaster, is a branch of the DfT and is responsible for investigating all accidents to shipping in UK territorial waters and to UK vessels throughout the World. MAIB does not apportion blame, establish liability, enforce laws, or prosecute. There are four MAIB investigation teams, each consisting of a principal investigator and three investigators drawn from the fishing industry, marine engineering, maritime architecture, or maritime industries. The remit of the MAIB is much broader than major incidents and includes incidents involving loss or abandonment, stranding or disabling of a ship, death, serious injury or loss of a person from a ship, material damage to a ship or maritime structure, or serious pollution. Following an incident, MAIB will prepare a report after visiting the vessels involved and interviewing appropriate individuals. Technical equipment may be used to survey sunken vessels. The report will identify causes and contributing factors to the incident, including recommendations for changes in future practice. A copy of the report is also sent to the next of kin of those who died in the incident.

Table 6.5 UK river and maritime incidents

Year	Incident	Effects	Type of incident
1987	Herald of Free Enterprise	193 fatalities	Capsize of roll-on-roll-off-ferry, Zeebrugge
1989	Marchioness	51 fatalities	Pleasure cruiser run down by dredger on the River Thames
1976	Piper Alpha	167 fatalities	Explosion and fire on offshore oilrig
1953	Princess Victoria	133 fatalities	Roll-on-roll-off ferry sank in North Channel

Maritime and Coastguard Agency (MCA)

The MCA has its headquarters in Southampton and offices and coordination centres along the UK coast employing in excess of 1000 people with approximately 3500 volunteers. It is responsible for the safety of all on board any vessel in UK waters and on UK flagged vessels. It will also ensure that equipment on board ship is fit for purpose, that seafarers carry the correct documentation, and certifies qualifications as well as inspecting dock facilities. Other responsibilities include the hydrographic accuracy of charts and environmental safety of coasts and waters, and leading the response to pollution incidents. Through HM Coastguard, the MCA is responsible for coordinating rescue at sea, and it will shortly take on full responsibility for the provision of air sea rescue when it is privatized in 2015 and the RAF withdraw from this capability.

HM Coastguard has over 300 *coastguard rescue teams* (CRT) around the UK manned by volunteer *coastguard rescue officers* (CROs). The teams are activated by *maritime rescue coordination centres* (MRCCs) which monitor all maritime distress radio frequencies. Rescue may be provided by CRT assets, lifeboats of the RNLI, search and rescue helicopters, emergency towing vessels contracted to MCA, or fire services (some cliff and coastal rescue). Emergency calls may also come via the 999 (112) system. (See Figure 6.3 for rank markings.)

When an incident occurs, the MCA will plot the position of the incident, broadcast information to alert vessels in the area, and establish communication with the affected vessel or installation commander to ascertain what assistance is required. They will then request the dispatch of air assets to the scene and identify and task specialist resources and personnel as well as informing the Royal Navy if required.

As part of the response to a maritime incident, a *salvage control unit* (SCU) may also be established and if necessary a *shoreline response centre* (SRC) may be set up if there are significant on-shore effects. Management of significant pollution will be directed by the *MCA Counter Pollution Branch*. The *Receiver of Wreck* (RoW) has the power to enforce return of washed-up materials which have been illegally removed and can insist that such wreckage is left *in situ* pending an official salvor.

Fulltime Coastguard ranks and insignia

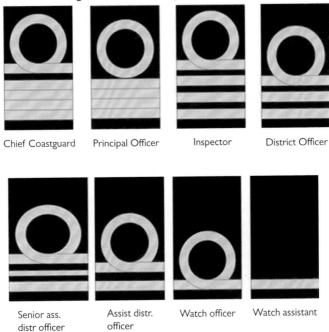

| Chief Coastguard | Principal Officer | Inspector | District Officer |

Senior ass.
distr officer
(Sr watch mgr)

Assist distr.
officer
watch mgr)

Watch officer

Watch assistant

Volunteer Coastguard ranks and insignia

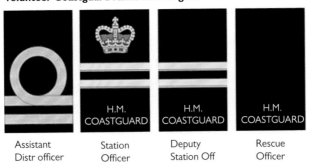

Assistant
Distr officer

Station
Officer

Deputy
Station Off

Rescue
Officer

Fig. 6.3 Coastguard rank markings and insignia.
Reproduced under creative commons licence from https://en.wikipedia.org/wiki/Her_Majesty%27s_Coastguard

Dealing with a suspect package ('white powder incident')

Suspect packages are a relatively common occurrence and can be as effective in causing disruption even when nothing toxic is subsequently identified. Very often, concerns will be raised after the discovery of an unknown substance, often referred to as a 'white powder incident'. In most cases, investigation will reveal that the substance is completely innocuous, left out of a malicious desire to cause panic or that the unexpected parcel has a perfectly innocent explanation. However, it is important that sensible advice is given to members of the pubic who find themselves in such a situation. Such advice will minimize disruption without causing unacceptable risks to public health.

Suspicious packages

Any of the following features may give cause for concern regarding the nature of a package:
- The presence of a threatening or suspicious message
- Incorrect spelling of common words or address details
- Handwritten addresses from an unknown source especially if marked '*personal*' or '*addressee only*'
- Absence of normal stamps, post marks or franking, excessive postage
- Oily stains
- Unusual or suspicious smells
- Unusually shaped envelopes
- Unexpected post from abroad.

Emergency services and medical professionals may be asked to provide advice regarding the management of such an incident. Appropriate advice is given in Box 6.7.

Box 6.7 Advice to the public regarding a suspicious package

Dealing with suspicious material in a closed environment

If a suspicious package has not yet been opened
- DO NOT OPEN IT, TOUCH IT, or MOVE IT
- Notify a manager and CALL THE POLICE (999)
- DO NOT take the letter or package to the police
- DO NOT take letter or package to an A&E department or other part of the health service.

If the package is already open
- Do not touch it or move it
- Do not clean up any spillages
- Do not brush powder from clothes (it should be removed with the clothes during decontamination)
- Call the police immediately (999)
- Shut windows and door and leave the room, leaving the package behind
- Remain apart from others but available
- Make sure that personnel from outside the room are evacuated as rapidly as possible
- Evacuate exposed individuals from inside the room separately and to a suitable location until appropriate medical care can be arranged
- Inform the building manager who should switch of the air conditioning and close all fire doors and windows.

Dealing with suspicious material in the open environment
- Do not touch it
- Call the police (999)
- Stay away from the material and ensure that others do not approach it
- Do not attempt to clear up any spilled material
- Do not attempt to remove powder or other contamination from clothing (this will be done during decontamination).

Risk assessment

The risk assessment is the responsibility of the police who will review the situation, assessing information from witnesses, carry out a scene assessment, and determine whether or not there is a credible threat. Only then will appropriate further action be taken.

No credible threat

If it is determined that there is no credible threat then the public and involved personnel can be reassured and no further action need be taken. (The police may commence an investigation into a hoax incident.)

Credible threat

If there is a credible threat, specialist assistance will be called upon. The package will be removed by the police and sent for analysis. The police will identify those who may have been exposed, who may have been in a room with the suspect material, have passed through a contaminated area, or have been in proximity to material in an open environment

These individuals will be decontaminated, their clothing removed and bagged, and alternative clothing provided. Patient data (including GP details) will be collated. Once they have been decontaminated, exposed people with symptoms should be directed by incident commanders to appropriate medical care for further advice and treatment as required. Suitable aftercare and reassurance will be necessary and eventually personal items will need to be returned.

Affected buildings or areas will remain closed until the laboratory results are available. Heating and air conditioning must remain off. It may be possible to use other parts of larger buildings. If there is any risk of exposure to anthrax, prophylactic antibiotics will be provided.

Further management of a suspicious material incident

If there has been no exposure to a hazardous substance, that is to say the results of analysis are negative, exposed persons can be contacted (usually by the CCDC) and reassured, post-exposure prophylaxis can be ended, and personal items returned. Cordoned areas will be returned to normal use.

If the results are positive and exposure to a chemical or biological agent is confirmed, exposed persons and their GPs will be contacted and informed and appropriate treatment commenced where appropriate. Cordons will remain in place while a forensic investigation of the scene is commenced. Once this investigation is complete, decontamination can be carried out. Contaminated possessions will be destroyed by burning. In all such cases, careful release of information and appropriate handling of the media are essential.

Communications

Introduction

Effective communication is essential in managing the complexities of a major incident. Communication failures have repeatedly been identified in the public enquiries that invariably follow such events: examples include the *Kings Cross* and *Clapham Junction* incidents. The result has been more robust communications systems and an emphasis on effective transmission and recording of information. However, the possibility of communication failure remains for a wide variety of reasons including equipment incompatibility, loss of coverage of telecommunications, lack of capacity, individual failure to give a clear, concise, unambiguous message, and lack of awareness of command structures. It is undoubtedly the case that the more complex and technical a system, the more likely it is to fail under the challenge of a major incident. For this reason, simple methods such as runners with messages and the use of whistles or hand signals retain their place as means of communication during the complexity of a major incident.

This section covers the methods of communication available to those responsible for responding to such an incident (Box 7.1). The role of the media is covered in Chapter 15. The key features of a robust communications system are given in Box 7.2 and of an effective communication in Box 7.3.

Box 7.1 Methods of communication at a major incident

- Radio systems
- Telecommunications:
  - Mobile
  - Land lines
- Runners
- Pagers
- Whistles
- Hand signals
- Public information announcements and warnings.

Box 7.2 Key features of a robust communications system

- Identify and ensure essential communications and processes
- Identify the potential weaknesses and failure points in the systems they use
- Establish robust methods of communication by:
  - use of alternative communication methods
  - diverse technical solutions
- Have effective fallback arrangements
- Ensure interoperability with other agencies
- Ensure that staff are trained appropriately.

Box 7.3 Key features of an effective communication

- Intelligible
- Accurate
- Timely
- Unambiguous
- Concise
- Recorded (logged).

Planning

Each Local Resilience Forum has a *telecommunications sub-group* (TSG) tasked with ensuring robust and effective telecommunications in the event of an incident. The *Emergency Planning College* provides training for the members of these groups. Nationally, the *Electronic Communications – Resilience and Response Group* (EC-RRG) led by the *Department for Business Innovation and Skills* leads the development and maintenance of effective electronic communications structure by means of government–industry liaison (Box 7.4). Through the *National Emergency Plan for Communications*, the EC-RRG plans telecommunications responses in the event of an incident which are operated through the *National Emergency Alert for Telecommunications* (NEAT) scheme. It is an absolutely essential component of any plan that immediate access is available to all necessary telephone numbers and this information is regularly reviewed and updated. The UK government provides detailed and highly technical advice regarding communications resilience (see http://www.gov.uk/telecoms-resilience).

Box 7.4 Membership of the EC-RRG

- Network operators
- Representatives of the Internet sector
- Airwave (see p. 212)
- Ofcom
- Department for Business Innovation and Skills
- Civil Contingencies Secretariat
- Centre for the Protection of National Infrastructure (CPNI)[a]
- Department for Culture, Media & Sport
- MOD
- Representatives of the devolved governments.

[a] The CPNI (part of MI5) is a government agency which protects the national infrastructure (*communications, emergency services, energy, financial services, food, government, health, transport and water*) by providing advice to government departments, and public and private bodies in the areas of cyber, personal, and physical security so as to mitigate the threat from espionage, terrorism, or cyberattack. CPNI also provides advice in the area of business continuity planning.

Resilient communications

A major incident will result in an increase in demand for both fixed and mobile communications by responders, the public, and media organizations alike. For example, during the terrorist incident in London on 7 July 2005, demand for use of the GSM (Global System for Mobile Communications) mobile networks greatly exceeded capacity with the result that callers experienced difficulty in making and receiving calls up to several hours after the incident.

There is no single solution to achieving resilient communications. Processes and organizational issues are as much a part of robust communications as the technical means itself. Relying on a single means without adopting a layered 'fallback' approach will lead to significant risk of communication failure. The general consensus from post-incident reviews and investigations is the importance of diversification.

Main implications

Access to public land mobile networks (PLMNs) cannot be guaranteed. Responders should consider the following key messages:

- GSM networks are not scaled for abnormally high demand.
- Do not rely on the invocation of privileged access.
- Unless privileged access is invoked, a registered SIM (subscriber identity module) card offers no entitlement.
- Privileged access only applies to outgoing calls from a handset.
- If you are entitled to privileged access ensure that your registration is current.
- Understand the limitations of GSM communications.

Options for diversification

There are a number of 'fixed' and 'mobile' options (see Table 7.1).

Team responses: three-step process for reducing reliance on GSM networks
The following guidance has been produced and published by the Civil Contingencies Secretariat, Cabinet Office:

Step 1. Identify your existing critical communications processes:
This step might have identified a process that involves office call-in staff requesting the presence of senior staff at a fallback facility. Staff that need to be contacted tend to spend a significant amount of time away from the office, not necessarily 'on the road' but also visiting other offices. Standing instructions state that a call placed to a mobile phone will be used to specify the location of the fallback facility and obtain the individual's availability and an estimated arrival time.

Step 2. Identify your communications requirements:
This step might identify that the actual amount of information that needs to be communicated could be relatively small. At a bare minimum, this information could be 'pushed' to the recipient (such as by a text message). The recipient might be on the move or in a building and acknowledgement of the request is required.

Step 3. Modify process or technology requirements:
This step might identify that by modifying the process and adopting pre-determined procedures the bare minimum information that could be communicated is a single 'codeword' to which the recipient fully understands the response. This opens up more possible technologies beyond those providing voice communication. These might include a SMS text message, e-mail to a fixed or mobile device, and pager message. SMS text messages may appear attractive but are dependent on availability of the GSM PLMN, e-mail could be sent to fixed or mobile devices (such as an e-mail-enabled mobile phone or Blackberry by using mobile data services) although mobile devices typically use GPRS services which share GSM network infrastructure. There are two pager services which appear to have good resilience and signal penetration in buildings.

Table 7.1 Options for diversification

Fixed	Mobile
Fixed line public voice/data network (PSTN)	Public wide-area paging systems (Vodafone & Pageone)
	Digital Private Mobile Radio (e.g. TETRA/Airwave, Tetrapol)
Virtual Private Network (sharing PSTN capacity)	CB (Citizens Band) radio
Private voice/data network (e.g. GSI)	Raynet (Radio Amateurs' Emergency Network)
	Satellite voice/data service
Internet-based services (e.g. web pages, e-mail, voip)	Private mobile radio (e.g. two-way VHF, UHF)
	Data service (GPRS)-enabled communicator ('pocket PC', 'smart phone' or Blackberry type device)
	Third-generation mobile network
	WiFi (wireless local area networks)
	Wireless data networks (e.g. BT Transcomm, PacNet)

The original process also required the recipient to acknowledge the conversation. If the PLMN were unavailable, acknowledgement could be achieved using a number of means including a fixed-line telephone or e-mail. These means could impose delay, firstly by the originator seeking confirmation that the message has been received and secondly by the responder replying.

The procedure could be further modified to mitigate this delay. Central call-in staff might work down a contact list in sequence and only if mobile phone conversations resulted in no available responder being able to reach the fallback.

Communication requirements

For any situation or set of circumstances, responders should consider the following three key questions:
• Where and how the communication is initiated
• Where and how the communication is received
• Intended outcome of the communication.

Responders should also consider the two factors that may have an impact on effective communication: the location of the responders and the nature of communication.
    Location of responders:
• Urban or rural
• Inside or outside buildings
• Whether the locations are permanent or mobile.

Nature of the communication:
• 'Two-way' conversation involving two or more parties (radio net or conference call)
• 'One-way', and whether the information is:
    • 'pushed' (such as when an e-mail or text message is sent) or broadcast to the recipient or
    • 'pulled' by the recipient (as when a voice mail message or a web page is retrieved).

In order to build a truly resilient communications capability, a number of complex issues need to be appreciated:
• The degree of dependence of one solution on others
• Reliance on third-party networks
• Dependence on electrical power
• Diversity of commercial suppliers
• Geographic coverage
• Interoperability.

Radio systems

Personnel from the ambulance and uniform services will be accustomed to using radio telecommunications systems, other clinicians and managers will need to ensure that they are familiar with and practised in the use of whichever system they may be required to use at an incident. Health service communications at the scene of an incident will be provided by the ambulance service and prior experience with them will significantly improve communications. Radio equipment will include fixed (vehicle-based) and hand-held radios and facilities will exist for communication between the scene, ambulance control, and receiving hospitals. Due to their pitch, in general, women's voices are more intelligible by radio than men's.

Radio voice procedure

Inevitably during a major incident there will be a great deal of radio communication which risks overwhelming the network. It is essential that such communications are only made when necessary and chatter must be avoided. Necessary communications should be:
● clear
● accurate
● brief.

During each call the caller (in order) will:
● state the call sign being called
● state their own call sign
● give the message
● end with *over*.

Radio voice procedure terms

A list of standard radio voice procedure terms is given in Box 7.5. All users must be familiar with these. Following the exchange of call signs, *go ahead* or *send* are used to indicate readiness to receive the reply, *over* means please speak. *Roger* and *OK* confirm that the message has been understood, but if it is not clear, *say again all after ...*, *say again all before ...*, or just *say again* or alternatively *please spell* may be used to clarify. *Spell* may also be used by a speaker to indicate that the following word or phrase will be spelt out using the phonetic alphabet and is commonly used for less familiar names. Similarly, *numbers* should be used to indicate that a series of numbers (e.g. a map reference, telephone number or casualty figure) will follow.

Box 7.5 Common radio voice procedure terms

Over	Begin talking
Go ahead	I am ready for your message
Send	I am ready for your message
Roger	I understand
OK	I understand
Say again	Repeat ('say again all after'/'say again all before')
Spell	Either: (a) indicates that the following word will be spelt out using the phonetic alphabet, or (b) to request the spelling of a difficult or unclear word
Acknowledge	Please confirm that you have received my message
Numbers	Said before a list of numbers such a map reference or telephone number
Out	The exchange is finished [call sign] out to you the communication with a particular member of a radio net is concluded
Wait	I am unable to speak to you for a few seconds, please wait (may be repeated once, then 'wait out') ('wait one' = wait one minute)
Wait out	I am unable to speak to you but will contact you later
Standby	Be aware further information will follow
Wrong	If the speaker recognizes an error, repeated then followed by the corrected version

Acknowledge at the end of a message is a request for confirmation of receipt and understanding. If the speaker recognizes that they have made an error, they should say *wrong* and then give the correct version. *Difficult* is used to describe a message which can be understood but is not clear, *broken* when a message can only be heard in part, and *unworkable* when only fragments can be heard or interference is so bad as to make the message undecipherable. *Nothing heard* means what it says.

Once the exchange is finished, *out* is used to indicate the end of that particular exchange. The phrase *[a particular call sign(s)] out to you* can be used if communication is concluded with one or more call signs of a network, but the others are still required for further transmission of information. If, for any reason, having started a message the speaker is unable to continue, *wait* should be used; however, this should only be used to cover a few seconds and should not be repeated more than once. If a longer pause is needed, *wait out* is used and the communication is terminated. The communication can then be recommenced at a convenient time. *Standby* indicates that the listener should be alert for further messages which will follow shortly.

Phonetic alphabet and numbers

In order to ensure clarity, especially of names and numbers, it is essential that all those who may be called on to pass information at a major incident (and not only by radio) learn and practise the phonetic alphabet and numbers (see Tables 7.2 and 7.3).

Table 7.2 The phonetic alphabet

A	Alpha	N	November
B	Bravo	O	Oscar
C	Charlie	P	Papa
D	Delta	Q	Quebec
E	Echo	R	Romeo
F	Foxtrot	S	Sierra
G	Golf	T	Tango
H	Hotel	U	Uniform
I	India	V	Victor
J	Juliet	W	Whisky
K	Kilo	X	X-ray
L	Lima	Y	Yankee
M	Mike	Z	Zulu

Table 7.3 Phonetic numbers

1	Wun	6	Six
2	Too	7	Seven
3	Thuree	8	Ate
4	Fower	9	Niner
5	Fiyiv	0	Zero

Performing a radio check

A radio check begins with the call signs of the stations being called followed by the caller's own call sign followed by *radio check, over*. (*Yankee 1, Yankee 2, Yankee 3 from Yankee 4, radio check, over.*) Once all the call signs have checked in, the initiator ends the call with *OK, Out* (*Yankee 4 OK, out*).

If the radio-check message is poorly heard or there is interference, then the response should reflect this in order to make it clear to the caller that their transmission may not be properly received. The response from this call sign should reflect either that the message was not fully heard ('difficult') or interrupted ('broken'). This may signify to either the sending or receiving call sign that they may need to move position to obtain a better signal or reception.

Airwave

Airwave is a secure, restricted, and resilient mobile telecommunications system used by the emergency services and other organizations involved in emergency response, offering coverage of over 99% of the UK. Although primarily for the police, ambulance, and fire and rescue services, the system is also available to organizations with whom the emergency services need to communicate when responding to emergencies. Examples include acute receiving hospital emergency departments or local authority emergency planning units. Applications to use Airwave are made through Ofcom, the telecommunications regulator. The Multi Agency Airwave User Group represents the non-blue light Airwave users and is open to all public safety organizations either using Airwave or interested in taking up the service.

Since 2011, all LRFs have identified a multiagency Airwave Senior Responsible Officer (SRO) to champion development of a standard operating procedure (SOP) for local Airwave use across the responder community. The key theme is that of interoperability, in order to fully realize the advantages of having a common radio platform for responders as recommended by the Civil Contingencies Secretariat.

Risks from radio transmission

Some terrorist explosive devices may be detonated by radio waves. Therefore radio usage must be carefully controlled in these circumstances. In general, personal radios should not be used within 15m of a suspect device or vehicle radios within 50m. Specific instructions from relevant bodies (e.g. bomb disposal team) given at the time must always be followed. Some systems, including digital phones, transmit continuously and must be switched off or placed into 'flight mode' within a 50m radius of a suspect device. Where there is a risk of secondary devices following a detonation, the same rules apply.

Telecommunications

Land lines

Within hospitals and other buildings, such as emergency services and public body head-quarters, landlines ('fixed' lines) will be the main means of communication. It is important to remember that a major incident will put considerable strain on normal communication systems and calls must therefore be kept as brief as possible or avoided altogether if not essential. Wherever appropriate, the use of other methods such as pagers and face-to-face meetings should be considered. The subtle nuances of non-verbal communication can sometimes be missed, especially at times of stress, and the importance of clarity and brevity cannot be overemphasized. In some cases, regular planned meetings will reduce the need for calls as much of the transfer of information will not be urgent and can be held over. Most major incident plans will provide extra phone lines for use in a major incident, especially for special facilities, for example, the police casualty bureau or hospital emergency department. It is particularly important that hospital plans have arrangements in place to assist the hospital switchboard in dealing with the increased number of calls a major incident will invariably generate. In the event of a prolonged major incident, communications providers may be able to install additional landlines. Field telephones may be used at the scene of an incident to facilitate communications between the major elements of the emergency response. The armed forces may be able to facilitate effective field communications.

High-Integrity Telecommunications System (HITS)

HITS provides a satellite-based, robust communications system between central government, devolved governments, and Strategic Coordination Centres (Strategic / gold) which is designed to function independently should national landline (PSTN) fail. It is delivered in partnership with Atrium and the MOD and can transmit voice and data communications up to *RESTRICTED* level. HITS is fully inter-operable with conventional telephone systems—such sites with dual capability are known as hybrid sites.

HITS has been designed from the start to interoperate fully with ResilienceDirect. All police forces have been offered ResilienceDirect for use over HITS, giving the ResilienceDirect national coverage.

Transportable (deployable) satellite terminals were withdrawn from service at the end of 2013 and are no longer available to support operations or exercises. A new mobile element to support the fixed site provision may be available in due course.

Government Telephone Preference Scheme (GTPS)

GTPS was established in the late 1950s, at a time when the threat of nuclear war may have led to the destruction of significant parts of the national infrastructure.

Currently, GTPS is provided and managed on a national basis by BT plc, Cable and Wireless plc, and, in the Hull area, by Kingston Communications. In essence, the system is designed to limit outgoing calls from landlines if the network is overloaded during an emergency. When activated, the majority of unregistered customers will lose access to the 'dial tone' thereby preventing them from making outgoing calls (including 999/112). Only registered users will be able to make calls from the telephone connected to a registered line. All customers will still be able to still receive calls. GTPS is rarely used because of the implications of restricting access to fixed network for the majority of the general public. For this reason, registered responders should not see the scheme as a panacea for ensuring resilient communications in the event of a major incident.

Mobile Telephone Privileged Access Scheme (MTPAS)

As mentioned already, mobile phones will inevitably be subject to a greatly increased call frequency during a major incident which is likely to mean that the system will become unreliable or non-functional. MTPAS is intended to preserve access to mobile networks by those engaged in an emergency response when network capacity is under pressure. This is achieved via installation of a special privileged SIM card which is only available to CCA Category 1 and Category 2 responders and their partner agencies, government departments, and the devolved administrations. In the event of an incident, the police *strategic (gold) commander* will activate an agreed protocol notifying all network operators whose responsibility it then is to activate MTPAS. Authorization at this level is mandatory in view of the significant consequences of closing down networks and a standard form of words is used to initiate the process. As a result, mobile phone cells adjacent to an incident will be identified and only MTPAS phones will be allowed access to the network. Other phones will receive a fast bleep tone (*fast busy signal*). If other phones receive an engaged tone or a message that all lines are in use, MTPAS has not been activated. Access to MTPAS is in tranches so that access can be allowed to specific groups of responders without necessarily allowing access to all. Calls to an emergency number (999, 911, or 112) will bypass MTPAS. MTPAS will not work with mobile phones registered on foreign networks.

ACCOLC (Access Overload Control) was the UK national system designed to restrict mobile telephone usage in the event of a major incident. Only enabled numbers were allowed access. *ACCOLC* was replaced by *MTPAS* in 2009.

ResilienceDirect

ResilienceDirect is an online private network for the use of emergency responders and planners during the planning, response, and recovery phases of a major incident. The main intent is to facilitate multiagency collaboration through the sharing of key material such as emergency plans, guidance, and briefings as well as assisting communication between government, planners, and emergency responders (see Box 7.6). Access is granted by the Cabinet Office and is available to all Category 1 and 2 responders, government departments, emergency services, and other key organizations in the UK resilience community.

ResilienceDirect is a web-based service built on a secure platform, accessible via the standard Internet and accredited networks used by the public sector (e.g. GSi and PNN). It is also accessible via HITS.

Volunteer radio nets

RAYNET, the UK radio amateurs' emergency network, is a national voluntary communications service provided for use during emergencies by licensed radio amateurs. RAYNET has around 2000 members and uses a range of equipment types, operating systems, and frequencies. Volunteers use their own equipment, usually to pass on voice messages, although increasingly data can be transmitted. Members are authorized to pass messages between and on behalf of a wide range of agencies including the emergency services, coastguard, local and central government agencies, utility services, voluntary aid societies, and charities and will usually have local knowledge of the area in which an incident has occurred. RAYNET has a regional and national structure and is actively involved in major incident planning and exercises as well as providing assistance at sporting, social, and other mass gathering events. Arrangements for activating such assistance should be agreed, confirmed, and rehearsed in advance.

Further information is available at http://www.raynet-uk.net/main/index.asp. The 24-hour emergency contact telephone number for RAYNET is 0303 040 1080.

Box 7.6 Activities of ResilienceDirect

- Sharing emergency plans among LRF members, national/sub-national partner organizations, and neighbouring LRFs
- Maintaining awareness of forthcoming exercises, events, and meetings including relevant agendas and minutes
- Sharing situation reports and briefings between local responders, and sharing this with the public as appropriate
- Communicating situation reports to LGDs and/or COBR
- Gathering and reviewing comments on new policies or plans before publication
- Collating lessons learned following events
- Managing contact information to ensure a single, up-to-date version of distribution lists
- Issuing news and guidance from central government to local responders via the Resilience Gateway.

Public information, announcements, and warnings

Public information announcements and warnings can be issued via radio, television, the Internet, loudspeaker vans, or house-to-house calls, for example, when needing to advise people to leave their homes.

Social media

Social media has soared in popularity in recent years, offering a compelling option and potential channel through which to release important information to the public in the event of an emergency.

The Defence Science and Technology Laboratory was commissioned by the CCS to conduct a project to better understand how responders can most effectively use social media to communicate with the public in an emergency. An accessible guide for emergency responders has been produced and is entitled 'Smart Tips for Category 1 Responders using Social Media in Emergency Management'. This is available via the http://www.gov.uk website.

Telemedicine

If the facilities are available, the use of telemedicine may allow the virtual attendance of experts offering advice and experience at the scene of an incident, or to offer specialist support to responders remotely. Although the relevant technology is already available, limited capacity and bandwidth is likely to prevent the use of routine means during the response phase, such as mobile telephone networks, and a bespoke telecommunications system would be necessary. The provision of 'nodes' may be possible, utilizing existing public infrastructure such as community centres, healthcare facilities, or libraries.

Alternative methods of communication

Runners

Providing the scene is safe and sufficient personnel are available, the use of runners is an effective way of sending information. Messages should be sent in written form to avoid the phenomenon of *Chinese whispers*. Runners must be fully aware of exactly whom they are giving the message to and must be instructed to inform the original sender when they have returned. Members of the armed forces, or on occasion volunteer members of the public, may be used as runners.

Pagers

In some circumstances personal pagers may be used to pass information, but if a reply is required, means must be available for this to occur.

Whistles

The fire service uses repeated whistle blasts to indicate the presence of imminent danger and the need to evacuate an area. As a consequence, whistles are not normally used for other communication purposes.

Hand signals

Although semaphore is now obsolete, several professional groups use systems of hand signals. These include members of the armed forces and those controlling the movement of aircraft. Although effective within the groups that use them, such signals should not be used more widely or by those unfamiliar with them. Improvised signals are meaningless and should be avoided.

Information sharing

Sharing information is a key function for effective cooperation required to fulfil the full range of civil protection duties including emergency planning, risk assessment, and business continuity management. Information sharing should not be thought of only as a formal process and should occur as part of everyday cooperation. Under the Civil Contingencies Act 2004 (CCA), Category 1 and 2 responders have a duty to share information with other Category 1 and 2 responders. The CCA does not contradict the Data Protection Act 1998. (See Box 7.7 for definitions.)

Consideration of information sharing for formal planning, response, and recovery purposes should include three main types of information:
- Personal data
- Emergency plans
- Commercial or sensitive data.

Sensitive information

The CCA allows exceptions from the supply of some sensitive information. There are broadly four kinds of sensitive information:
- Information prejudicial to national security
- Information prejudicial to public safety
- Commercially sensitive information
- Personal information.

The CCA also offers safeguards that make clear that sensitive information can still be shared between Category 1 and 2 responders for emergency planning purposes—specifying that the information may only be used for the purpose for which it was requested. The focus of the Data Protection Act 1998 is on personal data.

A number of enabling conditions must be met by organizations who wish to share data about any living individual, if the information could be used to identify that individual. Briefly, the conditions that must be met include the following:
- The legal basis to share the information (either express powers, implied powers, or common law)
- Ensuring that the processing of the data is fair to the individual
- Meet one of six conditions to process personal data under Schedule 2 of the Data Protection Act 1998
- Meet one of a number of further conditions to process sensitive personal data under Schedule 3 of the Data Protection Act 1998.

Box 7.7 Information sharing: definitions

Information sharing refers to any information that is non-personal such as plans, schematics, and commercial or business data.

Data sharing refers to information that can be used to identify a living individual, and usually comes under the remit of the Data Protection Act 1998.

Personal data is defined as data relating to a living individual who can be identified from the data or from those data and other information which is in the possession of (or is likely to come into the possession of) the data controller.

Sensitive personal data is defined as data relating to a person's ethnic origins, political opinions, religious beliefs, trade union membership, health, sexual life, and criminal history.

Maps and symbols

The Civil Contingencies Secretariat has worked with the Ministry of Defence and Ordnance Survey to create a set of common map symbols which are linked to the common terminology of the civil protection lexicon. A set of core symbols was published in 2012 as a statement of good practice, the adoption of which aims to promote interoperability and facilitate shared situational awareness between emergency responders.

The current core symbol set is restricted to those elements referred to in civil protection multiagency guidance documents rather than the elements specific to individual emergency responder organizations or their single service doctrine (see Box 7.8). The document is available through the http://www.gov.uk website.

Generic examples

Core items

The core symbol set is founded on a small number of basic building blocks which represent:
- incidents and hazards
- command, control, coordination, or communication (C4) sites
- assets
- infrastructure
- cordons, zones, and areas.

These are illustrated in Figure 7.1.

Zone boundaries and cordons

All cordon symbols are comprised of a line or lines, which may be solid or dashed, and with or without castellation. For example, the inner cordon is drawn with castellation inside while the outer cordon is drawn with castellation outside, as shown in Figure 7.2.

Exclusion zones

These will mark the area of a specific threat or danger zone, and will usually be annotated appropriately (see Figure 7.3).

Access and egress

See Figure 7.4 for general access and egress points
The example shown in Figure 7.5 demonstrates a section of inner cordon with the access and egress points, including the scene access control point (SACP).

Chemical, biological, nuclear, or radiological hazard boundaries

The examples in Figure 7.6 show how the existing zone cordons are modified with different threats.

Box 7.8 Core map symbol set: key design principles

- Based on common UK civil protection terminology, and multiagency civil protection doctrine
- Coherent wherever possible with key existing symbol sets, notably the international standard NATO APP-6
- Simple in design form and based around a small number of basic building blocks which are generally geometric, rather than pictorial or associative
- Rapidly appreciable to users with a basic grasp of the primary acronyms and abbreviations
- Suitable for drawing by hand as well as through a software-embedded symbol set
- Not requiring colour as an essential component of their basic form, although it may enhance the distinctiveness of certain features.

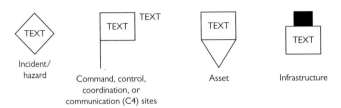

Fig. 7.1 Illustration of the four main symbols.

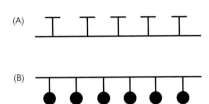

Fig. 7.2 Illustration of inner (A) and outer (B) cordons.

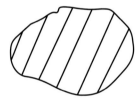

Fig. 7.3 Illustration of an exclusion zone.

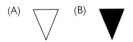

Fig. 7.4 Generic access (A) and egress (B) points.

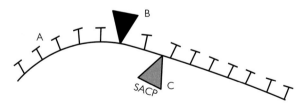

Fig. 7.5 Illustrated example of an inner cordon (A), egress point (B), and SACP access (C).

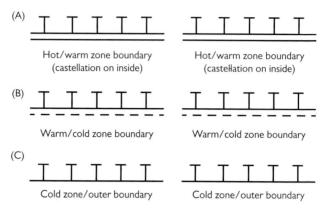

Fig. 7.6 Illustration of the symbols, in both colour and black and white, for cordons between each of: (A) hot/warm, (B) warm/cold, and (C) cold/outer Zone.

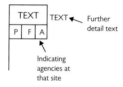

Fig. 7.7 Generic building block for single service command and control sites.

Command, control, co-ordination, or communication (C4) sites

The generic symbol for a C4 site is a flag as shown in Figure 7.1, with the specific type annotated with the use of text, both within the flag and surrounding it. The three main types are classified as:

- multiagency coordination sites
- single-agency command and control (C2) sites
- co-located command and control sites.

Single-service command and control

(See Figure 7.7.) The text inside the main flag indicates the level or type of C2 site, the banner beneath the flag is used to indicate whether it relates to any or all of police (P), fire and rescue (F), and ambulance (A) services, and the free text to the right of the flag can record further attributes such as acronyms or abbreviations of additional agencies (e.g. LA for local authority) at that site or the specific responsibility held at that C2 site.

For examples see Figure 7.8, Figure 7.9, and Figure 7.10.

Assets and infrastructure

An asset may be broadly defined as any resource relevant to an emergency response. They are likely to be either a deployable asset, such as High Volume Pumping (HVP) equipment, or a physical location that has been designated with a specific role such as a Rendezvous point (RVP) or a Helicopter Landing Site (HLS). The generic symbol for an asset is shown in Figure 7.1 p. 223. Examples of symbols for commonly utilized assets are shown in Figure 7.11.

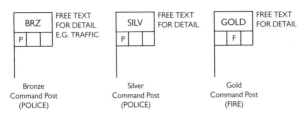

Fig. 7.8 Illustrative examples for Operational/bronze (BRZ), Tactical/silver (SILV) and Strategic/gold (GOLD) levels showing how single-service C2 sites are drawn.

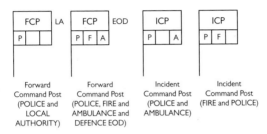

Fig. 7.9 Illustrative examples for forward command posts (FCP) and incident command posts (ICP), showing how co-located C2 sites are drawn.

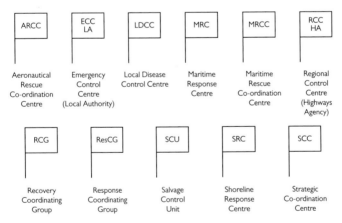

Fig. 7.10 Illustrations showing range of additional, specific C4 multi-agency sites as a variant on the basic flag symbol.

(A)

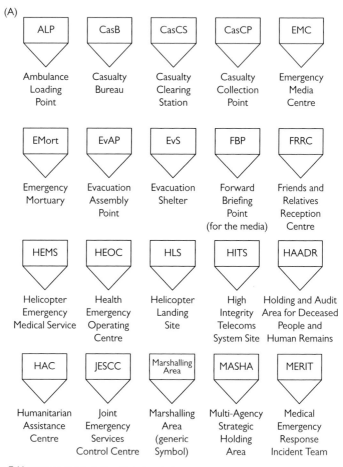

Fig. 7.11 Examples of commonly used asset symbols.

(B)

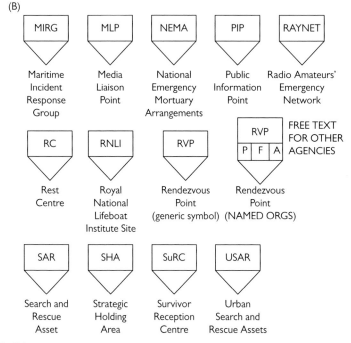

Fig. 7.1 (*Contd.*)

Infrastructure is broadly defined for the purposes of the symbol set to include buildings, points and elements of networks that have a primary use relevant to the emergency and are geographically fixed. As such, they do not include highly mobile or deployable units such as vehicles, boats and aircraft. The generic symbol for infrastructure is shown in Figure 7.12. Examples of symbols for common infrastructure items are shown in Figure 7.13.

Infrastructure includes key items that may be impacted by an emergency, such schools or critical infrastructure that supports essential services, and those features that will provide resources to emergency responders, such as hospitals.

Risk and readiness status
For any given infrastructure or asset, a Red/Amber/Green status may be used to indicate the degree to which that feature is either at risk (for infrastructure), or to the degree that it is functionally operational (for assets). Some examples are shown in Figures 7.11, 7.12, and 7.13, .

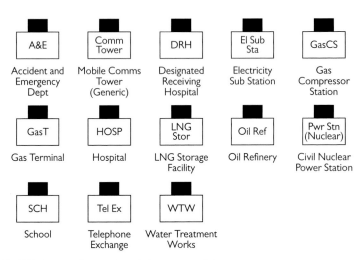

Fig. 7.12 Examples of commonly used infrastructure symbols.

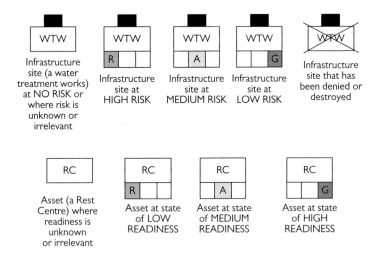

Fig. 7.13 Examples of infrastructure and asset risk and readiness annotation.

Further information

For further information see http://www.cabinetoffice.gov.uk/cpsymbology

Chemical Incidents

Chemical incidents

The majority of major incidents which arise from exposure or potential exposure to toxic chemicals occur as a consequence of an accidental release. However, the possibility of a deliberate, terrorist release incident cannot be excluded. This may be as the result of obtaining and intentionally releasing one or more industrial chemicals, or through the sabotage or destruction of such a facility. *De novo* creation of a toxic chemical is possible but much more challenging.

Accidental release

The majority of significant incidents involving exposure to harmful or potentially harmful chemicals will result from accidents during the manufacture, transport, or use of chemicals intended for normal industrial or other use. Potential causes include human error, transport accidents, and fires. These incidents may be complicated by the presence of multiple chemicals which may react with each other to generate further toxic products.

Deliberate release

Inevitably, unless an announcement has been made by those responsible, recognition of a covert release is likely to be delayed until casualties start to present in large numbers. If the release is associated with an explosion or the release is in a public area, such as the sarin attacks on the Tokyo underground, recognition should be much more rapid. Onset of signs and symptoms of chemical agent poisoning may be very rapid, as in the case of cyanide or nerve agent poisoning, or of more gradual onset. It must be remembered that associated traumatic injuries may be more rapidly lethal than most chemical agents, with the exception of cyanide.

The following features may raise the suspicion of a deliberate release:
- A known or threatened incident
- Unexplained death or loss of consciousness in an otherwise healthy adult
- The casualty reports unusual smells, tastes, or vapours/smoke
- A number of casualties describe similar symptoms
- Similar symptoms occur in a large group with common exposure
- The unexplained death of outdoor animals such as birds is identified.

Toxic industrial chemicals

A toxic industrial chemical (TIC) is defined as:

> an industrial chemical which has a LCt50 (50% lethal vapour concentration) value of less than 100,000 mg/min/m^3 in any mammalian species and is produced in quantities exceeding 30 tonnes per year at one production facility.

This definition differentiates TICs from highly toxic specialized chemicals which are only produced in very limited volumes and used under very close supervision.

TICs which pose an acute inhalational hazard are of the greatest concern. Following a release, the toxic cloud may remain concentrated downwind from the release point and in low-lying areas where there is little air circulation. If the conditions are windy, however, there may be rapid distribution over large areas. The distribution of chemicals will also be affected by sunlight (which may cause degradation), rain, and temperature inversion. Because antidotes are available for only a minority of TICs, effective decontamination and general supportive care are the cornerstones of therapy in the majority of cases.

Initial response to a chemical incident

If a chemical agent is suspected, the first priority is to ensure the safety of medical personnel by using the 'STEP 1–2–3' principle (see Table 8.1). The initial management of a suspected accidental chemical incident or deliberate chemical release should be carried out in the following sequence:

- Command and control
- Safety
- Cordons
- Communication (not discussed separately in this chapter)
- Assessment
- Triage
- Decontamination
- Treatment and initial resuscitation
- Toxicological testing
- Transport
- Specific treatments.

The *STEP 1–STEP 2–STEP 3* system (Table 8.1) offers an approach to the initial response to a possible chemical incident and is widely used. It is essential that responders do not risk their own safety or that of their colleagues or members of the public.

Command and control

The initial response to a chemical incident is established by local emergency services and coordinated by the police. Specialist agencies that would also be involved at an early stage include Public Health England (incorporating the Public Health Laboratory Agency and National Poisons Information Service) and the Environment Agency. In Scotland, this role is taken by the Scottish Environment Protection Agency. Command and control is discussed in more detail in Chapter 5.

Safety

There are three components to scene safety:

- Safety of self (PPE)
- Safety of the scene (ensuring accessibility and safe egress for responders and safe working conditions)
- Safety of the casualties (mitigating risks associated with the incident).

Using this approach will minimize the risk of primary chemical exposure, or of further exposure, not only to emergency personnel but to casualties at the scene. Scene safety is often a significant problem due to the potential spread of contamination as a result of:

- movement of bystanders, spectators, casualties, and emergency personnel
- wind speed and direction
- use of dispersal materials such as water or foam
- secondary devices placed to hamper the emergency response (during a deliberate release).

Cordons

The early and effective establishment of cordons is an important component of command and control as well as being crucial in ensuring scene safety and reducing the risk of injury or contamination. The police are generally responsible for establishing and enforcing cordons, but will take advice from the fire and rescue services. Positioning of the cordon will require careful consideration of:

- the suspected agent involved
- any dispersal methods used
- local environmental factors including temperature, wind speed and direction, and layout of the surrounding streets and buildings.

Table 8.1 The STEP 1–2–3 safety principles for emergency personnel

STEP 1	ONE CASUALTY	Approach using NORMAL procedures
STEP 2	TWO CASUALTIES	Approach with CAUTION Maintain a low index of suspicion Report on arrival, update control
STEP 3	THREE CASUALTIES or MORE	Do NOT approach IF POSSIBLE: Withdraw Contain Report If contaminated—isolate yourself Send for specialist help METHANE/CHALET assessment ASAP

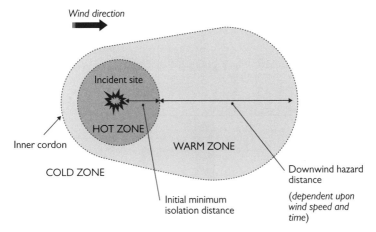

Fig. 8.1 Zones and cordons at a chemical incident site.

The cordons are intended to contain the incident within a fixed area and to prevent any unauthorized entry or exit. The inner cordon contains the immediate vicinity of the incident site and suspected edge of the contaminated area.

Outside the inner cordon, movement of personnel and unaffected individuals should be able to continue without any significant risk of contamination or injury. The outer cordon will be placed to contain the entire incident scene and emergency responses. There may be more than one contaminated area. Cordons must consist of an effective visual and physical barrier. Environmental conditions must be monitored in order that the cordon can be moved if necessary. Similar changes may be required as further information becomes available about the agent or agents concerned. (See Figure 8.1.)

Assessment

Appropriate and regularly updated scene assessments must be carried out to ensure an optimal and safe response.

Triage

Triage for chemical casualties follows the same basic principles as for any other group of patients and is discussed in detail on pp. 148–52. The aim is to ensure that the most serious casualties are decontaminated first so that clinical management can be initiated. Figure 8.2 outlines triage at a chemical incident.

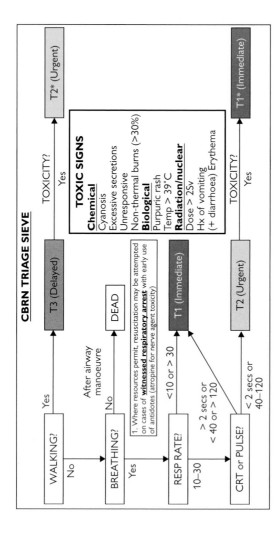

CBRN TRIAGE SIEVE

WALKING?
No → (continue)
Yes → **T3 (Delayed)** → **TOXICITY?** Yes → **T2* (Urgent)**

BREATHING?
No → After airway manoeuvre → **DEAD**
Yes → (continue)

1. Where resources permit, resuscitation may be attempted on cases of **witnessed respiratory arrest** with early use of antidotes (atropine for nerve agent toxicity)

RESP RATE?
10–30 → (continue)
<10 or > 30 → **T1 (Immediate)**

CRT or PULSE?
> 2 secs or < 40 or > 120 → **T1 (Immediate)**
< 2 secs or 40–120 → **T2 (Urgent)** → **TOXICITY?** Yes → **T1* (Immediate)**

TOXIC SIGNS
Chemical
Cyanosis
Excessive secretions
Unresponsive
Non-thermal burns (>30%)
Biological
Purpuric rash
Temp > 39°C
Radiation/nuclear
Dose > 2Sv
Hx of vomiting
(+ diarrhoea) Erythema

Fig. 8.2 Triage at a chemical incident.

Decontamination

Full individual decontamination should be carried out as soon as possible to enable any necessary resuscitation to take place and to prevent further absorption of the chemical agent. Immediate decontamination may be life-saving although is only likely to be possible where such facilities already exist, such as emergency decontamination stations within industrial sites.

Decontamination is best performed at the border of the inner cordon, upwind of the threat and in close proximity to the treatment facility. It should only be carried out by trained personnel wearing appropriate PPE. Ambulatory casualties should be directed to self-decontamination facilities. Removal of clothing alone will reduce exposure to chemical contaminants by 80–90%. Clothing should not be pulled off over the head and must be disposed of appropriately. If specialized decontamination units are initially unavailable, improvised methods may be utilized using the equipment listed in Boxes 8.1 and 8.2. However, *no* attempt should be made to carry this out until appropriate PPE is available. Local procedures may be in place by which some hospital are designated as 'dirty' receiving hospitals with decontamination facilities whereas others will only receive either non-contaminated or decontaminated casualties. However, contaminated casualties may still self-present to local hospitals. Good security arrangements are essential and appropriate facilities for decontamination must be available to reduce the risk to emergency department staff and patients.

Following removal of clothing, the principal method is dry decontamination by blotting with absorbent materials such as paper towels. Dry decontamination is proving to be a safer, more effective method of decontamination even for large-scale incidents. Clothing, eyewear, and jewellery must be removed and carefully double-bagged to prevent exposure from off-gassing. Wet decontamination should be reserved for caustic chemical contamination. Suggested lists for dry and wet decontamination equipment/resources are shown in Boxes 8.1 and 8.2, respectively.

Box 8.1 Dry decontamination equipment and resource list

- Scissors (to aid removal of clothing)
- Brushes/sponges/paper towels
- Scrapers, e.g. spatulas (to remove gelatinous/viscous compounds)
- Absorbents, e.g. Fuller's earth/flour/baking powder
- Adsorbents, e.g. detergent
- Clothing and valuables bags and ID tags
- Replacement clothing.

Box 8.2 Wet decontamination equipment and resource list

- Running water (ideally warm/tepid) supply
- Mild detergent solution
- Buckets/brushes/sponges
- Spray devices (low pressure)
- Facilities to collect/isolate water run-off—or safe disposal into waste water
- Shelter/drying facilities
- Changes of clothing.

Wet decontamination

RINSE–WIPE–RINSE
- Step 1: gently wash affected areas with water to dilute the contaminant and remove particles and water-based chemicals.
- Step 2: wipe affected areas gently but thoroughly with sponge, soft brush, or washcloth to remove organic chemicals and petrochemicals. A mild detergent solution may help to adsorb and remove oily/greasy compounds.
- Step 3: gently rinse affected areas with copious amounts of water.

Treatment

Clinical care of casualties should take place upwind of the incident site and recommended minimum distances observed at all times. Equipment 'pods' may be called forward from their storage at key locations such as public transportation hubs or industrial sites. These are intended for pre-hospital use and contain resuscitation equipment for conventional or CBRN clinical management.

Early decontamination may be the only 'treatment' required following chemical agent exposure. Only interventions necessary to save life should be undertaken in the 'hot zone,' as listed in Box 8.3. Casualties should be extracted to specific treatment areas within the 'cold zone' as rapidly as possible according to the priority they are assigned at triage.

At least one centralized treatment area should be located in between the hot and cold zones, and ideally upwind of the incident site—the 'warm zone'. All casualties must be evacuated through this area in order to prevent inadvertent cross-contamination from potentially 'dirty' to established 'clean' areas. Each treatment area must be divided into 'dirty' and 'clean' with a decontamination barrier between the two. Ideally T3, or 'walking wounded' casualties should be directed to a separate area for decontamination and later treatment.

Box 8.3 Life-saving interventions in high-risk CBRN areas
- Control of catastrophic, external haemorrhage
- Basic airway management ± adjuncts
- Bag–valve–mask ventilation +/- airway adjuncts or LMA/iGel
- Intramuscular/intraosseous antidotes
- Decompression of tension pneumothorax.

UK Reserve National Stock

Arrangements are place for the NHS to access the UK reserve national stock for major CBRN incidents. Stockpiles of drugs and equipment are placed at strategic locations in England, Scotland, Wales, and Northern Ireland which would be used for mutual support in the event of a deliberate or accidental release of CBRN materials. The processes to be followed in the event that access to the stockpiles is required by the NHS in England are outlined below.

Obtaining nerve agent, cyanide, and botulism antidote supplies

NHS Trusts, NHS Foundation Trusts and NHS England Regional Teams should access the following items by contacting their local NHS Ambulance Service Trust Emergency Control Room:

- Nerve agent antidote pod: for treatment of nerve agent poisoning (90 people)
- Obidoxime injection: further treatment for nerve agent poisoning
- Dicobalt edetate pod: for treatment of cyanide poisoning (90 people)
- Botulinum antitoxin: for treatment of botulism.

NHS ambulance services in England either initiating their own requests or responding to requests from NHS Trusts, NHS Foundation Trusts, or NHS England Regional Teams should contact NHS Blood and Transplant as follows:

- Primary number: 0208 201 3827
- Secondary number: 0845 850 0911

The NHS England EPRR Duty Officer must also be informed via 0844 822 2888: ask for 'NHS 05'.

Obtaining antibiotic, radiation, and other antitoxin 'pods'

Several types of 'pod' are available, as listed in Box 8.4. NHS Trusts, NHS Foundation Trusts, and NHS England Regional Teams should access these via the NHS England EPRR Duty Officer:

- Primary number: 0844 822 2888: ask for 'NHS 05'
- Secondary number: 0845 000 5555.

Callers should clearly give the details of the incident, the number of pods requested and their contact details.

The decision to request any of these medical supplies should be made in consultation with the Health Protection Consultant from the local Public Health England (PHE) Centre and/ or the local Director of Public Health.

Box 8.4 Medical supply 'pods' for post-exposure prophylaxis, available through NHS England National EPRR Duty Officer

Post-exposure prophylaxis for anthrax, plague, or tularaemia
Oral ciprofloxacin for 10 days—three types of pod available:
• 250 adults and children aged 12 years and above (500mg tablets)
• 250 children aged 8 to less than 12 years (250mg tablets)
• 50 children aged 0 to less than 8 years (250mg suspension)

or
• Further stocks of unpodded oral ciprofloxacin and doxycycline

or
• Ciprofloxacin intravenous injection.

For post-exposure treatment of plague
Gentamicin intravenous/intramuscular injection.

To block the uptake of radioactive iodine
Potassium iodate tablets, information leaflets for the public.

For the treatment of thallium and caesium poisoning
Prussian blue capsules.

For the treatment of opioid poisoning
Naloxone injection.

Clinical syndromes

The clinical presentation of each agent is not considered in detail and readers are referred to 'Further Reading' (Appendix 1) for more information. Figure 8.3 outlines the early diagnosis of chemical poisoning based on characteristic groups of presenting features. These syndromes are often referred to as *toxidromes*.

Patient group directions

The Department of Health has developed patient group directions (PGDs) in order to allow some chemical and biological countermeasures to be rapidly and widely administered in emergency situations.

PGDs allow the legal administration of countermeasures to groups of patients (e.g. in a mass casualty situation) without individual prescriptions having to be written for each patient. They empower staff other than doctors (e.g. paramedics and nurses) to give the medicine in question. Examples include ciprofloxacin, doxycycline, and potassium iodate.

The exemptions provided by Article 7 of the *Prescription Only Medicines (Human Use) Order 1997* (the POM Order) mean that PGDs are not required for the following countermeasures when given by anyone in an emergency to save life:
• Atropine sulphate injection
• Dicobalt edetate injection
• Glucose injection
• Pralidoxime chloride injection.

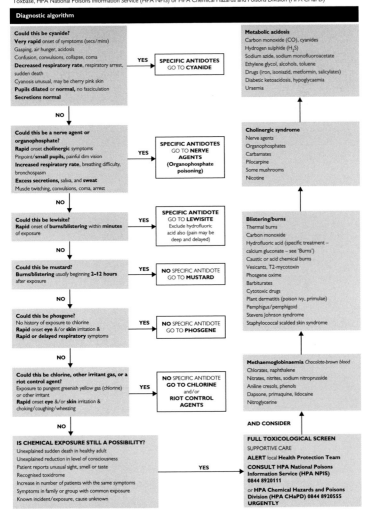

Fig. 8.3 Chemical syndrome (toxidromes).

Reproduced under the Open Government License from Heptonstall J, Gent N, CRBN incidents: clinical management & health protection, Health Protection Agency, London, November 2006 (Revisions v4.0 September 2008), www.gov.uk/government/uploads/system/uploads/attachment_data/file/340709/Chemical_biological_radiological_and_nuclear_incidents_management.pdf

Toxicology and forensics

Toxicological testing will be required in order to determine or confirm which chemical agent is implicated. Emergency departments should ensure that appropriate analysis kits are available for use in the event of a chemical incident: suggested contents are given in Box 8.5. The samples required are listed in Table 8.2. If specialist containers are unavailable, samples may be taken into normal specimen containers with plastic or metal-lined tops. Tubes which contain gel separators or have rubber bungs should not be used as they may leak or interfere with assays. An empty specimen bottle of the same type and from the same batch should be sent with every specimen to act as a control for background chemical contamination. If nothing else is available, the minimum standard for toxicological sampling required is 30mL of urine without preservative.

Samples should be taken as soon as possible after the completion of decontamination and ideally before treatment is started but not if it will delay life-saving measures. Standard precautions for handling clinical specimens should be used. When taking blood samples, the venepuncture site should *not* be cleaned with alcohol swabs as this may also interfere with assays. All samples should be labelled as *high risk* with the casualty's details along with the date and time. Chemical incident analysis request forms (see Figure 8.4) must be completed, included with the samples, and delivered to the nominated laboratory services according to local protocol.

Box 8.5 Suggested contents of a chemical analysis kit

- 1 × 10mL plastic lithium heparin tube
- 1 × 5mL glass lithium heparin tube
- 1 × 4mL EDTA tube
- 1 × 60mL universal container for urine (without preservative)
- 1 × chemical incident analysis request form per patient (see Figure 8.4)
- 1 × double plastic bag for form and samples
- Needles and syringes
- Gloves.

Table 8.2 Required samples for blind toxicological screening, in order of importance

Adults	Children
10mL blood in plastic lithium heparin tube5mL blood in glass lithium heparin tube	5mL blood in glass lithium heparin tube5mL blood in EDTA tube
10mL blood in plastic EDTA tube	30mL urine without preservative
30mL urine without preservative	

Chemical incident analysis request form

Unless you are certain which samples are required and to which analytical toxicology laboratory they should be sent, please check first with HPA Chemical Hazards and Poisons Division (HPA CHaPD) 0844 8920555
READ THE NOTES ON TOXICOLOGICAL TESTING BEFORE YOU TAKE A SAMPLE
PLEASE COMPLETE THIS FORM IN BLOCK CAPITALS

REFERRING LABORATORY:				ANALYTICAL TOXICOLOGY LABORATORY:	
PATIENT DETAILS					
Surname:				First name:	Sex:
Hospital number:				Date of birth:	Age:
Hospital/Trust:				Ward/Unit:	
Analysis requested by:				Consultant:	
SAMPLE DETAILS				Name and address for report	
Sample date	Sample time	Sample type	Req Lab No	ATL No (specalist lab use only)	
		Heparinised blood (10ml)			
		Heparinised blood (5ml)			
		EDTA blood (4ml)			
		Urine (30ml)			

EXPOSURE DETAILS		
Place of exposure:		Unknown:
Date (dd/mm/yy) of exposure:		Unknown:
Time exposure occurred (24 hr clock):	:	Unknown:
Exposed to (give name of chemical):		Unknown:
Length of exposure (estimate duration in minutes):		Unknown:

Clinical features (please describe these as fully as possible, and give time and date of onset for each symptom or sign):

Telephone number:
Telephone number for urgent results:
Name and address for invoice:

Telephone number:

DO NOT WRITE ON THIS FORM – USE IT AS A MASTER TO MAKE PHOTOCOPIES

CHAIN OF EVIDENCE FORM	A form has been completed and accompanies these specimens (Yes/No):

BEFORE REFERRING THESE SPECIMENS, please NOTIFY the ANALYTICAL TOXICOLOGY LABORATORY PHOTOCOPY the COMPLETED REQUEST FORM and GIVE THE PHOTOCOPY to the TOXICOLOGY CO-ORDINATOR

Fig. 8.4 Chemical incident analysis request form.

Reproduced under the Open Government License from Heptonstall J, Gent N, CRBN incidents: clinical management & health protection, Health Protection Agency, London, November 2006 (Revisions v4.0 September 2008), www.gov.uk/government/uploads/system/uploads/attachment_data/file/340709/Chemical_biological_radiological_and_nuclear_incidents_management.pdf

Chain of evidence

For forensic purposes, there must be a chain of evidence for all samples which allows it to be clearly demonstrated that no possibility of tampering or contamination could have occurred. A suitable form (Figure 8.5) must be used and every time a sample changes hands, starting with the individual first taking the samples, a new form must be completed. The forms should be kept together and numbered in sequence.

Any break in the chain of evidence documentation may compromise the evidential value of the sample and jeopardize future criminal proceedings. A senior clinician must sign the form as soon as practically possible. Receiving laboratories will have their own local protocols for who is sufficiently senior to authorize sample handover and these should be adhered to in all cases.

Fig. 8.5 Example of a chain of evidence form.

Reproduced under the Open Government License from Heptonstall J, Gent N, CRBN incidents: clinical management & health protection, Health Protection Agency, London, November 2006 (Revisions v4.0 September 2008), www.gov.uk/government/uploads/system/uploads/attachment_data/file/340709/Chemical_biological_radiological_and_nuclear_incidents_management.pdf

Transport

Once appropriate decontamination measures have been taken, casualties should be removed from the scene as soon as is practical. It is vital that evacuation of all casualties, regardless of severity, takes place through a single location in order to reduce the spread of contamination. A specially adapted triage sieve for chemical casualties is shown in Figure 8.2, p. 234. Casualty movement from the scene should be carried out under the strict supervision of the emergency services ensuring that no contaminated casualties are inadvertently released to hospitals.

The ambulance circuits and loading points should be upwind of the incident site. The evacuation plan should also be coordinated at a higher level to ensure casualties are sent to appropriate hospitals and distributed so that no single hospital is overwhelmed if possible. In the event of a hospital receiving a significant number of contaminated casualties, the evacuation plan may have to be changed to redirect 'clean' casualties to alternative hospitals.

Public information

Appropriate warnings and information must be given out in the event of a chemical incident in order to prevent further members of the public being exposed and to allay potential anxiety. Details of the location, type of hazard, and surrounding exclusion zone should be released. General instructions should also be given along the following lines:

'Go in. Tune in. Stay in.'

Evacuation routes must be followed without exception and members of the public should be requested to report suspicious mists, fogs, low-lying clouds, powders, or liquids in the vicinity.

If any individuals are out in the open in the vicinity of a chemical release they should be advised to:
• cover their nose and mouth with a wet cloth if possible (dry is better than nothing)
• breathe lightly and calmly until out of danger
• keep their eyes closed and covered as much as possible
• leave the affected area immediately
• stay upwind and uphill of the incident scene
• keep car windows and air vents closed and the air conditioning turned off until out of the immediate area if driving.

Advice to individuals

Individuals who suspect that they have been exposed to a chemical agent should be advised to:
• remove all their clothing and bag it in a sealed bag
• wash with soap and water, then rinse with copious amounts of water
• flush eyes with water for at least 10–15 minutes
• seek medical attention immediately as instructed.

Details of 'dirty' hospitals or hospitals with decontamination facilities may be announced.
Individuals who are inside buildings in the vicinity of the incident should be advised to:
• move to, and remain in, an above-ground floor inner room (without windows if possible)
• turn off all ventilation systems and air conditioning
• close outside doors, windows, and air vents
• be ready to seal windows, doors, and vents shut if instructed to do so
• exercise caution with uncovered food supplies
• listen to television and radio broadcasts for further information
• be prepared to evacuate quickly if instructed to do so.

In some cases, although rarely, caution may be needed regarding drinking water and bottled water may be safer.

Personal protective equipment (PPE)

Personal protective equipment (PPE) exists in two basic forms: *splash and contact* protection and gastight suits. The latter suits offer *level A, B, or C protection* (Table 8.3). Ideally, PPE should allow effective work to continue without creating further safety issues such as heat stress or physical exhaustion. A balance has therefore to be met between protection and performance degradation in order to allow members of the emergency services to carry out their role with maximum efficiency.

Members of the fire service have specific PPE suits for use during chemical incidents. 'Level A' protection is required when active release may still be occurring or when the release has stopped but information is not available regarding ongoing chemical hazards from ground or airborne contamination. Initially *positive-pressure self-contained breathing apparatus* (SCBA) should be used with a vapour-tight suit until monitoring results allow for reduction in the level of protection.

The NHS has a stock of one-piece *powered respiration protective suits* (PRPS) that can be issued to ambulance crews and forward medical teams. These suits can also be issued to hospital emergency departments for use when dealing with potentially contaminated casualties. The armed forces have lightweight CBRN protective equipment which gives protection against a wide range of potential chemical weapons. Both the NHS and military PPE suits give 'level C' protection. 'Level D' protection also exists although it only consists of specific work clothing and eye (splash) protection.

Table 8.3 Levels of protective clothing

Level A	• Vapour-tight, providing total encapsulation and a high level of protection against direct and airborne chemical contact
	• Worn with an SCBA unit enclosed within the suit
Level B	• Not completely vapour-tight, therefore providing a lesser degree of protection than level A
	• Worn with an SCBA unit, which may be inside or outside of the suit, depending on the type of suit
Level C	• Includes coveralls or splash suits providing a lesser level of protection than level B
	• Typically worn with a respirator or gas mask only rather than an SCBA unit

Specific antidotes

Specific antidotes are available for certain chemical agents and are listed in Table 8.4. Managers, in conjunction with clinicians and scientific advisors, will be required to ensure that appropriate supplies are available. Clinical details are available in standard texts.

Table 8.4 Specific antidotes

Agent	Toxic substance
Oxygen	Urgent treatment of any acutely sick, *contraindicated in paraquat poisoning*
Pralidoxime	Nerve agent or organophosphate poisoning
Atropine	Nerve agent or organophosphate poisoning
Diazepam	Anticonvulsant for nerve agent or organophosphate poisoning
Combi-pen (contains atropine, pralidoxime, and a diazepam precursor)	Nerve agent or organophosphate poisoning (issued to members of HM Forces)
Dicobalt edetate	Cyanide poisoning
Sodium nitrite/sodium thiosulphate	Cyanide poisoning (given together as an alternative to dicobalt edetate)
Hydroxocobalamin	Cyanide poisoning as an alternative to dicobalt edetate or sodium nitrite and sodium thiosulphate
Physostigmine	Some specific incapacitating agents
Dimercaprol (British anti-lewisite, BAL)	Lewisite and some arsenic compounds
Naloxone	Opiates

The hospital response to a chemical incident

The generic hospital response to a major incident is covered in Chapter 12. This section considers aspects of such a response specific to a chemical incident.

The hospital may be warned of a chemical incident by the emergency services, by an industrial site, the military, or a central government source. In some cases, however, where it has not yet been formally established that a chemical release has occurred, casualties may end up bypassing community or pre-hospital care services and arrive at hospital unannounced. In this event, the emergency department will usually be the first to recognize features of a chemical release incident. Once it is recognized that an incident involving chemicals has taken place, the key components of the hospital response are:

- protection of staff and existing patients (including appropriate PPE)
- effective and safe patient flow
- provision of decontamination facilities and avoidance of contamination of clinical areas
- diagnostics and clinical management of casualties
- information cascade
- maintaining the chain of evidence
- access to toxicological analysis
- case reporting.

All of these elements should be incorporated into hospital major incident plans.

Managing contamination at receiving hospitals

As soon it is suspected or established that casualties have resulted from a chemical release, the safety and protection of hospital staff and patients becomes paramount. All casualties and emergency service personnel who arrive at the hospital from the scene of a suspected chemical incident must be considered to be contaminated unless they have been decontaminated at the scene. Individuals who may be contaminated must not be admitted to clinical areas until they have been decontaminated. 'Chemical' PPE/PRPS must be worn by all personnel dealing with casualties suspected to be contaminated and decontamination measures must be carried out for all patients arriving from the suspected release area if this has not already been done.

All non-incident patients must be removed from the emergency department using the normal procedures developed for conventional major incidents. Among casualties who have already arrived in the department, there may be patients who were not involved in the incident but who have come into contact with contaminated casualties. Clinical areas may need to be divided into 'clean' and 'dirty' areas to ensure that unaffected patients do not become contaminated themselves. Decontamination should be carried out in specifically designated areas or outside the hospital in NHS decontamination units.

The senior clinician on duty for the emergency department must ensure that all necessary PPE and decontamination resources are made available.

Diagnosis and clinical management of multiple casualties at hospital

Ideally, primary triage using the triage sieve will be carried out on arrival, *outside* the emergency department, and prior to decontamination. Sometimes decontamination will need to be carried out as management of critically unwell casualties requiring advanced life support. Once decontamination is complete, clinical management should be carried out according to standard principles. Children are more likely to exhibit greater toxic effects than adults for an equal exposure to any given chemical. This should be considered during triage.

Information cascade

Individual hospital major incident protocols should be followed. Information about the incident must pass up the clinical and management chain so that adequate resources can be made available and extra support obtained (see Figure 8.6). Senior clinical staff must remain alert to the arrival of casualties with unexplained symptoms or unexpected numbers of casualties presenting with similar symptoms or signs. The Local Health Protection Team and Public Health England must be informed. All advice given should be recorded on a suitable form (Figure 8.7).

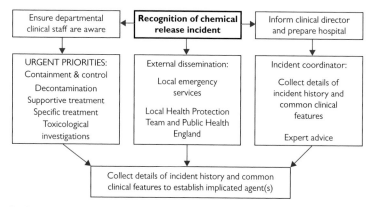

Fig. 8.6 The information cascade for a chemical incident.

Incident advice record form

Hospital/Trust:		Department:		Date:	
Type of incident:		Place of incident:		Number of casualties:	
Task/query	Advice received and action taken (Details of the advice/action, your name and signature)		Source of advice (Name, date, time)	Telephone number	
Staff protection/PPE					
Operational lockdown					
Turning off air-conditioning					
Patient containment					
Decontamination					
Patient investigation					
Patient treatment					
Post exposure prophylaxis					
Environmental sampling					
Who to inform					
Other					
Other					
Other					
Other					
Other					
Other					
Other					
Other					
Other					

DO NOT WRITE ON THIS FORM – USE IT AS A MASTER TO MAKE PHOTOCOPIES

Fig. 8.7 Specimen advice record paperwork for a chemical incident.

Reporting chemical exposure cases

A suitable chemical exposure record form should be used to document each individual case. An example is given in Figure 8.8. Once completed, the form should be forwarded to Public Health England. A copy of the completed form should also be kept in the patient's hospital notes.

Government Decontamination Service (GDS)

The GDS assists local and regional authorities in carrying out decontamination and recovery following a deliberate or accidental CBRN release. It also advises central government on the UK's capability to respond to such incidents. The GDS provides both generic and incident-specific advice on decontamination including of the open and built environment and other infrastructure. Decontamination of people is the responsibility of the Department of Health and the emergency services. Further information regarding GDS can be found by visiting the website: https://www.gov.uk/government/groups/government-decontamination-service

Local management plans

The Department of Health takes overall responsibility for public health and for offering advice designed to limit the public health consequences of chemical incidents. Within each designated Police Authority area, the director of public health and the clinical commissioning groups will establish arrangements appropriate for the coordination of the health response to chemical incidents.

Water contamination

For incidents that involve water contamination, the initial management is the responsibility of the water supply companies and the Environment Agency (EA) or Scottish Environmental Protection Agency (SEPA). Water companies are legally required to notify health and local authorities if an incident has occurred which has the potential to lead to a significant health risk. The EA (SEPA in Scotland) would take action to respond to the ecological effects of any water contaminant.

Other organizations involved in the management of a chemical incident

The Ministry of Defence (MoD) will be involved in any incident involving counterterrorism although it may be called in to assist in other incidents through the provision of manpower or equipment. CBRN expertise can be made available via the Defence Science and Technology Laboratories (Dstl) at Porton Down or the Defence CBRN Centre, Winterbourne Gunner. The Health and Safety Executive (HSE) is responsible for industrial sites and workplace use of potentially harmful chemicals, and oversees the provision of appropriate on-site emergency planning. The Department of the Environment, Food and Rural Affairs (DEFRA) takes overall responsibility for management of environmental contamination

Chemical exposure record form

PATIENT DETAILS This section may be completed by the patient, or a clerk, volunteer, or health professional					
Hospital/Trust			Date of arrival		Time
Hospital number			EMD number		
Surname			First name		
Male	Female	Age (years)	Date of birth		
Home address					
Town					
Country			UK resident?		Yes No
Postcode		Telephone number (include STD code)			
Name of GP (if patient UK resident)			PCT		
This section completed by	Patient	Clerk	Other (specify)		

EXPOSURE and DECONTAMINATION This section (and the rest of the form) must be completed by a health professional				
Has the patient been chemically contaminated?	Yes		No	Not sure
If yes, date and time of contamination?	Date			Time:
If yes, where was the patient when contaminated?				
Was the contaminant?	Solid	Liquid	Vapour/gas	Not sure
Route of exposure?	Inhaled	Eaten	On skin	Not sure
Name of chemical (or other detail, eg UN number):				Not known
Was the patient decontaminated at the scene?		Yes	No	Not sure
Has the patient been decontaminated in the EMD?		Yes	No	Time:

EXPOSURE-RELATED SYMPTOMS and MANAGEMENT					
Has the patient developed any symptom/s?		Yes	No		Not sure
If yes, please list the symptom/s:					
Date and time of onset of the first symptom?	Date			Time:	
Triage category at scene?	Not known	Immediate	Urgent	Delayed	
Triage category in EMD?	Not known	Immediate	Urgent	Delayed	
AVPU at scene?	Alert	Verbal stimulus response	Painful stimulus response	Unresponsive	Not known
Has any antidote been given?		Yes	No		Not sure
If yes, give name and dose of any drug given as antidote:					
Have specimen/s been taken for toxicology?	Blood		Urine		None

OUTCOME			
Has the patient been admitted to this hospital?	ITU	Ward	No/not sure
Has the patient been discharged?	Yes	No	Not sure
Given a follow up appointment at this hospital?	Yes	No	Not sure
Given instructions to see GP within 24 hours?	Yes	No	Not sure
Given an information leaflet?	Yes	No	Not available
Has the patient been referred to another unit?	No	Name of unit	
Did the patient die?	Date of death	No	
These sections completed by:	Name	Grade	Other

DO NOT WRITE ON THIS FORM – USE IT AS A MASTER TO MAKE PHOTOCOPIES

Fig. 8.8 Example of a chemical exposure clinical record form.

Reproduced under the Open Government License from Heptonstall J, Gent N, CRBN incidents: clinical management & health protection, Health Protection Agency, London, November 2006 (Revisions v4.0 September 2008), www.gov.uk/government/uploads/system/uploads/attachment_data/file/340709/Chemical_biological_radiological_and_nuclear_incidents_management.pdf

Chemical hazard labels

All vehicles transporting dangerous goods in quantity on journeys in the UK must carry appropriate information and warnings. These take the form of Hazchem plates (Figure 8.9) or Kemler plates (Figure 8.11).

Hazchem

Hazchem provides information about the hazardous substance carried, including the PPE requirement in the event of a release and necessary control and dispersal methods. Details are also given regarding whether the chemical can be flushed into normal drainage systems or whether containment is required. The UN number for the chemical and UN hazard warning is also given. The information on the card can also be deciphered using a Hazchem guide (Figure 8.10).

Kemler

The Kemler plate is the European system. The upper number is the Kemler code for the substance which is being carried, the lower number the UN substance identifying number. The first digit of the Kemler number shows the primary hazard, the second and third give secondary hazards. If a number is repeated, the hazard is intensified. A preceding X indicates that the substance must not be brought into contact with water.

TREM cards

A TREM card is a Transport Emergency Card. A4 sized, TREM cards are carried in the cab of road vehicles carrying dangerous substances. The cards give instructions and information required in the event of an incident (Figure 8.12).

Chemdata™

Chemdata™ is an interactive database of over 50,000 substances and more than 150,000 different chemical names, including generic and trade names. The fire and rescue services have access to this database through equipment carried on response vehicles.

Toxbase™

Toxbase™ is the information database of the *UK National Poisons Information Service*. It provides clinical information regarding a wide range of toxic and therapeutic substances. Access is for medical professionals only through individual or institutional subscription.

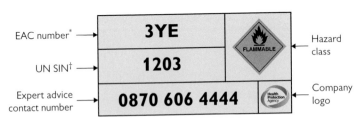

Fig. 8.9 The HAZCHEM warning label. * The Emergency Activation Code instructs emergency services on immediate actions. † The UN Substance Identification Number identifies the chemical.

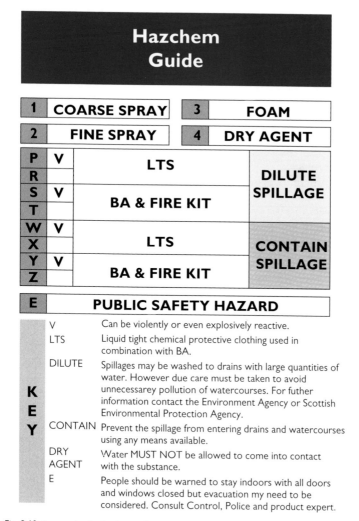

Hazchem Guide

1	COARSE SPRAY	**3**	FOAM	
2	FINE SPRAY	**4**	DRY AGENT	

P	V	LTS	DILUTE SPILLAGE
R			
S	V	BA & FIRE KIT	
T			
W	V	LTS	CONTAIN SPILLAGE
X			
Y	V	BA & FIRE KIT	
Z			

E	PUBLIC SAFETY HAZARD

KEY

V	Can be violently or even explosively reactive.
LTS	Liquid tight chemical protective clothing used in combination with BA.
DILUTE	Spillages may be washed to drains with large quantities of water. However due care must be taken to avoid unnecessarey pollution of watercourses. For futher information contact the Environment Agency or Scottish Environmental Protection Agency.
CONTAIN	Prevent the spillage from entering drains and watercourses using any means available.
DRY AGENT	Water MUST NOT be allowed to come into contact with the substance.
E	People should be warned to stay indoors with all doors and windows closed but evacuation my need to be considered. Consult Control, Police and product expert.

Fig. 8.10 An example of a Hazchem guide.

Reproduced with permission © Ricardo Energy & Environment 2016 (http://the-ncec.com/free-online-hazmat-hazchem-guide/).

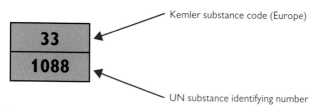

Kemler substance code (Europe)

33

1088

UN substance identifying number

Fig. 8.11 The Kemler plate.

Cefic Tremcard - Instructions in Writing

HAZSING1	
Class	8
PG	I
HI No	886
UN	1790

LOAD
Hydrofluoric Acid with more than 60% hydrogen fluoride

Name of substance(s): HAZCHEM HYDROSOL
- Usually colourless fuming liquid - Perceptible odour.
- Completely miscible with water.

NATURE OF DANGER
- Highly corrosive.
- Contact with liquid causes severe damage: to eyes, to skin, to air passages.
- May attack many materials and clothing.
- Attacks many metals with liberation of hydrogen which is flammable and forms explosive mixture with air.
- Toxic: by absorption through skin, by inhalation, by ingestion. Symptoms may develop after several hours.
- The vapour poisons: by inhalation.
- Heating may cause toxic fumes.
- Decomposes in a fire giving off toxic fumes: hydrogen fluoride.
- The vapour is heavier than air and spreads along ground.

PERSONAL PROTECTION
- Respiratory protective device enabling driver to escape e.g. escape hood or mask with combined gas particle cartridge.
- Goggles or face shield.
- Light protective clothing.
- Protective gloves.
- Protective footwear.
- Eyewash bottle with clean water.

INTERVENTION EQUIPMENT
- Not applicable.

GENERAL ACTIONS BY THE DRIVER
- Stop the engine.
- No naked lights. No smoking.
- Mark roads with self-standing warning signs and warn other road users or passers-by.
- Keep public away from danger area. Keep upwind.
- Notify police and fire brigade as soon as possible.

ADDITIONAL AND/OR SPECIAL ACTIONS BY THE DRIVER
- Put on your respiratory protective device and keep out of the danger area.
- If substance has entered a water course or sewer or been spilt on soil or vegetation, inform police.

FIRE (information for the driver in case of fire)
- Do not attempt to deal with any fire involving the load.

FIRST AID
- If substance has got into the eyes, immediately wash out with plenty of water. Continue treatment until medical assistance is provided.
- Remove contaminated clothing immediately and drench affected skin with plenty of water, then wash with soap and water.
- Seek medical treatment when anyone has symptoms apparently due to inhalation, swallowing or contact with skin or eyes.
- Persons who have inhaled the fumes produced in a fire or in a chemical reaction may not show immediate symptoms. They should be taken to a doctor with this card. Patient must be kept under medical supervision for at least 24 hours.

SUPPLEMENTARY INFORMATION FOR EMERGENCY SERVICES
- Consult an expert immediately.
- Keep container(s) cool by spraying with water if exposed to fire: Beware dangerous reaction with water if containers ruptured.
- Extinguish with waterspray, foam or dry chemical.
- Do not use water jet.
- Use waterspray to "knock down" vapour.
- Sewers must be covered and basements and workpits evacuated.
- Keep remaining cargo dry.
- Use dry plastic or stainless steel containers for repacking.
- Do not flush road with water.

Additional information
In case of Emergency Contact: David Howard
HazChem Systems Ltd
212-214, Katherine Street,
Ashton-Under-Lyne, Lancashire OL6 7AS

EMERGENCY TELEPHONE: 0161 339 0821

© Cefic Prepared by Cefic from the best knowledge available; no responsibility is accepted that the information is sufficient or correct in all cases
Cefic TEC(R) - 80S1790-I
1 01/01/2009

APPLIES ONLY DURING ROAD TRANSPORT ENGLISH
Cefic Revision 10/2004 Issue: ADR 2007.0

Fig. 8.12 Example of a TREM card.
Reproduced with permission © 2015 HazChem Systems Ltd (www.hazchemsystems.co.uk/tremcard.html).

Hazard warning symbols

The standard symbols used for dangerous chemicals are shown in Figures 8.13 and 8.14.
- Class 1: explosive, e.g. fireworks, ammunition, hydrazine: subgroups 1.1–1.6 include 1.1: mass explosion hazard, 1.4: no significant hazard
- Class 2: gases (2.1: flammable; 2.2: non-flammable, non-toxic; 2.3: toxic)
- Class 3: flammable liquids (e.g. diesel, xylene, methanol, alcohol)
- Class 4: flammable solids, e.g. barium, sodium (4.1: flammable solid; 4.2: spontaneous combustion risk; 4.3: release flammable gas on water contact)
- Class 5: oxidizers (5.1) or organic peroxides (5.2)
- Class 6: toxic (6.1: includes sarin, nerve agents, mustard, lewisite, pesticides) or infectious (6.2) substances
- Class 7: radioactive substances and articles (sources in nuclear industry, industrial radiography, military, nuclear medicine, radiotherapy)
- Class 8: corrosive substances (e.g. chlorine, fluorine, sodium hydroxide, nitric acid)
- Class 9: miscellaneous dangerous substances (e.g. pepper spray, F: mace, asbestos).

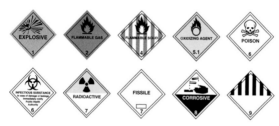

Fig. 8.13 UN hazard classes.

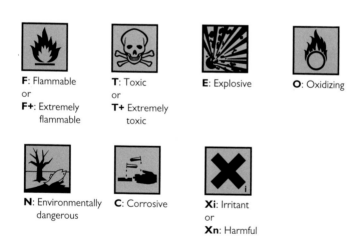

Fig. 8.14 EU standard chemical package labels.

Biological Incidents

Recognition of a biological incident

A biological incident is likely to take one of the following forms:
- Rapid epidemic spread of an infectious disease within or spreading from its normal geographic boundaries
- Accidental escape of a pathogenic disease-causing organism from a laboratory
- Deliberate release as part of terrorist or other malicious activity.

At the present time, the obvious examples of the first category include so-called *avian or bird 'flu'*, *swine flu*, or the recent threat of imported *Ebola* (viral haemorrhagic) fever. An example of the second is the outbreak of smallpox in Birmingham in 1980. The UK has yet to be affected by a known deliberate release of a pathogenic organism but the USA was subject to anthrax attacks in 2001.

Natural disease outbreaks

In general, a natural disease outbreak presents different challenges to those of a conventional major incident. Its onset is likely to be gradual and identification will generally follow recognition of clusters of typical clinical features identified by conventional surveillance methods. In the majority of cases, effective management will not require the implementation of major incident protocols or conventional local scene management, but will be achieved by the extension of established clinical and other methods. However, additional measures such as stockpiling of vaccines, changes in border controls, and treatments for specific threats may be required, as will plans to ensure availability of assets such as intensive care beds and infectious disease facilities (including isolation capability) depending on the analysis of possible threats.

Accidental release of pathogenic organisms

There is a theoretical risk of accidental release of a pathogenic organism from one of the high-security laboratories in the UK licensed to handle them. However, biosecurity measures have ensured that no such incident has occurred in the last 30 years.

Bioterrorism incidents

It is fortunate that biological weapons are, for the most part, sufficiently difficult and hazardous to produce that they are used less frequently than other methods such as conventional explosives and chemicals.

The US Centres for Disease Control and Prevention (CDC) has defined the *'Big Six'* main biological agents that threaten the most significant public health impact and have the greatest potential for large-scale dissemination and interpersonal transmission. These are considered *'Category A'* agents and are listed in Box 9.1. *Category B* agents are moderately easy to disseminate and have lower morbidity and mortality rates. Examples of these are listed in Box 9.2.

Category C agents are pathogens that could potentially be engineered for mass dissemination because of their availability, ease of production, and potential for high morbidity and mortality. Examples of these are listed in Box 9.3

Features of an intentional biological agent release

A bioterrorism attack is most likely to be initiated in a covert manner in order to disguise the release of the pathogen and avoid the recognition of the release and a timely response by the emergency services. Therefore, recognition of such a release will be more challenging and occur over a longer period of time during which the pathogen may be widely disseminated.

Possible scenarios include:
- spread of disease by an intentionally infected individual
- contamination of air or water via ventilation or storage systems
- contamination of foodstuffs or introduced via animal vector
- Intentional modification (e.g. genetic) of an existing pathogen.

Crucially, an intentional disease carrier is likely to actively avoid treatment, unlike a genuine victim who will seek assistance at an early opportunity. It is theoretically possible that an innocent individual might be forcibly infected with a pathogenic organism although no example has yet been recorded.

Possible early clinical and environmental indicators of an intentional biological agent release incident are in Table 9.4. Recognition by even the most effective public health surveillance systems will still be delayed until a sufficient number of cases appear and data is collected and analysed. Table 9.5 shows some of the public health surveillance indicators that may be seen.

Natural epidemic disease activity

The majority of natural disease outbreaks will occur against a background of a low but ongoing incidence of cases and may be affected by the uptake of population-based preventative measures such as vaccination. In general, these outbreaks are associated with morbidity rather than mortality, although deaths (e.g. from measles) can occur. Infectious disease outbreaks of this kind are controlled or managed using conventional public health processes. Conventional major incident structures are unlikely to be needed, at least at the local level, although national coordination may be required. The response of the public and media to a naturally occurring outbreak will be dramatically different to that to a suspected terrorist incident. Occasionally unusual imported infectious diseases do occur, but awareness of potential risk factors, such as travel to an area known to harbour the disease, together with clinical suspicion in the event of an unusual presentation will generally be effective in achieving control of any actual or potential outbreak. The remainder of this chapter will concentrate on deliberate release of infective agents, although in some areas (e.g. the hospital response), there will be considerable overlap.

Box 9.1 Category A agents (the 'Big Six')
- Anthrax
- Plague
- Smallpox
- Tularaemia
- Filoviridae—viral haemorrhagic fever (VHF)
- Botulinum toxin.

Box 9.2 Examples of category B agents
- Brucellosis
- Epsilon toxin of *Clostridium perfringens*
- Food safety threats (e.g. *Salmonella* species, *Shigella, E. coli*)
- Glanders
- Melioidosis
- Psittacosis
- Q fever
- Ricin toxin
- Staphylococcal enterotoxin B
- Typhus
- Viral encephalitis
- Water supply threats (e.g. *Cryptosporidium parvum*, cholera)

Box 9.3 Examples of Category C agents
- Nipah virus
- Hantavirus (VHF)
- Multi-drug resistant tuberculosis.

Box 9.4 Clinical indicators of an intentional biological agent release
- Unusual numbers of presentations of rare or non-endemic diseases
- Unusual age, occupational, or geographic distribution
- Unexpectedly high morbidity or mortality for known disease
- Unusual seasonal incidence
- Agent-specific clinical clues (e.g. smallpox rash)
- Predominance of respiratory symptoms among usually well individuals.

Box 9.5 Public health indicators of an intentional biological agent release
- Incidence demonstrating an epidemic curve with an 'explosion' of cases
- Simultaneous outbreaks of unusual diseases
- Tight geographical or occupational clustering
- Unusual resistance patterns or modes of transmission
- Numerous animal casualties as well as human
- Absence of a normal disease host or vectors.

Recognition of an intentional biological agent release

Non-contagious agents

Non-contagious agents, such as anthrax bacillus spores, will require an effective means of widespread dispersal in order to clinically affect large numbers of individuals, as the pathogen is not easily transmitted from person to person. Potential techniques may include the use of explosive canisters containing agent or spraying devices attached to vehicles or aircraft. Smaller numbers may be affected by material sent by post as in the US anthrax attacks of 2001. The outcome of dispersal of these agents is more predictable in that only those in the vicinity of the release will be affected. Prompt management should contain further spread of infection.

Contagious agents

Some agents, such as smallpox and plague, spread from person to person so rapidly that widespread dispersal may not be necessary. A small amount of agent dispersed and infecting only a few individuals will have the potential to start an epidemic affecting millions. Such a method is inherently unpredictable in its outcome, and could result in huge numbers of casualties spread over large areas crossing national boundaries.

Dispersal

Non-contagious biological agents are usually dispersed either by air in the form of fine particles (aerosols) or by contamination of food or water sources. Contagious agents can also be transferred by person-to-person spread from a deliberately infected individual. Once a deliberate release has occurred, the key factors in how the disease will spread are the ease and rapidity of its person-to-person transmission.

Bioterrorism surveillance

The sooner a deliberate biological release is identified, the more morbidity and mortality can be reduced by rapid containment and effective treatment. Disease activity monitoring in populations is a responsibility of public health services supported by central government agencies. Normally focused on routine infectious diseases of public health concern, such as tuberculosis or measles, or natural disease outbreaks, such as Ebola, the same systems are used to detect outbreaks which may be the result of bioterrorist activity. In the UK, the surveillance and response framework is coordinated by the Civil Contingencies Secretariat, Department of Health (DH), and Public Health England (PHE). General approaches to surveillance are listed in Box 9.6 and the features of an effective surveillance system are listed in Box 9.7.

Effective, robust communication networks and information technology systems are vital so that public health information can be shared rapidly and effectively. With the vulnerability of technology systems to a coordinated terrorist attack and limitations in infrastructure, resources may be insufficient to cope with the inevitable higher demands and activity during the response to a bioterrorist incident.

Detection

The UK detection system consists of local infectious disease epidemiology services staffed by *consultants in communicable disease control* (CCDC) working closely with local health services. Regional laboratories maintained by PHE provide diagnostic services and can also offer expert advice on the clinical and organizational management of outbreaks. PHE also maintains reference laboratories with expertise on specific pathogens.

Deliberate release

Deliberate biological releases may be declared or covert. The responses to a declared release will obviously be more rapid and will be coordinated centrally. Extra resources will be supplied as required to areas affected. Detection of a covert release will only be possible once the first cases of infection begin to arise and the pattern is recognized. The appearance of diseases that rarely occur in nature may alert the surveillance organizations to the possibility of a covert deliberate release. For example, current guidelines state that deliberate release should be considered as a cause in the event of even a single case of inhalational anthrax.

Contact tracing

Once the causative agent has been identified, every individual who has been, or may have been, exposed needs to be traced, decontaminated if necessary, and offered appropriate treatment. This response is coordinated via an outbreak control team consisting of a CCDC and other appropriate subject matter experts.

Box 9.6 General approaches to biological surveillance

- Clinical (case-based) surveillance
- Environmental surveillance
- Laboratory (sample)-based analysis.

Box 9.7 Features of an effective bioterrorism surveillance system

- Effective population monitoring
- Laboratory identification of potential agents with sufficient positive predictive value
- Effective and timely dissemination of public health information
- Adaptability to new or unexpected threats
- Financial and technological feasibility.

Biological agent biodromes

Particular groups of symptoms, or *biodromes*, can be associated with certain organisms. Therefore, the appearance of significant numbers of new cases presenting with a common biodrome or one or more cases of an unexpected or rare biodrome could indicate the release of a biological agent. Table 9.1 lists examples of such biodromes and their associated pathogens.

Table 9.1 Biological agent biodromes. Reproduced with permission from Greaves and Hunt, *Responding to Terrorism: A Medical Handbook*. Elsevier 2011

Principal symptoms	Potential pathogen
Fever + respiratory compromise	Pulmonary anthrax
	Plague
	Ricin
	Tuberculosis
	SARS
	Tularaemia
	Glanders
	Q fever
	Staphylococcus enterotoxin B
	Pneumonia, e.g. *Chlamydia, Legionella, Mycoplasma*
Fever + generalized rash	Smallpox
	Viral haemorrhagic fevers (VHF)
	Measles
	Scarlet fever
	Dengue fever
	Chickenpox
	Typhoid
Fever + skin blistering/localized skin signs	Cutaneous anthrax
	Tularaemia
	Glanders
	T-2 mycotoxin
Neurological features	Botulism
	Equine encephalitis
	CNS infections
Fever + shock/DIC	Viral haemorrhagic fever (VHF)
	Meningococcal septicaemia
	Malaria/dengue
	Anthrax
	Plague
	Tularaemia
	Smallpox
	Ricin

Initial management of a suspected biological agent release incident

In general terms, the initial management of a biological outbreak involves:
• clinical care of affected patients
• identification of the causative agent, source, and transmission route
• identification of at-risk groups and individuals
• decontamination and control measures as appropriate
• use of vaccines and/or antibiotics for public health protection
• provision of information to the public and the media.

Local clinical care of affected patients will be the responsibility of NHS acute hospitals and community clinical services. Coordination of more serious outbreaks will also involve regional directors of public health, regional PHE epidemiologists, and the DH.

General incident management principles

The vital difference between a biological incident and any other type of incident is the delay between time of exposure to the causative agent and the onset of symptoms and hence recognition. Unless the release of the agent is immediately obvious, or an announcement is made by those responsible, index cases may travel a significant distance from the point of exposure before being identified, thereby creating considerable difficulty with containment of the incident and later contact tracing. This could allow the rapid spread of infection throughout the population, especially where the organism is highly virulent. The conventional boundaries and cordons of a more conventional incident will not apply in these cases.

On the rare occasions that a release is overt, conventional command and control of the incident may be possible. In order to achieve this, rapid containment is essential to prevent spread of infection and to ensure the provision of initial treatment as well as facilitating post-exposure prophylaxis if available for the organism concerned.

The assessment and treatment of biological incident casualties will depend on the suspected agent, information which may well be unavailable immediately following the incident. Provisional identification of the agent will often rely upon recognition of characteristic clinical signs until specialist laboratory testing can confirm the organism's identity by serology or culture.

Universal (standard) precautions

Since the management of affected patients may involve the handling of body fluids, changing of dressings, and disposal of contaminated objects, it is absolutely essential that appropriate precautions are taken to prevent inadvertent transmission by exposure to potentially infectious body fluids, and to avoid injury by potentially contaminated sharp instruments.

Because it will not normally be possible to tell whether a casualty is carrying a disease, particularly in the early stages of an incident, a minimum level of precautions *must* be followed at all times. These are referred to as *universal* or *standard* precautions, as shown in Box 9.8.

Box 9.8 Universal, or standard, precautions

- Practise good basic hygiene with regular hand washing between patients
- Cover wounds or skin lesions with waterproof dressings
- Wear disposable gloves and gowns/aprons when attending to dressings or performing procedures that may involve handling or discharge of body fluids
- Avoid use of sharp instruments if possible—but where necessary, handle and dispose of these safely and appropriately
- Protect eyes, mouth, and nose from possible blood or other body fluid splashes with safety glasses or masks with visors
- Be familiar with local procedures following sharps injury or blood splash incident
- Clear up body fluids promptly and disinfect surfaces appropriately
- Dispose of all contaminated waste safely according to local guidelines, including how to dispose of soiled linen
- Clean, disinfect, and sterilize equipment as appropriate.

Personal protective equipment

There are three categories of PPE for use in biological incidents:
- Barrier PPE: gloves and gowns
- Droplet PPE: gloves, gowns, and eye protection (i.e. face shields)
- Aerosol PPE: gloves, gowns, and face masks/respirators.

The main route of infection spread between individuals is normally by direct contact. In addition to universal or standard precautions, additional contact precautions should be maintained to minimize transmission. Where facilities are available one means of achieving this is isolation. Gloves and a gown must be worn at all times. Face shields and eye protection should also be worn when conducting an examination or procedure that may involve aerosols or droplet formation, such as airway suctioning or the use of nebulizers. PPE should be removed between patients, and disposed of appropriately in marked clinical waste bins.

Airborne infection control and basic respiratory precautions

Small particles containing infectious pathogens may be formed by droplets expelled from the respiratory tract of an infected individual, or by intentional release in aerosol form. Close contact (generally accepted to be less than 1–2m) may not be required for transmission, although it may make person-to-person spread more likely. Prevention of airborne transmission requires a higher level of respiratory protection than can be offered by surgical masks (see Boxes 9.9 and 9.10).

Droplet spread involves larger, heavier particles (greater than 5 micrometres) requiring closer contact for transmission and may be protected against by wearing a surgical mask which reduces exposure and absorption via the mucosa of the upper respiratory tract and eyes.

Box 9.9 Basic respiratory precautions

In addition to standard precautions:
- Wear a surgical mask
- Protect against droplet spread
- Manage each patient in a single room or cubicle
- Discuss inpatient bed placement with the infection control team
- Ensure that *all* visitors must wear surgical masks
- Limit patient movement to that necessary for medical reasons only
- If the patient is moved from their room/cubicle ensure they wear a surgical mask
- The decision to discontinue basic respiratory precautions should be taken in consultation with the infection control team.

Box 9.10 Airborne infection precautions

In addition to basic respiratory precautions:
- Senior clinical staff and microbiologist should be consulted urgently
- Surgical masks should be immediately placed on each patient
- Patients should be placed in single rooms or side rooms, the door kept closed, and access strictly limited to essential medical personnel only
- Ideally, each patient should be admitted to a negative-pressure isolation room or isolation ward
- FFP3 masks must be worn as part of PPE.

Decontamination at scene

On rare occasions, a release may be identified while its effects are confined to a specific location. In such circumstances, immediate wet decontamination should be carried out, following local protocol. Further information regarding at-scene decontamination is shown on pp. 235–6. Mass decontamination may be required for large-scale incidents, and the decision to carry this out must take into account:
- the extent of the release
- the environment at the release site
- the risk of transmission
- the persistency of the suspected agent.

Forward medical teams with full PPE and specialized equipment may be required to deal with casualties within the hot zone, especially where conventional trauma has occurred or casualties are entrapped. This degree of protective equipment will inevitably reduce the level of medical interventions that can be performed. However, at-scene decontamination may not be carried out if the recognition of an event is delayed. Once careful contact tracing leads to the identification of the potential source or location of the initial release, quarantine and decontamination of the area may be appropriate. A number of biological agents are highly persistent, especially if the environmental conditions are favourable, and therefore an effective cordon will be required to deny access and prevent further spread. It should be remembered that patients attending hospital from such a scene will require decontamination before admission.

Isolation and quarantine

Current regulations define the isolation precautions required for health workers against the most contagious and virulent organisms, such as those responsible for VHF (including Ebola). In the case of infection with the higher airborne risk group of VHF (including Lassa, Marburg, and Ebola viruses), additional airborne precautions are recommended. Isolation and PPE recommendations for these agents are given in Figure 9.1.

Surge planning

Hospital major incident plans for biological incidents must ensure that there is adequate surge capacity in the event of multiple cases of infection by the most highly contagious or potential harmful organisms. These plans should include the identification of a specific zone or ward as an isolation area. In the largest incidents, a regional, or even national, response may be necessary to provide adequate numbers of high-dependency beds.

Public health information

Early dissemination of accurate information is the key factor in reducing public panic. As well as monitoring infectious diseases, PHE is required to provide support and advice on how infectious disease threats can be managed. Fact sheets are available for several likely public health biological threats including anthrax, plague, botulism, and smallpox. Regular meetings and conferences also take place to enable discussion of the latest developments in infectious disease threats, diagnostic tests, and new treatment.

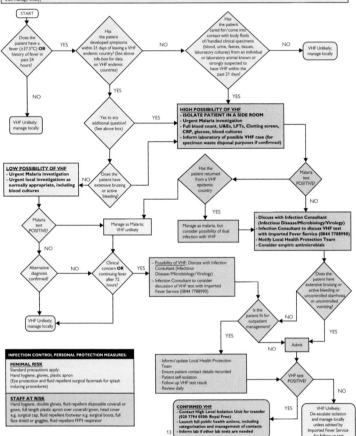

Fig. 9.1 Management algorithm for suspected viral haemorrhagic fever (VHF) presentation.

Reproduced under Crown Copyright from Advisory Committee on Dangerous Pathogens, Management of Hazard Group 4 viral haemorrhagic fevers and similar human infectious diseases of high consequence (November 2015) (www.gov.uk/government/uploads/system/uploads/attachment_data/file/534002/Management_of_VHF_A.pdf).

Biological agent transmissibility and public health impact

In order for a disease to be passed from individual to individual (transmitted), three main requirements have to be met—there have to be:
• an infectious individual (the source)
• a susceptible individual
• a means of contact between them.

Methods of transmission of an organism or biotoxin include droplet spread, direct physical contact, or airborne spread. Thus the exposure required for transmission will depend on the mode of transmission of the organism or toxin. In terms of public health risk, agents which are reliably transmitted by airborne spread are the most dangerous, and most difficult to protect against.

Virulence refers to an organism's ability to cause disease and relies on the initial number of infecting organisms or unit of biotoxin, the method or route of exposure, the defence mechanisms of the host, and the characteristics of the individual organism or biotoxin

A summarized comparison between biological agents in terms of their overall risk to public health is shown in Table 9.2.

Table 9.2 Comparison of biological agent by risk to public health. Reproduced with permission from Greaves and Hunt, *Responding to Terrorism: A Medical Handbook.* Elsevier 2011

Biological agent	Risk of P-P* transmission	Morbidity scale	Mortality scale
Anthrax	Low	Moderate	High
Brucellosis	Low	Low	Low
Food-borne pathogens	Moderate	Low	Low
Glanders	Low	Moderate	High
Melioidosis	Low	Low	Low
Plague	Moderate	Moderate	High
Psittacosis	Low	Low	Low
Q fever	Low	Low	Low
Tularaemia	Low	Moderate	Moderate
Water-borne pathogens	Moderate	Low	Low
Arenaviridae	Moderate	Moderate	Moderate
Bunyaviridae	Moderate	Moderate	Moderate
Encephalitides	Moderate	Moderate	Low
Filoviridae	High	High	High
Flaviviruses	Moderate	Moderate	Moderate
SARS	High	Moderate	Moderate
Smallpox	High	Low	Moderate
Aflatoxin	Low	Low	Low
Botulinum toxin	Moderate	Moderate	High
Epsilon toxin	Low	Low	Low
Staphylococcus enterotoxin B	Low	High	Low
T-2 Mycotoxin	Low	Moderate	Moderate

* Person-to-person.

Mathematical models of infection spread

The behaviour of infectious diseases can be modelled as a way of predicting disease outbreaks and refining responses. These models rely on certain assumptions, namely that the population can be subdivided into a set of distinct classes: Susceptible, Infectious, or Recovered. This is referred to as the SIR model. In order to understand the model, certain basic assumptions have to be accepted:
- All individuals are in the 'susceptible' class at birth
- Susceptible individuals are able to catch the disease (and become 'infectious')
- Infectious individuals spread the disease to 'susceptible' individuals
- Infectious individuals remain in the 'infectious' class for a given period of time (depending on the organism responsible)
- Infectious individuals may then recover, entering the 'recovered' class
- Individuals in the 'recovered' class may then be assumed to be immune for life (or at least against that particular strain of organism such as from an influenza epidemic).

Estimation of the effective contact rate in a given population is a key requirement for mathematical modelling of disease spread. This is the product of the total contact rate per unit time (effective or not) and the risk of transmission. However, there are limitations to this calculation as contact rates can vary widely between individuals and groups.

Transmission risks can only be determined from retrospective studies of previous outbreaks. These studies can also be useful in investigating the efficacy of a vaccination by comparison between vaccinated and unvaccinated groups for a specified organism.

Several software models are available to facilitate this process, as well as much more complex epidemic simulations, such as 'Epigrass'. However, the modelling of irregular events, such as deliberate release, is very difficult and often unreliable because of the assumptions involved and the extrapolation from historical data.

Reproductive ratio

The basic reproductive ratio, R_0, is defined as the average number of secondary cases occurring in a susceptible population. When R_0 is greater than 1, the disease is capable of infecting susceptible individuals and the number of cases will therefore increase. Conversely, when R_0 is less than 1, the disease will always fail to spread. Estimation of the R_0 can help to quantify the risk of a given disease to the population. Comparative examples of R_0 values are shown in Table 9.3.

Mass population models

Computer models are available to help predict disease spread in order to facilitate national, or even international, efforts to manage infectious outbreaks. The same models can also be used to generate scenarios for 'tabletop' exercises.

The Large-Scale Agent Model (LSAM) was developed by the National Centre for the Study of Preparedness and Catastrophic Event Response at the Johns Hopkins University, Baltimore, Maryland, USA. The LSAM can be used to plan for natural epidemics, and deliberate biological and chemical agent releases. This system involves complex computer simulation of communities representing real populations. One of the main focuses is on surge capacity, enabling scenarios to challenge available medical facilities in the event of a significant incident.

Table 9.3 Examples of R_0 values

Disease	R_0
AIDS	2–5
Smallpox	3–5
Measles	16–18
Malaria	> 100

Pre- and post-exposure prophylaxis

Pre-exposure prophylaxis

Pre-exposure prophylaxis is the treatment provided in advance of potential exposure to a specific, or suspected, organism. It may take the form of a vaccination schedule or medical therapy, such as an antibiotic. The aim is to target individuals who are identified as being at increased risk of exposure. This may include routine immunization of a national population at risk of endemic diseases such as yellow fever, widespread immunization in response to a perceived new threat (e.g. avian 'flu), or immunization of a more specific population (e.g. military personnel or health services staff).

Post-exposure prophylaxis

Post-exposure prophylaxis is the practice of providing treatment immediately after a suspected or confirmed biological agent release, in order to attempt to limit the duration, severity, incidence, and transmission of disease in asymptomatic individuals. The groups most likely to require post-exposure prophylaxis include:
• individuals exposed at the incident scene (including emergency responders)
• contacts of highly transmissible disease cases
• hospital medical staff and laboratory workers.

Guidance regarding suitable post-exposure antibiotic prescribing is available from PHE. National stockpiles are available for mass treatment and guidance for obtaining these, as well as PGD's for biological countermeasures, is outlined on pp. 238–9 and p240 respectively.

Use of vaccines

Vaccines may be used for both pre- and post-exposure prophylaxis. The smallpox vaccine can be used to limit disease severity post exposure. The anthrax vaccine is at the moment only provided to those at risk of exposure (veterinary staff, laboratory workers, and military personnel) and to reduce the risk of disease after exposure to anthrax in some cases.

The hospital response to a biological incident

Key elements of the hospital response to a confirmed, or suspected, biological release incident are listed in Box 9.11 and should be incorporated into hospital major incident plans.

Recognition

It is rare for a biological incident to be recognized by emergency services working at the scene, or for warnings to have been given of a deliberate release. Were such to be the case, the hospital incident plan could be activated allowing for preparation of facilities for decontamination and treatment before casualties start to arrive. However, due to the inevitable delay in developing symptoms, casualties will usually attend hospital services sometime after the initial release took place. This is referred to as a 'slow rise' event. In these circumstances, hospital emergency departments and inpatient medical teams may be the first to recognize the features of a biological incident. Equally likely is that recognition will result from wider surveillance processes.

Provision of PPE and decontamination facilities

Appropriate PPE/PRPS must be worn by all personnel dealing with casualties. Decontamination measures may be required if casualties have been overtly and recently exposed to particulate infective material such as anthrax spores. In general, there is no requirement for decontamination of casualties presenting sometime after an event for screening or of those with established clinical disease although, in both cases, precautions must be taken to avoid infection of healthcare workers. Decontamination should be carried out in specifically designated areas.

If the individual reports possible exposure at the site of a suspected, or confirmed, release, a risk assessment should be made as to whether there is any remaining contamination of body or clothing. Appropriate action may also be required to deal with contaminated clothing or other materials left at the individual's home or workplace.

> **Box 9.11 Key components of the hospital response**
> - A high level of awareness for potential outbreaks
> - Effective surveillance and recognition systems (clinical and laboratory)
> - Early request for PPE and decontamination facilities
> - Early requests for expert advice
> - Diagnosis and clinical management of affected patients
> - Effective communication and information cascade
> - Maintenance of the chain of evidence (if deliberate release is suspected)
> - Effective coordination and overall incident management.
> - Horizon-scanning and consideration of potential new threats.

Primary care

Primary and community care services may be involved in the response to an actual or potential biological incident in one or more of the following ways:
• Management of the ill in the community and referral to secondary care as required
• Management of exposed but unaffected individuals
• Provision of advice and information to local community
• Provision of prophylaxis under guidance from PHE
• Reassurance and advice for the 'worried well'.

Primary care health professionals should seek expert advice from PHE as early as possible if the potential features of an unusual outbreak are recognized. To ensure public safety and the safety of staff, invasive procedures and detailed patient assessment should be avoided. These can be more safely and appropriately performed after the patient arrives in hospital. PHE may advise on which hospitals are to be used in the case of specific biological incidents but advice should be sought from the hospitals before patients are transferred in case any special arrangements are required. In addition, it is vital that the ambulance service is warned, via their control, of any potential health and contamination risks. It is absolutely essential that comprehensive records of management decisions are kept in addition to contemporaneous clinical records. Details of actions taken, advice given, and those to whom information has been passed should be recorded. (See Table 9.4 and Box 9.12.)

Table 9.4 Distinguishing between an acute and delayed presentation

	Acute	Delayed
Detection by	Emergency services, emergency departments, general public	Primary healthcare professionals, general public, HPA surveillance
Timescale	Detection over minutes to hours	Detection over hours to days
Geography	Occurs in circumscribed area	May or may not occur in clusters
Commonality	May have a shared exposure	May or may not occur from a shared exposure
Aetiology	Also consider chemical agents, biotoxins and radiological threat	Consider radiological material causes

Box 9.12 Public health requirements during the response to a biological incident
• Care for the unwell and exposed well
• Identification of the source of the exposure
• Determination of the extent of the incident
• Prevention of further exposure
• Monitoring the effectiveness of measures taken
• Provision of information to the public
• Consideration of whether incident is result of deliberate action
• Management of mass sociogenic illness if necessary (see p. 408).

Cardinal signs and tips for key biological agents

The advice in Figure 9.2 and Figure 9.3 is designed to assist hospital clinicians in the initial management of suspected biological agent releases.

Unusual Illness, including Deliberate or Accidental Releases: Cardinal Signs and Tips for Key Biological Agents

If you see any of the following:
- New or unusual clusters of infections with a number of ill people presenting at around the same time
- Cluster of patients with a similar syndrome with unusual characteristics or unusually high morbidity and mortality
- Unexplained increase in the incidence of a common syndrome above seasonally expected levels or occurring in an unusual setting or key sector of the community
- Single case of disease with unusual or unusually severe symptoms and no history suggesting an explanation for illness

STOP/ THINK/ ACT!

! CONTACT:
- **Medical Microbiologist and/ or Infectious Disease (ID) Consultant through the hospital switchboard IMMEDIATELY**
- Director of Infection Prevention and Control (DIPC) through the hospital switchboard/ Infection Control Team
- Consultant in Communicable Disease Control (CCDC) at the local Health Protection Unit (HPU)
- 24hr Duty Doctor at HPA Colindale Tel. 020 8200 4400 or 6868

Key Documents

accessible at: hpa.org.uk/deliberate_accide ntal_releases/biological

CBRN Incidents

Emergency Clinical Situations Algorithm

Suspect Packages and Materials Algorithm

Key Biological Agents	Infection Control – Protection and Personal Protective Equipment (PPE) for health care workers caring for patients
Not or rarely transmissible person-to-person: **Anthrax (Inhalational), Botulism, Tularemia, Glanders, Melioidosis, Q-fever, Brucellosis**	**Standard precautions:** Always use standard infection control procedures according to local policy. PPE comprises: single-use apron or if risk of extensive contamination full-length impermeable gown, gloves, wear surgical mask and eye protection for taking blood and splash hazards.
Transmissible from person-to-person via respiratory droplets: **Pneumonic Plague**	**Respiratory precautions:** PPE comprises: PPE comprises: full-length gown or single-use apron, gloves, surgical mask, eye protection for taking blood and splash hazards.
Transmissible from person-to-person via airborne route and from contaminated fomites: **Smallpox, VHF**	**Airborne protection:** PPE comprises: single-use impermeable gown, apron, gloves, boots, head cover, correctly fitting respirator mask (ENV149 FFP3), face shield, visor, or goggles. Strict patient and environmental hygiene (washing, spillage management etc).
Decontamination of surfaces and/or spills: As per local protocol. Autoclave or incinerate clinical waste.	

For information on **accessing stocks or pods** (containers with sufficient equipment, antidotes and antibiotics to meet the needs of 100 people) for immediate response in a major incident: http://www.dh.gov.uk/en/Policyandguidance/Emergencyplanning/DH_4069610
Other modes of prophylaxis may also be available.
For links to **agent specific guidelines** and the **Investigation and Management of Unusual Illness** document: http://www.hpa.org.uk/Topics/InfectiousDiseases/InfectionsAZ/DeliberateReleases/

DH Department of Health

Fig. 9.2 Advice for dealing with an actual or potential biological incident.

RESPONDING TO SUSPECT PACKAGES AND MATERIALS – ACTIONS TO BE TAKEN

Further details in: Guidelines for health professionals dealing with suspected packages and materials

http://www.hpa.org.uk/infections/topics az/deliberate release/menu.htm

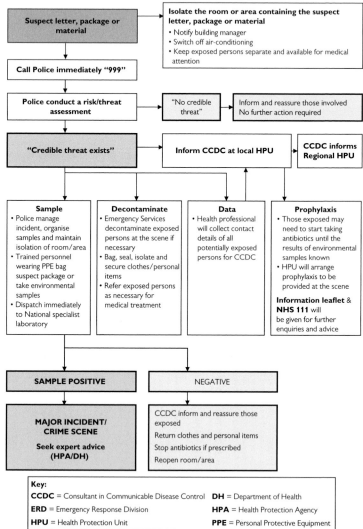

HPA Centre for Infections. Version 2.2 21 November 2006

Fig. 9.3 Responding to suspect packages and materials—actions to be taken.

Reproduced under Open Government License from Health Protection Agency, November 2006 (http://webarchive.nationalarchives.gov.uk/20140714084352/ http://www.hpa.org.uk/webc/HPAwebFile/HPAweb_C/1194947391200).

The role of hospital clinicians

Patient welfare is the first priority, but appropriate infection control measures must be instituted immediately in order to minimize exposure to staff. Clinicians must seek advice at the earliest opportunity from the usual hospital sources such as infectious disease specialists and microbiologists. Infection control teams must be informed as well as PHE locally. Further clinical responsibilities are summarized as follows:
• Assessment of risk of disease transmission to staff and other patients
• Protection of staff who may be exposed to the patient
• Assessment of the need for decontamination
• Initial triage and life-saving treatment
• Diagnose and formulation of a management plan
• Clinical investigations
• Effective communications.

A record must be kept of all staff (and anyone else), who has been in contact with infected patients (including personal contact details). It is also of vital importance to keep comprehensive records, not only of clinical decisions but also of management activity. Each entry must be dated, timed, and signed. A list of important information to document in case(s) of unusual illness is shown in Box 9.13.

Box 9.13 Information checklist for case(s) of unusual illness
• Name of clinician recording information with contact details
• Hospital
• Number of cases
• Is deliberate release suspected?
• Is there any information about others who might be exposed/ at risk (including staff)?

For each case:
• Name
• Address
• Sex
• Age
• Occupation
• GP details
• Date and time of presentation
• Mode of presentation (walk-in, ambulance, GP referral, etc.)
• Name of senior clinician in charge
• Ward
• Date/time of onset of symptoms
• Nature of symptoms/severity of illness
• Has there been an expert clinical assessment? By whom?
• Clinical findings (who performed assessment?)
• Any risk factors/exposures identified?
• Relevant past medical history/drug history?
• Vaccination status
• Samples taken
• Investigations undertaken and results available
• Working diagnosis
• Management: decontamination, treatment
• Outcome
• Post-mortem—if done where?
• Record all staff in contact with the patient with their personal contact details.

Information cascade

Individual hospital major incident protocols should be followed, ensuring that information is appropriately, rapidly, and effectively shared between clinical and managerial staff. At all times, senior clinical staff must maintain a high degree of awareness of the arrival of unexplained or unexpected numbers of individuals presenting with similar symptoms or signs, information which should immediately be passed into the management chain. Senior staff should also ensure that local emergency services and PHE have been informed. A nominated individual should be tasked with seeking expert advice regarding the suspected organism involved, correct identification, and microbiological testing as well as clinical management requirements.

The senior clinician on duty for the emergency department is responsible for ensuring that all necessary PPE and decontamination resources are made available. Other hospital departments which will need to be informed so that they can prepare to receive patients include the general wards, intensive care, or high dependency units. Infection control teams will need to be informed to ensure adequate numbers of isolation bed spaces are made available. Off-duty personnel may need to be called in and the responsibility for this will need to be given to a prior nominated individual (see Figure 9.4).

Maintaining the chain of evidence

In cases of possible intentional biological release, it is vital that patients' personnel effects, as well as medical samples, are kept appropriately packaged and documented to ensure that the chain of evidence is maintained. This is especially relevant where samples may pass between several different departments or laboratories. Every movement of a sample should be documented. Appropriate attention must at all times be paid to biosecurity and infection risk.

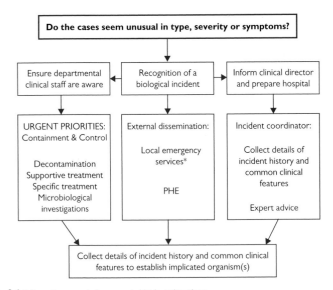

Fig. 9.4 Information cascade for suspected biological incidents.

* If a deliberate release is suspected, ensure the police have been informed if not already aware.

Microbiological testing

Where the cause of an unusual or unexpected illness is unknown or uncertain, guidance recommends that screening samples are taken including toxicological and microbiological investigations, as well as routine haematology and biochemistry. Instructions for microbiological blind testing are shown in Table 9.5. Samples must be taken as early as possible, and wherever possible before specific drug therapy has been administered as long as life-saving treatment is not delayed. Standard precautions should be used in all cases with additional PPE (e.g. double gloves, eye and face protection, and FFP3 mask) if relevant or where highly infectious causes are suspected. Specimens should be handled, labelled, and transported as high risk.

Table 9.5 Samples to be taken in a biological incident (actual or suspected)

Sample	For	Requirements
Blood cultures	Extended aerobic and anaerobic culture	Two sets of blood cultures immediately (from one bleed) with another two if possible within the first hour (also from one bleed). Document if antibiotics have been given prior to sampling
Sera	Serology and biological toxin assays	2 × 10mL clotted blood, for both acute (admission) and convalescent phases

Acute sample may be used for toxin assays, freeze and save any excess |
| Whole blood (EDTA) | Molecular investigations, e.g. PCR | 2 × 10mL or 4 × 5mL whole blood acute phase |
| Urine | Microscopy, culture, and storage | Clean catch into sterile container—optimal volume >20mL |

The unidentified biological agent and 'white powder' incidents

The unidentified biological agent

Several technologies with the potential to offer rapid, portable, and automated analysis and diagnosis of known biological agents are currently being developed. These may one day allow the performance of 'on-the-spot' identification of suspicious materials at the site of release. This would offer significant advantages not only in identifying 'harmless' materials in the event of negative testing, but also to enable rapid control of spread with effective infection control measures and early post-exposure prophylaxis. Otherwise, common sense precautions must be followed. The substance must not be touched or moved, air conditioning switched off, the area isolated and closed, and staff who have been exposed to it identified. Expert advice can then be sought regarding the nature of the substance. (See also 'Dealing with a suspect package ('white powder incident')', pp. 200–1 and flowchart on p. 280.)

Radiological and Nuclear Incidents

Introduction

Incidents involving radioactivity are fortunately rare. However, when they do occur, the consequences are likely to be very significant, both in terms of their health effects and environmental contamination. There is also a widespread fear of the consequences of radiation exposure, resulting from genuine concern combined with lack of knowledge and the highly charged moral, philosophical, and political context within which such issues and their potential for harm are commonly debated.

This chapter discusses, briefly, the physics and clinical presentation of radiation effects, aiming to dispel some of the myths most likely to handicap the response to such an incident. It then discusses in greater detail the operating and regulatory framework within which a response to a nuclear incident would be mounted. It should be remembered that, almost uniquely, radiation incidents may be associated with significant effects, including death, for many years after the incident.

Definitions

A *nuclear* incident is one in which fission occurs. As a result, many different radioisotopes are released. Such an incident will involve either a nuclear explosive device (nuclear bomb) or a nuclear reactor (see Table 10.1). The levels of radiation released will be very high and isotopes such as strontium, caesium, and iodine will be emitted as well as neutrons (see p. 294).

A *radiation* incident occurs when one or more individuals are exposed to the potentially harmful effects of ionizing radiation. There will commonly only be exposure to one radioactive isotope. Such events, which require only the presence of a radioactive substance, are more likely to occur than nuclear incidents.

Table 10.1 Historical radiation incidents

Nuclear installation incidents

2011	Fukushima, Japan	Meltdown triggered by a tsunami. Massive land and sea contamination. In excess of 300,000 evacuated. INES level 7[a]
2004	Fukui Prefecture, Japan	Steam explosion, four killed, seven injured
1986	Chernobyl, USSR	Explosion, fire, and meltdown; 31 immediate deaths, 300,000 evacuated, and potentially tens of thousands of excess cancer deaths. INES level 7
1979	Three Mile Island, Pennsylvania, USA	Partial core meltdown with release of radiation. INES level 5
1957	Sellafield (formerly Windscale) UK[b]	Fire destroyed the core and released an estimated 750 terabecquerels of radioactive material. INES level 5
1957	Kyshtym, USSR	Steam explosion. About 70 metric tons of highly radioactive material were carried into the surrounding area and 22 villages were affected with deadly doses. INES level 6

Incidents involving civilian exposure to radiation[c]

2013	Mexico City, Mexico	Theft of a cobalt-60 medical radiation source in transit presumed to have led to a fatal dose for the thieves
2010	New Delhi, India	Cobalt-60 incorrectly disposed of among scrap metal, one death, six hospitalized
2006	Glasgow, UK	Massive therapeutic overdose of radiation leading to death of a child[d]
2006	London, UK	Murder of Alexander Litvinenko with polonium-210.
2001	Georgia, former USSR	Three woodcutters keep warm using three warm cylinders which turn out to be strontium 90 generators
2001	Thailand	Seven injuries and three deaths from exposure to a stolen source
1987	Goiânia, Brazil	Caesium source left in an abandoned hospital stolen by thieves and left in scrap yard, 249 contaminated, four deaths. INES level 5

[a] As of 2016, there have only been two INES level 7 incidents.

[b] To date, Sellafield/Windscale has suffered five INES level 4 and one level 5 incidents.

[c] Most such incidents are not true major incidents, although the steps necessary, for example, to trace victims and locate missing sources may be on a considerable scale.

[d] Given as an example, therapeutic errors and malfunctions, rather than major incidents are by far the most common events associated with radiation.

Types of incident

The majority of incidents of radiation exposure involve small numbers of individuals and are due to human error, equipment, or procedural failures at units using radiation for therapeutic purposes or at nuclear installations, usually power plants. However, incidents involving radiation may have a more malign intent. While it is true that effective security makes a significant attack on a nuclear installation unlikely, and the technical complexity of handling and producing a device makes the construction and use of an *atomic bomb* an improbable event, neither can be ruled out as the action of a so-called *rogue state*. In addition, significant harm can be caused either by maliciously ensuring exposure to a radioactive source placed by a terrorist and unknown to those at risk, or by the production of a so-called *dirty bomb* or *radiological dispersion device* (RDD).

Radiation units

Radioactivity is measured in *becquerels* where 1Bq = 1 disintegration per second. Absorbed energy (per unit mass of tissue) is measured in *grays* where 1Gy = 1 joule per kg of tissue. The equivalent dose of radiation, which uses a weighting factor to reflect the sensitivity of a tissue to radiation effects, is measured in *sieverts* (Sv). The unit *curie* (1 curie = 37GBq) is obsolete. Conventionally (and confusingly) the sievert is not used for high levels of radiation producing deterministic effects (see p. 296), which are measured in grays.

Classification of radiation and nuclear incidents

These incidents are classified according to the *International Nuclear and Radiological Event Scale Level* (INES) (see Figure 10.1).

Level 7: major accident

Major release of radioactive material with widespread health and environmental effects requiring implementation of planned and extended countermeasures There have only been two such events to date: Chernobyl (1986) and Fukushima (2011).

Level 6: serious accident

Significant release of radioactive material likely to require implementation of planned countermeasures. There has been only one such event to date: Kyshtym in 1957—a failed cooling system at a military nuclear waste site.

Level 5: accident with wider consequences

An incident resulting in release of radioactive material likely to require implementation of some planned countermeasures, several deaths from radiation, and severe damage to the reactor core. Release of large quantities of radioactive material occurs within the installation with a high probability of significant public exposure.

Level 4: accident with local consequences

Minor release of radioactive material unlikely to result in implementation of planned countermeasures, other than local food controls, but at least one death from radiation. Damage to the installation will result in release of significant quantities of radioactive material within an installation with a high probability of significant public exposure.

Level 3: serious incident

These incidents result in exposure to greater than ten times the statutory annual limit for workers, producing non-lethal deterministic health effects (see p. 296) Exposure rates of more than 1Sv/h will occur in the operating area with severe contamination in a limited area but with a low probability of significant public exposure.

Level 2: incident

Such an incident is defined by the exposure of a member of the public to radiation in excess of 10mSv including exposure of a worker in excess of the statutory annual limits. There will be radiation levels in an operating area of more than 50mSv/h. and significant contamination within the facility into an area not expected by design. Significant failures in safety provisions will have occurred, but without actual health consequences.

Level 1: anomaly

These consist of overexposure of a member of the public in excess of statutory annual limits or minor problems with safety components with significant defence-in-depth remaining.

Level 0: deviation

No safety significance.

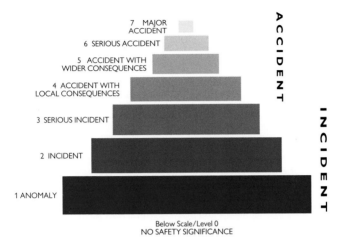

Fig. 10.1 Levels of a radiation incident.

Reproduced with permission from The International Atomic Energy Agency (www-ns.iaea.org/tech-areas/emergency/ines.asp).

Basic radiation physics

Ionizing radiation is a form of emitted energy. Most substances are stable and do not emit radiation. However, some are capable of emitting radiation and are described as *radioactive*. Energy from radiation, like any other form of energy, is capable of causing harm to living tissue.

Radiation is a natural phenomenon. It occurs all around us, from cosmic rays, from the earth, and in food and water. Box 10.1 gives some values for *background radiation* levels. As well as medical sources, manmade uses of radiation include mining, food sterilization, radiography of pipes luggage and buildings, as well as nuclear power and weaponry.

This section contains only enough physics to ensure a basic understanding of the radiation and nuclear threat and the essential components of an effective response.

Particulate radiation

Alpha (α) particles are identical to helium nuclei, consisting of two neutrons and two protons. Because of this, they are heavy and this, together with their charge, means that they can only travel short distances and cannot penetrate human skin. Alpha particles, therefore, are only dangerous if they are inhaled, ingested, or absorbed, for example, through a wound. However, when they do interact with living tissue, their mass and charge means that they will cause significant damage.

Beta (β) particles are electrons. They are lighter and react less strongly with tissue than alpha particles. As a result they are capable of travelling further and are more penetrating. They are capable of passing through skin, but some protection will be offered by clothing or standard PPE. Prolonged exposure may cause radiation burns but beta particles are usually only harmful when inhaled, ingested, or absorbed through a wound. In this respect, they behave similarly to alpha particles. Protection is offered by aluminium or Perspex®.

Because *neutrons* are uncharged, they have a long range and are capable of penetrating everything except thick concrete and hydrogen-rich material such as water. Fortunately, they are usually only emitted as a result of a nuclear detonation or accident.

Electromagnetic radiation

Both *gamma* and *X-rays* are forms of electromagnetic wave. As the wavelength of these waves decreases, their energy increases. Gamma and X-rays both lie at the low-wavelength, high-energy end of the spectrum of electromagnetic radiation. Both are highly penetrating and they can only be stopped by significant thicknesses of lead, concrete, or water. X-rays are usually man-made but gamma rays are produced as radioactive materials decay. (See Figure 10.2 and Table 10.2.)

Box 10.1 Background radiation levels

Polar flight from UK to Japan	50–7µSv
Annual background dose (UK)	2mSv
Annual occupational limit (general public)	1mSv
Annual occupational limit (radiation worker)	20mSv
Threshold for ARS[a]	0.5–1Sv
$LD_{50}/60$ without supportive therapy[b]	3.5–Sv
$LD_{50}/60$ with supportive therapy	5–6Sv

[a] Acute radiation syndrome. Radiation units are described on p. 291.

[b] $LD_{50}/60$ is the dose of radiation that will kill 50% of an exposed population within 60 days.

Reproduced with permission from Greaves and Hunt, *Responding to Terrorism: A Medical Handbook*. Elsevier 2011.

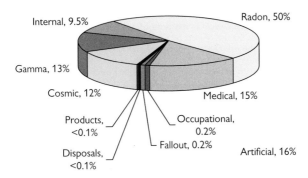

Natural, 84%

Internal, 9.5%

Radon, 50%

Gamma, 13%

Cosmic, 12%

Medical, 15%

Products,
<0.1%

Occupational,
0.2%

Fallout, 0.2%

Disposals,
<0.1%

Artificial, 16%

Fig. 10.2 Contributions to the average UK annual radiation dose.

Reproduced under Open Government License from S.J. Watson et al, HPA/-RPD-001, *Ionising Radiation Exposure of the UK Population: 2005 Review*; Health Protection Agency, Centre for Radiation, Chemical and Environmental Hazards, Chilton.

Table 10.2 Summary of radiation types

Type	Penetration	Nature	Protection
α particles	Do not penetrate skin	2 protons +2 neutrons	Skin
β particles	Penetrate the dermis	Electrons	Clothing/PPE (partial) 1mm lead
Neutrons	Everything except thick concrete and water	Neutrons	
γ rays	Highly penetrating	Electromagneticradiation	7.6cm lead

Stochastic and deterministic effects of radiation

When cells are irradiated, in the majority of cases there will be no effects on the health of the individual either because there was no damage to the cells or because the cells repaired themselves correctly. However, as the dose of radiation increases, the risk of damage increases and so does the risk of incorrect cellular repair. These cells, may, in the long term, be associated with the risk of development of cancer. These dose-dependent effects are referred to as *stochastic effects* and may occur with any dose of radiation; no dose of radiation is too small to cause at least a marginal increase in cancer risk.

In some cases, the dose of radiation may be sufficient to cause cells to die. There is, therefore, a threshold dose below which these *deterministic effects* will not occur as long as this threshold is not reached. Deterministic effects include hair loss and sterility.

Types of device associated with radiation and nuclear incidents

Radiological dispersion devices

Radiological dispersion devices (RDDs), sometimes called *dirty bombs* will usually involve a radiological source such as cobalt, caesium, or iridium acquired from a bona fide industrial or medical setting. Alternative possible sources for the radioactive component of a RDD include fuel rods from a nuclear reactor and radioactive waste. Combined with conventional explosive, the result is a RDD. Inevitably, the detonation of such a device—with its connotations of a nuclear bomb—is likely to result in alarm; however, large numbers of radiation casualties are unlikely. The spectrum of injuries will range from irradiation alone to irradiation and contamination with radioactive fragments energized by the conventional detonation. Early deaths from acute radiation sickness (ARS) are likely to be limited due to the limited radiation exposure. RDDs or dirty bombs *do not* involve a nuclear detonation.

Covert release of radiation

Similar sources of radiation without explosives may also be associated with cases of acute radiation exposure if their presence is not recognized. Deliberate releases without explosives (covert releases) may be used as a terrorist weapon although their lack of immediate impact makes this option less attractive to the terrorist. They could potentially be placed to contaminate food or water supplies or target areas of high-density occupation. Such events are more likely to be accidental or the result of petty crime without awareness of the consequences. In 2006, Alexander Litvinenko was murdered using polonium-210, the only known such case in the UK to date. (See Table 10.3 for threats.)

Improvised nuclear devices

Although improvised nuclear devices can be created, it is difficult to obtain sufficient fissile material and technically complex as well as hazardous to prepare such a device and to ensure nuclear detonation. The device may 'fizzle' or the conventional explosive may detonate, effectively producing an RDD but failing to initiate a nuclear detonation. Mortality is likely to be higher than with a 'dirty bomb'. Such an event is unlikely, although it cannot be ruled out in the context of a failed state or takeover of an installation by those with a terrorist agenda.

Nuclear installation incidents

The majority of major incidents due to radiation are likely to arise as a result of an incident at a nuclear installation. Such an incident is most likely to be due to a procedural or equipment failure, but the Fukushima incident arose from extreme weather conditions and terrorist activity is possible. Nuclear power plants use fuel rods containing uranium to generate electricity by heating gas or water which is used to drive turbines. Some nuclear plants such as

Table 10.3 Summary of radiation and nuclear threats

Threat	Likely number of casualties	Involving acute trauma?	Contamination?	Radiation	
				Dose >0.5Sv	Type(s)
Nuclear detonation	10^4–10^5	Yes	Yes	Yes	α, β, γ, n
Attack on a nuclear reactor	0–10^2	Yes	Yes	Yes	α, β, γ (n)
RDD plus explosive	0–10^3	Yes	Yes	Yes	α, β, γ
Covert exposure	0–10^2	No	Yes	Yes	α, β, γ

Adapted with permission from Bland SA. Mass casualty management for radiological and nuclear incidents. *J R Army Med Corps* 2004; 150: 27–34.

Sellafield in Cumbria, also process spent nuclear fuel rods. Nuclear reactors are also found in submarines and surface vessels where they are particularly useful for powering vessels without the necessity for frequent refuelling.

Any event involving a nuclear installation has the capability to result in both contaminated and irradiated casualties as well as conventional trauma cases. Because the nuclear material at a power plant is not sufficiently confined, incidents involving nuclear power stations *do not result in nuclear detonation*. However, the potential for both local and distant contamination means that the consequences may be devastating.

Nuclear weapons

Nuclear weapons are considered briefly because there is a small, but nonetheless real chance of such an event occurring as a result of the actions of a terrorist group or failed state. Fortunately, the likelihood of any terrorist organization being able to obtain or develop and use a devastating nuclear weapon without detection is very small. However, were such an event to occur, the consequences are likely to be so devastating as to require a response on an unprecedented scale and beyond the conventional mechanisms described in this book.

Fission weapons

Nuclear fission weapons use material such as uranium or plutonium. Atoms are bombarded by neutrons and split creating a chain reaction of nuclear splitting, releasing more energy as well as gamma and neutron radiation and fission products. Casualties will be injured by any combination of blast, heat, and radiation. In addition, any nuclear detonation is associated with the release of energy as an electromagnetic pulse (EMP) which is capable of rendering unshielded electronic devices such as communications and medical equipment inoperable.

Fusion weapons

Fusion weapons (also referred to as hydrogen bombs) derive their energy from the process by which nuclei fuse at very high temperatures to form a larger nucleus. The commonest use fusion of hydrogen isotopes (deuterium and tritium) to form helium (hence the alternative name). The destructive potential of these devices is much greater than that of fission weapons.

Combined weapons/neutron bombs

Weapons which use both fission and fusion have been tested. Neutron bombs use fission to initiate a fusion reaction, resulting in limited blast and heat but massive amounts of radiation.

> Initial levels of radiation will have fallen by about 90% by 7 days after a nuclear detonation.

Useful advice for the public following a radioactivity incident

Basic common-sense advice should be offered to the general public in the period immediately following an incident. Initial public advice is outlined in Box 10.2.

Box 10.2 Initial advice to the public during a radiation incident

- Reduce the duration of exposure to radiation.
- Get as far away as possible from the source and stay there.
- Get behind as thick a barrier as possible.
- Go inside and stay inside.
- Cover the mouth and nose with (preferably wet) fabric.
- Remove *all* clothes and seal in double plastic bags and shower as soon as possible with lots of soap and water.
- Turn the radio or television on and follow the advice as given.
- Turn off ventilation systems including fans and air conditioning.
- Avoid food which might have been contaminated.

Acute effects of a nuclear explosion (detonation)

One can only hope that a nuclear detonation on UK soil never happens, although sadly the possibility cannot be completely excluded. It is perhaps more likely that UK responders and subject matter experts will be called to respond to an incident in a more geopolitically unstable area than that such an event will occur at home. A key component of ensuring that people are kept informed after a *radiation* incident is explaining the difference between a radiation incident and a nuclear detonation. As a brief guide, therefore, as well as releasing radioactivity, a nuclear detonation will also result in the following:

- *Flash*: intense light may cause blindness (temporary or permanent) and 'afterimages.
- An *electromagnetic pulse* (EMP): effecting electrical equipment.
- *Heat*: producing a range of effects from vapourization of bodies close to the detonation to burns at greater distances. Light-coloured clothing offers some protection. The environment may catch fire.
- *Blast wave*: a nuclear blast wave is the same as a conventional blast wave but whereas the blast wave of a conventional explosion takes a few milliseconds to pass a point, a nuclear blast wave may take hundreds of milliseconds and is consequently more likely to cause injury.
- *Seismic shock*: ground movement may occur if the detonation is sufficiently large.
- *Blast wind*: the mass movement of air and products of combustion referred to as the blast wind will occur in nuclear just as it does in conventional explosions.

In general, smaller yield devices will produce a greater proportion of irradiated casualties compared to blast casualties.

Managing a radiation (or nuclear) incident

Management of contaminated casualties

Definitions
Exposure can be said to have occurred when a part or all of a body is irradiated. Patients who have been irradiated, like those who have had an X-ray or a computed tomography scan, present *no risk* to rescuers or healthcare personnel. The seriousness of an exposure is affected by the duration of the exposure (the shorter the exposure, the lower the dose), distance from the source of the radiation (according to the inverse square law: *doubling* the distance reduces the exposure by *a factor of four*), and whether the victim is shielded from the radiation.

Contamination occurs when radioactive material is deposited on the skin (*external contamination*), contaminates a wound, or is ingested or inhaled (*internal contamination*).

Fortunately, radiation is relatively easy to detect and every receiving hospital medical physics or radiotherapy department has the necessary equipment and skills. Appropriate equipment and training has now been provided to all Emergency Departments in the UK (see Box 10.3).

Decontamination

It is important not to forget that removal of obvious contamination and *all* clothing (including underwear) will remove up to 90% of external contamination. The patient should be provided with a face mask during decontamination in order to reduce the risk of them inhaling radioactive material. Life-saving interventions can be performed at the same time. The skin should be more formally decontaminated using the *rinse–wipe–rinse* technique with large quantities of warm water with or without detergent. It is important to avoid breaking the skin, especially by scrubbing. Nasal and ear swabs should be taken to assess internal contamination. Decontamination is covered in more detail in Chapter 5, pp. 156–9 and p. 320.

Box 10.3 Personal protection for clinical staff dealing with irradiated or contaminated patients

- Waterproof apron
- Surgical gown or chemical suit
- Theatre cap
- Face mask (FFP3 or equivalent)
- Waterproof shoe covers
- Double gloves.

Triage of radiation (and nuclear) casualties

Pre-hospital triage

An adapted version of the conventional triage sieve may be used as the basis for triage in a radiological or nuclear incident involving mass casualties. The aim is to ensure that patients who have received a significant dose of radiation have their triage priority raised. Patients categorized as *T2* or *T3* using the conventional triage sieve should be upgraded to *T1* or *T2* respectively if they have:

- received a dose >2Sv (threshold may be increased if resources are limited)
- vomited within 4 hours
- diarrhoea
- pyrexia >38°C
- altered conscious level
- erythema (reddened skin indicative of radiation burns)
- obvious wound contamination.

Prodromal symptoms are those which occur in the early stages after radiation exposure and herald the onset of ARS (pp. 304–7). They can be used to give a guide to the severity of exposure (Table 10.4) and hence have some value as a planning tool.

Use of the expectant category

The expectant category is unlikely ever to be used in the UK and its use would imply a nuclear catastrophe. There have, however, been a small number of incidents overseas where it could have been employed as a means of concentrating limited resources on those most likely to benefit. Authorization would be needed at the highest level. However, the following are signs which suggest that the degree of radiation exposure is likely to be unsurvivable:

- Radiation dose >8Sv (may be altered depending on available resources)
- Vomiting with 1 hour after exposure *and* diarrhoea *or*
- Altered consciousness/coma *or*
- Hypotension (in the absence of another cause such as trauma)
- Lymphocyte count at 8–12 hours <1000/mm³ (may be increased to 1700/mm³).

Initial management of casualties

For the purposes of initial management, casualties may be sorted into the following groups:

- Irradiated only
- Externally contaminated only
- Internal contamination possible
- Contaminated wounds
- Combined: contaminated and injured ± irradiated.

Table 10.4 Symptoms as a guide to radiation exposure

Probability of ARS	Unlikely	Probable	High
Nausea	–	++	+++
Vomiting	–	+	+++
Diarrhoea	–	+/–	+/– to +++
Headache	–	+/–	+/– to +++
Hyperthermia	–	+/–	+ to +++
Hypothermia	–	–	+ to +++
Erythema	–	–	– to ++
Central nervous system dysfunction	–	–	– to ++

–, Absent; +, present; ++, severe; +++, very severe.

This logical approach aims to impose structure on what is potentially a confused and anxious process for victims and rescuers alike.

Irradiated only

Once contamination has been excluded, these casualties present no risk to clinical staff and can be treated in a completely normal manner. Further management will depend on the magnitude of their radiation exposure.

External contamination only

These casualties must be decontaminated as soon as possible, priority being given to those who also have conventional injuries. Once decontaminated, they can be managed normally.

Internal contamination possible

External decontamination is essential but further assessment including whole-body monitoring may be needed following a risk assessment. Swabs, urine, and faeces samples should be taken. Further management is discussed on p. 306.

Contaminated wounds

All wounds must be decontaminated and appropriately dressed. In some cases, surgical debridement may be needed in order to ensure that all radioactive material has been removed.

Combined: contaminated ± irradiated and injured

These are patients with conventional trauma and radiation exposure and they must be the first priority for treatment which should not be delayed for decontamination. Removal of clothing as part of the resuscitation process will reduce exposure. Initial management is limited to life-saving interventions (see Box 10.4).

Box 10.4 Key principles for managing the acutely irradiated patient

- Assume contamination until it is excluded by monitoring.
- If contamination is present, decontaminate *but* assume the patient is *also* internally contaminated.
- Remove *all* the patient's clothing, double bag, label, and store it.
- Follow protection guidelines on p. 310.
- Do not allow pregnant staff to work with contaminated patients.
- Whenever possible, stay as far away from the patient as possible.
- Give symptomatic treatment.
- If the radiation dose is >1Sv, surgery (if required) should take place before 48 hours or after marrow recovery.

Radiation and the body

The effects of radiation on the human body are predictable and range, according to the degree of exposure, from the minor to the rapidly fatal. Unlike other forms of tissue damage, however, the long-term effects of radiation mean that all those exposed to it will require long-term follow-up and monitoring for delayed effects. The clinical effects are described here in brief to a level helpful in the context of major incident planning and response; readers are referred to standard texts for greater detail.

Acute radiation effects

High doses of radiation (>2Sv) cause tissue damage and may cause the death of the victim. Doses of this magnitude will result in *acute radiation sickness* (ARS), which usually follows external exposure of all or most of the body to large doses of penetrating radiation (gamma rays, X-rays, or neutrons). ARS has four phases:
- Prodromal phase
- Latent period
- Manifest illness.
- Recovery or death.

Prodromal phase
This is characterized by non-specific symptoms such as nausea and vomiting (see Table 10.5) which are not generally life-threatening. If they have not occurred within 6 hours of exposure, significant ARS is unlikely although as in all cases of radiation exposure, long-term effects cannot be excluded and monitoring will be required.

Latent period
This is a period of apparent symptom-less good health of varying length before the onset of established ARS (*manifest illness*). With increasing radiation dose, both the *prodromal phase* and the *latent period* (the period before ARS is established) shorten and the severity of the resultant ARS increases.

Manifest illness
Radiation syndrome is a spectrum from asymptomatic exposure to neurovascular syndrome with a very poor prognosis. Early symptoms of severe acute radiation syndrome include nausea and vomiting, diarrhoea, loss of appetite, headache, and tiredness. Patients with ARS and trauma have a worse prognosis than those with one or the other.

Recovery or death
Fifty per cent of patients who have received 3.5Sv or more of radiation will be dead within 60 days without treatment ($LD_{50}/60$). This LD_{50} dose increases to >6Sv with expert medical intervention.

Classification of acute radiation syndrome

The clinical features are described according to the system of the body that is affected according to dosage. The approximate dose ranges shown in Box 10.5 illustrate probable symptoms and ARS severity.

Table 10.5 Radiation dose and ARS

Dose (Sv)	Expected effects	Syndromic dysfunction	Probability of ARS
<1	Below threshold		Unlikely
1–2	Mild		Probable
2–4	Moderate	Haematological dysfunction likely	
4–6	Severe (LD$_{50}$)[a]	Gastrointestinal dysfunction likely	
6–8	Very severe		Inevitable –severe
>8	Lethal		
>20	Lethal	Neurological dysfunction likely	

[a] Without medical treatment.

Box 10.5 Acute radiation syndromes

Dose <1Sv: usually asymptomatic
- Nausea and vomiting in the first 48 hours (<10% of patients)
- Mild delayed effects on results of blood count.

Dose 1–8Sv: haematopoietic syndrome (blood cells)
- Anorexia, nausea, vomiting, and tiredness 1–4 hours after exposure
- Latent period: 2 days to 4 weeks
- Bone marrow depression
- Effects on blood cells in the first 48 hours predict severity
- Hair loss at 2–3 weeks (3–4Sv).

Dose >6–20Sv: gastrointestinal syndrome
(In addition to the above.)
- Early nausea, vomiting, diarrhoea, and tiredness
- Latent period: hours to 1 week (shortens with higher doses)
- Severe abdominal pain, diarrhoea, and gut haemorrhage
- Fever
- Bone marrow depression.

Dose >20Sv: central nervous system/cardiovascular system syndrome
(In addition to the above.)
- Almost immediate projectile vomiting, explosive bloody diarrhoea, headache, collapse, confusion, loss of consciousness, agitation, sensation of burning skin
- A lucid interval of several hours may not always be present
- Neurological and cardiovascular symptoms predominate (convulsions, coma, hypotension, and shock)
- Death follows within 2–3 days.

Management of acute radiation syndrome

Immediately life-threatening injuries should be treated before decontamination has been carried out using conventional resuscitation processes and ensuring appropriate protection for staff. Although irradiated casualties pose no threat to clinicians, contamination should be assumed until it is ruled out by testing using the contamination monitors available to every A&E department. *If* contamination is confirmed, decontamination should be carried out but *internal* as well as *external* contamination should be assumed. In hospital, a range of blood tests, urine and faeces tests, and swabs will be taken to help assess the level of exposure, need for immediate treatment, and likely prognosis.

Management of internal contamination

Decorporation
Decorporation is the removal of internal contamination. This is often achieved by exploiting the chemical properties of the isotope, by using an agent which binds to it to produce a compound which can safely be excreted. A list of common agents is given in Table 10.6. Other methods include bronchial lavage and whole-bowel irrigation to wash out contamination.

Radioiodine treatment
Radioiodine is produced from uranium and plutonium during the process of fission. Once absorbed, it concentrates in the thyroid where it increases the risk of thyroid cancer, especially in children. Iodine tablets can be used to saturate the thyroid with safe iodine, preventing the toxic build-up of the radioactive isotope. Those exposed should receive potassium iodate as soon as possible after exposure (recommended doses: adult 170mg, child under 3 years 42.5mg, child 3–12 years 85mg). Planners must ensure that this is available in sufficient quantities. UK Reserve National Stock is discussed on pp. 238–9.

Medical management

Management of ARS has two components, supportive treatment and definitive treatment. Both are considered only briefly.

Supportive treatment
Supportive treatment is treatment of the patient's symptoms. This will include antiemetic therapy for nausea and vomiting, pain relief (analgesia), and treatment of brain swelling (cerebral oedema). Antibiotics should be given for infection which is more likely if the patient is immunocompromised as a result of the radiation, in which case blood component replacement may be needed. For the sickest patients, intensive care management will be required, including cardiorespiratory support. Health service plans for a radiation incident must identify intensive care capacity and effective means of matching capacity with demand.

Definitive treatment
This is specific and often highly technical and complex treatment for the syndromes associated with acute severe radiation exposure. Haematopoietic syndrome, if severe, will require treatment in a specialist haematological or transplant centre and will include prevention of infection by scrupulous hygiene, barrier nursing, air filtration, selective gut decontamination, treatment of infection, replacement of blood components, and potentially bone marrow transplantation. The requirement for such highly specialist beds *must form part of the planning process*: capacity, location, and patient allocation systems being essential. Surgery may be required for blast or penetrating injury to the abdomen or elsewhere and full supportive therapy may be necessary for those patients who develop overwhelming infection (sepsis). Barrier nursing may be needed for those with immune compromise. The presence of the neurological syndrome indicates a very poor prognosis. There is usually no latent period before the onset of neurological syndrome and the prognosis is exceptionally poor.

Table 10.6 Common decorporating agents.

Radioisotope	Decorporating agent
Americium	DTPA[a], EDTA[b]
Caesium	Prussian blue
Cobalt	Penicillamine
Iodine	Stable iodine (see text)
Plutonium	CaDTPA
Strontium	Aluminium, calcium
Tritium	Hydration, dieresis
Uranium	Bicarbonate

[a] Diethylenetriamine penta-acetic acid (by nebulizer). [b] Ethylenediaminetetraacetic acid.

Chronic effects of radiation

Following any radiation exposure there is an increased risk of developing cancer. This is due to damage to DNA within cells rather than cell death which occurs at higher levels of exposure. Skin and gastrointestinal cancers are the most frequent. Ongoing monitoring of patients is essential, probably including colonoscopy and removal of premalignant tumours. Lung fibrosis may also occur following radiation exposure. The normal average lifetime cancer risk is 25% for those who have not been exposed to radiation (beyond 'normal' background levels). For every 1000mSv, there is a 5% increase in the chance of developing cancer.

Planning to respond to a nuclear or radiation incident

Planning for a potential incident can be divided into *on-site, off-site, transit,* and *national* components. Unsurprisingly, given the potential consequences of an incident, the legislative and guidance framework which mandates the planning necessary to avoid an incident or deal with one is exceptionally thorough.

Nuclear sites are granted a licence to operate under the *Nuclear Installations Act 1965* and an emergency plan is required by the *Office for Nuclear Regulation* (ONR) before a licence is granted. Military nuclear facilities are exempt from the Act, but overseen by the *Defence Safety Agency*—DSA (formerly by the *Defence Nuclear Safety Regulator,* DNSR). An onsite exercise must be held every year, concentrating primarily on the role and responsibilities of the operator.

The REPPIR regulations (*Radiation (Emergency Preparedness and Public Information) Regulations 2001*), again regulated by the ONR, require local authorities to prepare plans for the offsite response to an incident if there is an appropriate facility in their area of responsibility. The at-risk area identified in and covered by the offsite plan is known as the *detailed emergency planning zone* (DEPZ). The main aim is to ensure the adequacy of the local emergency response lead by the authority. Each year, one off-site response is chosen for a national exercise testing the involvement of a wide range of responders including central government. Each licensed site must undergo an off-site exercise at least every 3 years and every 6 years a full exercise must be undertaken.

Regulations also demand that plans designed for each area of significant risk (the DEPZ) are capable of being extended to deal with a larger-scale incident. This is referred to as *extendibility.* Standard scenarios are available against which plans may be compared to ensure extendibility and compatibility with other off-site plans. There are no statutory requirements for the frequency of extendibility testing exercises. The REPPIR regulations contain the statutory guidance for those involved in the response to a radiation incident, clearly indicating the responsibilities of individual agencies including licensed operators and the legal and regulatory framework within which a response must be planned and potentially carried out. REPPIR applies to premises and transport operations involving radioactive materials (with some specified exemptions).

Planning at civil nuclear sites

Every facility handling nuclear material must have an emergency response plan in place. Such plans must include the management of a zone around the installation in order to ensure the protection of the public from foreseeable effects. The size of this zone will depend on the nature of the facility. The plan must include means to ensure:

- rapid alerting of responders
- rapid control of the incident
- protection of responders, including from dangerous doses of radiation
- minimization of risks to the general public
- coordination between responding agencies at all levels
- provision of information to government, the media, and the community
- plans for escalation of the response if this is required.

Plans must be regularly reviewed and updated and should follow a similar framework to other major incident response plans in order to increase interoperability with the emergency services. Each site must identify a *site emergency control centre*. The risk of an incident at a nuclear incident must be included on all relevant risk registers. Given the public perception of nuclear incidents, engagement with media organizations and with the local community is essential.

National arrangements

Originally established in 1990 as the *Nuclear Emergency Planning Liaison Group* (NEPLG), since 2012, the responsibilities of the NEPLG have been the responsibility of the *Nuclear Emergency Planning Delivery Committee* (NEPDC). The NEPDC brings together, under the chairmanship of the Department for Energy and Climate Change (DECC) a wide range of bodies including (as standing members):

- DECC
- Office of Nuclear Regulation (ONR)
- Civil Contingencies Secretariat of the Cabinet Office
- MOD
- Defra
- DH emergency planning
- Home Office
- Government Office for Science
- Nuclear Decommissioning Authority
- Devolved governments
- Local Government Association.

Other agencies such as the Met Office, Civil Nuclear Constabulary, and site operators attend as necessary. The NEPDC is charged with the development of national guidelines regarding response to a radiation or nuclear incident including preparedness, response, and recovery. NEPDC also coordinate the guidelines for the UK response to an event overseas. The NEPDC reports to the *Nuclear Emergency Planning Board* (NEPB) and is also responsible for risk registers, advice to ministers on resourcing, and review of site response plans. It overseas a number of working groups dealing with issues such as transport incidents, recovery, scientific advice, communications, and international liaison.

Principles of radiation protection

Radiation protection principles aim to ensure that wherever possible, doses are kept below the threshold level for deterministic effects and as low as possible to minimize the risk of stochastic effects.

The basic principles of radiation protection are *justification*: any exposure must be justified by benefit to the individual concerned, to another individual (e.g. a casualty requiring rescue), or to society; *optimization*: the exposure must be As Low As Reasonably Practical (*ALARP*); and *limitation*: unless emergency exposures (see p. 311) have been authorized, exposures must be kept below the threshold for deterministic effects. Radiation doses are reduced by four means:

- *Time*: the length of exposure must be strictly limited
- *Distance*: increasing the distance from a source reduces the radiation exposure according to the inverse square law (i.e. doubling the distance decreases the exposure fourfold)
- *Shielding*: wherever possible, materials that absorb radiation should be used to protect individuals
- *PPE*: appropriate PPE must be worn.

The *ERIC-PD* principles should also be followed:

- *Elimination*: wherever possible, a source should be removed or alternatives used, for example, in training
- *Reduction*: where elimination of a hazard is not possible, exposure should be as low as possible
- *Isolation*: where possible, the source should be isolated from contact with people
- *Control*: procedures should be in place to manage and reduce exposure
- *PPE*: PPE should always be used
- *Discipline*: staff must be trained to deal with radiation incidents and must follow established procedures.

Civil Nuclear Constabulary

The *Civil Nuclear Constabulary* (CNC), established in 2004 under the Energy Act, provides protection for civil nuclear sites (or within 5 miles of them), nuclear materials, and operators throughout the UK. In some respects, its role is more that of a guard service than a police force. The functions and performance of the CNC are overseen by the *Civil Nuclear Police Authority* (CNPA). The CNC are responsible for policing at all *UK Atomic Energy Authority* (UKAEA), *British Nuclear Fuels* (BNFL), and *URENCO* (a uranium enrichment and nuclear fuel supply company) sites and of all nuclear materials in transit. Most CNC officers are armed. CNC headquarters are at Culham in Oxfordshire and personnel are distributed around seventeen locations across the UK. Nuclear weapons and military nuclear installations are guarded by the Armed Forces and Ministry of Defence Police.

Atomic Weapons Establishment (AWE)

The AWE is responsible for provision and maintenance of the UK's Trident nuclear warheads and is operated under licence by a number of companies including SERCO and Lockheed-Martin. AWE offers expert advice to UK government.

Emergency exposures

During a radiation emergency, it may be necessary and is permissible for individuals to exceed established dose limits in exceptional circumstances such as saving life or maintaining vital infrastructure. Such individuals must be *informed volunteers* who have had the risks explained to them. A dose of up to 100mSv for intervention in a nuclear plant aimed at rescue or prevention and reduction of future doses, and of 500mGy for the purpose of saving life may be permitted. In all such circumstances, the ALARP principles must be followed— radiation dose must be *As Low As Reasonably Practical*.

The decision to allow emergency exposures and hence to override *REPPIR* regulations must be taken by an appropriately trained senior officer or manager, usually in conjunction with the RPA. Those who undertake to receive emergency exposures should be identified in advance and must undergo training appropriate to their role. When an incident occurs, careful checks must be made to ensure that these individuals are fit for the role, are appropriately equipped, and are fully informed. Managers of sites where REPPIR applies are required to provide the necessary information to ensure a safe and effective response in the event of an incident. Strict regulations regarding medical surveillance apply to all personnel who have received a significant dose of radiation whether as an authorized emergency exposure or as a result of the incident itself. REPPIR also requires those who receive emergency exposures to agree without pressure, to be appropriately briefed, to have the opportunity to ask questions, and to change their mind at any time. Pregnant or breastfeeding women and those under 18 should not receive emergency exposures.

The police response to a nuclear or radiation incident

The police have overall responsibility for the coordination of activity at any radiation (or other CBRN) incident. Radiological expert advice is provided to the police by scientists from the AWE. The police will also appoint an internal *radiation protection advisor* (RPA) responsible for the provision of expert advice including the appropriateness of levels of PPE as well as a number of *radiation protection supervisors* (RPSs) who will manage the technical aspects of the response to an incident. The roles of the police at an incident are divided into:
• category 1: personnel who undertake routine activities in the cold zone
• category 2: personnel who deploy inside the inner cordon but do not receive emergency exposures (p. 311)
• category 3: personnel who consent to receive emergency exposures.

Types of irradiation incident attended by the police include:
• nuclear site incidents
• non-nuclear (radiation only) site incidents
• CBRN incidents including potential terrorist incidents
• transport incidents involving radiation sources
• management of 'found' or lost (genuine or suspected) sources.

In the event of an incident involving a nuclear submarine, the MOD will coordinate the response with expert technical advice from the AWE. The schematic organization of a radiation emergency is shown in Figure 10.3.

Cordons
Cordons must be clearly marked and access/egress strictly controlled and recorded. Appropriate signage must be available at the access point. Appropriate dosage monitoring should begin as soon as possible within both cordons. Decontamination of equipment which has been in the hot zone may not be technically easy or quickly achievable. As a consequence, only essential equipment which is not likely to be needed elsewhere should pass the inner cordon.

Response plans and RADSAFE
In general, the majority of nuclear or radiation incidents will occur at identifiable sites of risk covered by the REPPIR regulations and the emergency services will have been involved in preparing response plans. Both the *Nuclear Emergency Planning Delivery Committee* (NEPDC) of the *Department of Energy and Climate Change* and *National Police Nuclear Group* (NPNG) of ACPO may also have been involved in this process. At such sites, the police will work with the operators to manage an incident in accordance with pre-agreed local plans. Both operators of nuclear sites and employers at radiation sites have a responsibility to provide the necessary information to police forces to allow optimum management of an incident. In the event of a civilian transport radiation emergence, RADSAFE, a private company founded to provide mutual aid in the event of such an incident, will provide advice and assistance (http://www.radsafe.org.uk).
RADSAFE offers a response at three levels:
• Notification/communication service with provision of generic safety advice provided by the CNC
• Advice and support at the incident scene
• Consignment owner response and clean up.

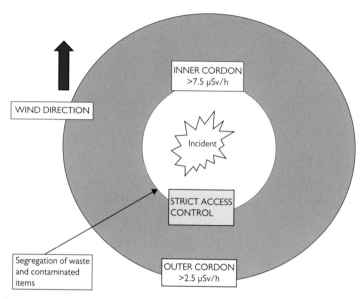

Fig. 10.3 Cordons at a radiation incident.

The roles of the police RPA and RPS

Roles of the police RPA

The police RPA must be appropriately trained and senior enough to take the necessary decisions. They are responsible for:
• provision of radiation advice for training, routine operations, and emergencies
• radiation training and protection advice.

They must also be consulted with regard to:
• management of and working within high-risk or hazardous areas
• assessment of radiation plans including site safety
• regular assessment of site emergency plans and safety mechanisms.

Role of the police RPS

The police RPS must be appropriately trained and will provide:
• advice on operations or at an incident
• advice regarding planning review and management of tasks involving radiation
• initial radiation advice and liaison with the RPA.

The essential roles of the police at a radiation or nuclear incident include:
• saving and protecting life
• overall coordination of the emergency response
• protection and preservation of the scene for evidential purposes
• investigation of the incident with regard to criminal liability
• communication with the public
• collation and dissemination of casualty information
• identification of victims (on behalf of HM Coroner)
• working with other agencies to restore normality.

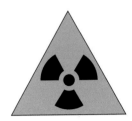

Fig. 10.4 The conventional radiation hazard warning sign.

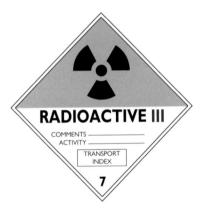

Fig. 10.5 The ADR transport warning sign for radiological material.

The site operator at a radiation incident

The licensed operator of a site which might be involved in an incident is responsible under REPPIR for the preparation of risk assessments (which must be sent to the HSE) and for its on-site emergency plan and the implementation of that plan should an incident occur. Such planning is carried out under the oversight of the HSE. Similarly, the carrier of radioactive material is responsible for the planning and implementation of their own effective emergency plan. Operators are required to work closely with the emergency services and other agencies in implementing the emergency plan on site and off and for transport incidents. All the agencies involved in the off-site response must be consulted by the operator in preparing the plan and their own employees must receive appropriate training which is regularly refreshed. The company will provide responders with a *company technical advisor* (CTA) supplemented by experts from the company's central administrative structure until the arrival of the government technical advisor (GTA) who will take over this role. In the case of an incident during transit, it is inevitable that plans will be more generic, but consultation must occur with representatives of all the different types of agency likely to be involved in the response.

The components of an operator's plan must include:
• pre-incident training
• guidance regarding when and how to call the emergency services
• command structures and responsibilities
• response procedures
• specialist technical procedures for foreseeable problems
• provision of resources
• sources of information and advice.

Fire and rescue services response to a radiation incident

Obviously, the primary duties of the fire and rescue service at any incident are controlling and extinguishing fires, prevention of escalation of a fire, and search and rescue. Fire services will manage the inner cordon in liaison with the police, controlling and recording those permitted to enter. Although decontamination of patients is a health service responsibility, under appropriate circumstances, fire services may undertake mass decontamination of large numbers of casualties.

Role of local authorities in a radiation incident

Local authorities have a legal duty to ensure that emergency plans for facilities in their area are in place and are regularly tested and revised. They have overall statutory responsibility for the off-site plan around a fixed installation which must be tested at least once every 3 years. *Extendibility* (see p. 308) must be built into the plan. In addition, because of the considerable impact of a radiation incident on the local community, the local authority will have a number of very important roles in responding. These are listed in Box 10.6. The local authority will take the lead role in post-incident recovery.

Box 10.6 Roles of the local authority in responding to a radiation incident

- Road signage, closure, and access/egress management
- Establishment of reception centres for the evacuated or minor casualties
- Coordination of voluntary sector responders
- Provision of information to the public
- Liaison with the media
- Provision of emergency mortuary facilities
- Establishment of a fund for charitable donations (if appropriate)
- Welfare support to victims and the evacuated
- Provision of emergency feeding (and enforcement of restrictions on foodstuffs where necessary)
- Emergency transport facilities
- Waste disposal facilities
- Provision of emergency accommodation
- Monitoring of domestic and private water supplies for contamination
- Provision of advice and enforcement of environmental health standards
- Provision of heavy plant for engineering purposes.

Role of Public Health England in a radiation incident

Public Health England has a key role in ensuring the provision of expert advice and personnel during the response to a radiation incident. PHE will provide staff for a radiation monitoring unit (see p. 319) as well as at the scene of an incident and will coordinate the collection and analysis of data from its Chilton (Oxfordshire) emergency centre. Areas for expert advice will include radiation protection, levels of exposure below which intervention is unnecessary, environmental monitoring, and criteria for specialist treatment.

National arrangements for incidents involving radioactivity (NAIR)

The NAIR scheme is led by PHE and provides assistance for incidents involving radioactivity. There are two stages of a NAIR response depending on the magnitude of the event.

Stage 1

A radiation expert with monitoring equipment is provided to advise whether a radiation incident has occurred and to provide advice regarding any necessary actions.

Stage 2

Provided by major nuclear establishments, a stage 2 response consists of a well-equipped team able to deal with a larger incident. In the event of a very significant incident, NAIR will supply larger teams of experts, drawing from the wider nuclear community.

NAIR and RADSAFE are both contactable using the same 24-hour telephone number (0800 834 153).

Radiation monitoring units

If there is a radiation emergency of sufficient magnitude, it may be necessary to establish a *radiation monitoring unit* (RMU). This decision will usually be taken by the NHS locally in conjunction with PHE and the local authority. The RMU will determine levels of human contamination among the population and provide advice regarding necessary medical management. The role of the RMU is the management of contamination, not irradiation. NHS planning guidance requires the identification of potential sites for RMUs as well as clear details regarding who will provide them. A wide range of bodies including local councils and the charitable sector will be involved in planning for the establishment of an RMU.

The RMU should ideally be co-located with a local authority reception centre, with good access and where it is not likely to be at further risk of exposure or the need for evacuation. Such a centre will also be able to provide food, shelter, and sanitary facilities. Safely decontaminated individuals will be able to move from the RMU to the reception centre. The ideal location will be rapidly or immediately available in the event of an incident.

Arrangements must be in place for the provision of basic and specialist monitoring equipment. The RMU manager will be a senior medical physicist with a deputy manager, radiation protection advisor (where available), radiation protection supervisors, personal monitoring team leaders, and monitoring staff. Consideration should also be given to deploying a suitably experienced medical practitioner to the RMU. Staff will be needed to marshal and direct members of the public, record information, and carry out decontamination (in teams). Security must be maintained by the police and personnel should be available to handle media and other information enquiries including those from concerned members of the public. The requirements for a RMU are shown in Box 10.7.

Initial monitoring will take place on entry to the RMU, usually using a portal monitor in the form of a frame through which patients walk, similar to X-ray machines at airport security. This will be followed by monitoring for external contamination, with decontamination where appropriate, and finally with monitoring of internal contamination. Hand-held monitors are usually used for external contamination, but assessment of internal contamination will require more specialized equipment and analysis of samples such as urine. During an incident, action levels for decontamination, referral for medical assessment, and more specialist treatment for acute radiation syndromes will be provided by PHE. Appropriate scoring systems are available online. These levels will be incident and nuclide specific.

All those monitored by the RMU should be given the results of their measurements. Standard forms are available. Information should also be provided for those who are potentially contaminated or found to be contaminated: pre-prepared information sheets are available. Although this information is confidential, data necessary for effective management must be made available to those coordinating the incident. This information will usually consist of the numbers involved and levels of contamination rather than individual patient data.

Box 10.7 The requirements for a RMU

- Space for those awaiting monitoring
- An area for external contamination monitoring
- Facilities for external decontamination
- Space for internal contamination measurement
- An area of approximately 300 square metres of indoor and 300 square metres of outdoor space.
- Suitable access and egress to maintain separation of contaminated groups.
- Facilities for recording and reporting information including communications facilities
- Private areas for counselling
- Toilet facilities (separate for pre and post monitoring where possible)
- Heat, light, and power
- Storage for contaminated and clean clothing
- Staff welfare and rest facilities
- Supplies of PPE for staff (on the advice of the nominated RPA).

The Government Decontamination Service

Available on a 24-hour helpline (0300 1000 316) or through Defra, the *Government Decontamination Service* (GDS) has responsibility for:

- overseeing decontamination and recovery of contaminated land, buildings, and infrastructure including the appointment of contractors
- provision of advice, guidance, and assistance on decontamination to responsible authorities during planning for, and response to, CBRN incidents
- ensuring that responsible authorities have access to necessary specialist supplies
- advising central government on:
  - the national capability for the decontamination of building infrastructure, transport, and the environment
  - national and regional preparedness
  - national risk assessment programmes
  - relevant areas of the national counter-terrorism strategy.

If requested to do so, members of GDS will attend strategic coordinating and recovery coordinating groups as well as the STAC for the provision of expert advice. GDS is based at MOD Stafford and provides an on-call team 24/7, 365 days a year, ready to provide advice and guidance following a CBRN incident. GDS covers England, Wales, Scotland, and Northern Ireland.

Central government response to a radiological or nuclear major incident

The central response to a significant nuclear incident will be coordinated by a strategy group meeting in the cabinet office briefing rooms (formerly the *National Security Council subcommittee on threats, hazards, resilience and contingency*, now *Strategy Group*). Administrative support is provided by the Cabinet Office Secretariat. For civil incidents, the LGD is the *Department for the Environment and Climate Change* (DECC). For a military incident the LGD will be the *MOD* and, for a terrorist incident, the LGD will be the *Home Office*.

Devolved regions

The Scottish government would lead the response to an incident in Scotland. The Welsh assembly has specific responsibilities in the event of an incident and the Northern Ireland assembly would coordinate local responses to an incident outside its borders (Northern Ireland has no nuclear power stations).

Nuclear Emergency Briefing Room (NEBR)

In the event of an incident, a NEBR will be established in London. The DECC as LGD will ensure the availability of adequate information to inform cross-department central government responses as well as monitoring the response and identifying potential lessons for the future and policy implications. It will contribute to informing the public (in association with the *Cabinet Office News Coordination Centre*) and support and inform ministers and the COBR committee.

DECC is also responsible for liaison with the nuclear and other industries and for informing overseas agencies and governments. DECC will appoint a *government liaison officer* (GLO) to support the *government technical advisor* (GTA) appointed by the *Office of Nuclear Radiation* (ONR) and provide secretarial support to the *SAGE*.

The ONR is responsible for monitoring the response to the incident and ensuring that operators are taking all necessary steps to return to normality.

Summary of COBR committee responsibilities in response to a radiation or nuclear incident

- Preparation and dissemination of advice to the media and public
- Coordination and monitoring of the overall response
- Coordination and prioritization of the actions of central government departments
- Consideration of the need for scientific research into the most appropriate actions
- Preparing summaries of 'actions so far' and the unfolding of the incident
- Monitoring of public health and environmental issues
- Predicting likely future effects and coordinating the response to concerns
- Ensuring the initiation of a recovery plan
- Considering financial and legal issues
  Ensuring international cooperation and spread of information.

The government technical advisor

The *government technical advisor* (GTA) is a senior member of the ONR and is an appointee of the Secretary of State at the DECC. The GTA provides advice regarding countermeasures to protect the public and responding agencies and the course of the emergency and the effects of the release. The GTA will also provide advice and information for media briefings and ensure through the GLO that the LGD remains fully informed. The GTA will liaise closely with responding agencies through the SCC, providing advice to the emergency services and other agencies and working closely with the STAC. A *health advisor* is appointed to work alongside the GTA.

Public Health England Centre for Radiation, Chemical and Environmental Hazards (PHE-CRCE)

The PHE-CRCE is responsible for coordinating the activities of all organizations involved in radiation monitoring following an incident involving radiation release.

An *impact management group* (IMG) may be established under the direction of COBRA to provide a single point of contact (POC) within central government for management and other issues, identify potential future effects of the incident, and coordinate the central cross-department response allowing effective integrated decision-making. Scientific advice will be provided by the *SAGE*.

Depending on the nature of the incident, the LGD will activate its own emergency response centre. In the event of a civilian incident, DECC will activate their response centre in the NEBR. Coordination between national and local levels is the responsibility of the Department for Communities and Local Government Response Coordinating Group (ResCG). Thus they will ensure effective coordination with the local response coordinated from the Strategic Coordinating Group at the Strategic Coordination Centre (Strategic / gold) which includes the *STAC*. As soon as is practically possible, a *Recovery Working Group* will be established as part of the strategic coordination centre, which will work with the IMG. The response structure for Wales is the same as that for England, and for Scotland is similar except that the Scottish government undertakes the role taken by DECC in England and Wales and the legal framework is different (see Figure 10.6).

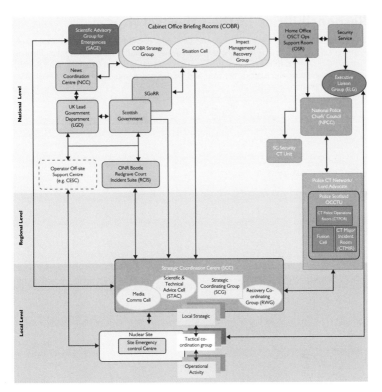

Fig. 10.6 The organizational structure for responding to a nuclear incident in England and Wales.

Responsibilities of the other services

The responsibilities of the other organizations were defined by the Nuclear Emergency Planning Liaison Group (NEPLG), now subsumed within the Nuclear Emergency Planning Delivery Committee (NEPDC) (see p. 309). They reflect legislation (REPPIR, HSWA, IRR), statutory regulation, and custom, practice, and experience. A summary of the roles of other services is shown in Table 10.7.

Table 10.7 Roles of the agencies and services at a radiation or nuclear incident

Service	Roles and responsibilities
Ambulance service	Coordination and management of on-scene response
	Triage, treatment, and transport of casualties
	Liaison with other off-scene health assets
	Ensuring availability of health services assets
Civil Aviation Authority	Restriction of access to airspace
	Expert advice to civil aviation industry
Department of Communities and Local Government – Resilience and Emergencies Division (DCLG-RED)	Formation of a link between central government and resilience communities
	Provision of government liaison officer to SCG
	Ensuring appropriate passage of information to government
	Coordination of the availability of national assets
	Facilitation of mutual aid requests
	Management of VIP visits
Department for Energy and Climate Change	*LGD for radiation incidents* (see text)
Department of Health	Support of local health agencies
	Liaison with central government
	Representation of the health 'voice' at all levels
Department for the Environment, Food and Rural Affairs (Defra)	Protection of animal welfare
	Minimization of radiation effects on the environment, farming, and food production
Environment Agency	Provision of advice on environmental contamination to responding organizations and to government departments
	Provision of advice to the public
	Management of water supplies to minimize impact
	Determination of whether the operating company/agency has breached legislation or authorization
	Advice regarding disposal of radioactive waste
	Monitoring of the environment for contamination
Food Standards Agency	Assessment of the risk of radiation to food supplies
	Elimination of contaminated food from the food chain
	Provision of advice on precautionary measures and to agencies such as the Environment Agency
	Monitoring of food for contamination
Government Office for Science	Ensuring the best possible scientific advice is available to planners, responders, and central government.
Local health providers (CCGs)	Coordination of the health services response to an incident (a lead CCG may be appointed if the incident affects more than one area)
	Provision of health advice at all levels of response including STAC
	Monitoring of people for contamination
Hospital trusts	Provision of trained staff
	Provision of space for assessment, decontamination, and treatment
	Provision of specialist equipment including monitoring
	Provision of specialist radiation advice to clinicians
Met Office	Provision of meteorological advice in the event of an atmospheric release of radiation
MOD	*LGD for an incident at a Defence establishment*
	Military Aid to the Civil Authorities
	Provision of technical assistance to civilian responders (if requested)

Dealing with the media following a radiation incident

Generic aspects of dealing with the media are covered in Chapter 15. This section covers aspects of media interaction specific to nuclear or radiation incidents. Guidelines for handling the media in the event of such an incident have been developed by the *NEPDC Communications Working Group*.

The REPPIR regulations require the operator of a nuclear installation to provide education to the public regarding risks and preparedness and the local authority to establish arrangements for the dissemination of information if an incident has occurred or is likely. REPPIR requires specific information to be made available to the public. In the event of an incident a *strategic media advisory cell* (SMAC) and *media briefing centre* (MBC) will be established to ensure the dissemination of accurate and consistent information.

A *forward media briefing point* may also be established nearer the incident, depending on safety considerations. The responding organizations will usually ensure that each has an appropriate media spokesperson. The SMAC will advise the SCG on effective communication with the media. In the event of a very significant incident, spokespersons will be made available by the LGD and a *news coordination centre* may be established centrally.

Mass fatality CBRN events

Fortunately there has not yet been such an incident in the UK, although in the current political climate a terrorist atrocity is at least theoretically possible. Were this to happen, bodies and remains would be placed in body bags rather than attempting decontamination at scene, and access to them strictly limited. The remains would then be disposed of through burial, cremation, or other arrangements taking into account the wishes of the bereaved families where possible.

Recovery

Major incident recovery is considered in detail in Chapter 14. Specific aspects of recovery from a CBRN incident are discussed here.

In general, the amount of decontamination and the need to restrict access to contaminated areas for safety reasons are both likely to be limited. Options for post-incident management include decontamination as well as temporary relocation while the risk disperses due to decay of radioactive material. There may, however, be a need to consign to waste significant amounts of contaminated foodstuffs. The recovery phase is usually coordinated by the local authority; were there to be an incident on a huge scale, central coordination at national level might be required. All bodies and agencies likely to be involved must ensure that plans are in place for a coordinated and effective recovery process which ensures that disruption to those involved is minimized. DECC remains the LGD for the recovery phase.

The period following an incident would normally see the establishment of a *recovery working group* (RWG) or *recovery advisory group* (RAG) as soon as it became clear that off-site contamination had occurred. The RWG/RAG operates during the incident under the authority of the SCG and in conjunction with the SCAT and GTA to ensure an effective transition between the response and recovery phases. Once the incident is over and the response phase changes to the recovery phase, responsibility will be assumed by the *Strategic Recovery Coordinating Group* (SRCG) activated by the local authority.

The SRCG will usually have a number of subgroups including:
- finance and legal
- communications
- business and economic recovery
- environment and infrastructure
- health and welfare
- monitoring
- community recovery committee.

Detailed recommendations are available for the composition and responsibilities of these groups which must be clearly established and practised in each region before an incident occurs (see https://www.gov.uk/government/uploads/system/uploads/attachment_data/file/252750/neplg_ch_18.pdf).

Membership of a Recovery Working/Advisory Group (RWG/RAG)
- Local authorities
- Police
- Health services including commissioning groups/providers
- Water authorities
- The relevant licensed nuclear operator(s).

Plus representation from the following national bodies:
- Public Health England
- Environment Agency
- Office of Nuclear Regulation
- Defra
- MOD
- Government Decontamination Service
- Government liaison team including GTA
- HSE—nuclear directorate
- CNC
- The emergency services, utility companies, and voluntary organizations will attend as required.

Both the RAG and SRCG will operate at least initially from the strategic incident control centre (Strategic / gold). The Environment Agency (or equivalent in the devolved regions) will provide advice regarding the means of disposal of radioactive waste and PHE will coordinate radiation exposure data.

Representation on the SRCG

- Local authorities
- Environment Agency
- Food Standards Agency
- NHS England
- Social care providers
- PHE
- Utility companies including water
- MCA (where appropriate)
- Emergency services
- MOD where appropriate
- Natural England
- Licensed nuclear site operators
- HSE
- Chairs of subgroups (see p. 328)
- Government Decontamination Service
- Animal health agencies (where appropriate)
- Voluntary organizations representative
- Transport companies
- Chair of Community Recovery Committee (if established).

Nuclear incidents overseas

It is unlikely that an incident overseas would result in contamination at a level sufficient to cause immediate risk to life or health, although widespread low-level contamination is possible (and has occurred in the past). The DECC is the LGD for such an incident and responsibilities fall exactly as they would for a UK-based incident.

The response to an overseas incident has three phases:
- Alert, notification, and classification
- Response
- Recovery.

During the first phase, a decision regarding the likely impact and necessary level of response will be made by DECC and ONR before plans are activated.

The UK response to an incident abroad is covered by a number of international agreements. The *Convention on Early Notification in the Event of a Nuclear Accident* requires any signatory country to inform the *International Atomic Energy Authority* (IAEA) in the event of an incident which might have consequences beyond its borders. Within the EEC, the EURATOM Treaty enforces the same requirement. The UK is part of the IAEA's Global Response and Assurance Network (RANET) under which it agrees to offer assistance in the event of an incident overseas in a signatory country. Warning of an event overseas may also come through RIMNET.

A nuclear event overseas may be classified, for UK response purposes as the following:
- Level 1. *Significant emergency*: probably requiring little more than DECC advice.
- Level 2. *Serious emergency*: risk of widespread or prolonged impact. COBRA-led response required together with SAGE and IMG. DECC in consultation with other central bodies will consider establishment of a recovery group.
- Level 3. *Catastrophic emergency*: severe and widespread impact requiring an immediate central government response and central coordination.

RIMNET

RIMNET was established following the Chernobyl incident in 1986, as a nuclear radiation monitoring and emergency response system and to monitor the consequences for the UK of a nuclear incident overseas.

Radiation dose rate readings are taken every hour at 96 sites in the UK and checked for any indication of abnormal increase over background levels. Any evidence of an incident of radiological significance for the UK would result in an alert.

Conventional Weapons: Explosives and Ballistics

Introduction

The term *conventional weapons* is usually used to refer to bombs and firearms. Although the injuries inflicted by these weapons and their mechanisms of wounding have some aspects in common, the resulting incidents may be very different. Explosions (which may not, of course, be the result of terrorist activity and are more likely to be due to human error or failure, either in the home or in an industrial setting) may well be associated with all the characteristic features of a major incident, particularly the presence of multiple casualties. Shooting incidents, however, may be over before a formal emergency response has been mounted, are likely in general to involve fewer casualties, and will not usually approach the status of a major incident, although the tasks facing the police particularly may be complicated and prolonged. There are, of course, exceptions to this, the 2010 incident in Cumbria in which Derrick Bird killed twelve people and wounded a further eleven at a series of random locations, being an example. We are fortunate in the UK that with the exception of the shootings at Dunblane in 1996, we have not suffered the school killing incidents so common in the USA. Where such firearms incidents do occur, in many cases a standoff develops (with or without hostages). In such cases the response will involve the police and ambulance services for real or potential casualties, but again, a full major incident response will not be required.

On the other hand, guns are readily available in modern society and commercial explosives can be relatively easily obtained or improvised explosives produced 'at home' using information from the Internet. In addition, the wounds that result from these weapons, and especially from explosive devices, all too horribly bring home the true terror that perpetrators wish to inflict and therefore it is essential that an appropriate response to such incidents is available when needed.

This chapter begins with a brief description of blast and ballistic injury with, as in other chapters, just enough science to underpin an informed professional response to an incident. For details of medical management of victims, readers are referred to 'Further Reading' (Appendix A).

Responding to terrorist incidents

Incidents related to terrorism often involve weapons such as handguns or rifles as well as explosives, either improvised or manufactured. The marauding firearms incident, involving one or more individuals indiscriminately shooting into a crowd or taking opportunistic shots while moving from place to place, is an example of a terrorist attack that may result in multiple severe casualties and deaths. Attacks are often planned to strike at a high-profile location for maximum media attention although the protection of such sites often leads to the selection of more accessible, less well-protected ('soft') targets. More likely sites of attack are therefore large public spaces such as theatres or cinemas, shopping centres, sports stadium, or leisure centres. The intention of the terrorist is just as the name suggests—to cause terror. The result is often panic and indecisiveness which may compound the incident and even lead more victims into danger.

Due to the non-permissive nature of the incident there are often significant delays to professional medical assistance reaching casualties. Practical exercises have previously demonstrated delays of anything from 1 to 2 hours before responders are able to safely reach the injured at the scene of an incident. This increases the risk of death from potentially treatable causes, especially external haemorrhage from gunshot or blast wounds and amputations. A number of initiatives have been developed in order to improve public awareness and provide information on how to act in the event of a terrorist attack involving firearms or other weapons. One such endeavour is CitizenAID which provides a clear and simple series of immediate actions providing guidance for anyone on how to react to an incident safely based on decades of military experience. It also details how to provide vital information to the emergency services, to help organize others at the scene and to give life-saving care while waiting for professional medical responders to arrive. It is free to the UK public via a downloadable App and also available to purchase as a quick-reference pamphlet. Important messages also include the use of tourniquets to control bleeding when other measures have failed, which can be a life-saving intervention when used appropriately.

Public advice from the National Police Chiefs' Council regarding how to react to a terrorist incident involving firearms follows the simple slogan of "RUN HIDE TELL". For further information and guidance see: "http://www.npcc.police.uk/staysafe"

Recent experience has also led to the realization that terrorists may utilise any method to cause death and injury in often spectacular fashion. The use of 'kinetic' weapons such as heavy goods vehicles, utility vehicles, and similar to simply drive into crowds of people or buildings to cause damage and shock. Responders and the emergency services must therefore be prepared for large scale incidents involving multiple blunt trauma cases with resulting patterns of injury, not just penetrating or blast-related mechanisms. Current mass casualty planning includes the requirement for scaled logistic stores of items such as external fixators for fractures and hospitals must be prepared to rapidly increase emergency and critical care capacity.

Injury from bullets

The study of the effects of bullets (or to be precise, missiles in general) on the body is termed *wound ballistics*. From the point of view of the treating clinician, a thorough understanding of wound ballistics is essential for the optimal management of patients. What is given here is a brief introduction. Bullets (and weapons) are often referred to as *high* or *low velocity*. As a simple rule, handguns fire low-velocity and rifles high-velocity rounds, although there are exceptions. In fact, it is better to refer to rounds (or bullets) as *high* or *low energy*. All missiles have kinetic energy and it is this, which, when transferred to the target, produces injuries or death. The kinetic energy of a missile is proportional to the mass of the missile and to the square of its weight, thus the energy can be increased by having a greater mass, but will be increased more effectively by having a faster speed. Manual weapons fire one bullet with each compression of the trigger, automatic weapons continue to fire until pressure on the trigger is released and as long as ammunition is available.

Energy and injury

If a bullet is stopped when it strikes a body, the energy available for damaging tissue is the total kinetic energy of the missile. If the missile passes through the body, slowing as it goes, only part of the energy available will be lost and the damage reduced: in this case the energy which causes damage will be the difference between the kinetic energy on entering the tissue and that on leaving it. The amount of damage done by any projectile will depend on the available kinetic energy (and hence its mass and to a greater extent, velocity), tissue factors, missile features, and finally the aerodynamics of the missile.

Bullets are often divided into *high-energy* and *low-energy* missiles: the most important factor for injury potential is the amount of energy transferred rather than simply the velocity. The key clinical distinction is that low-energy rounds produce tissue damage effectively confined to the track of the missile whereas the passage of a high-energy round is associated with the phenomenon of *cavitation*. When a high-energy round passes through tissue, it generates a shock wave which pushes tissues away from the missile track creating a temporary cavity many times the diameter of the missile. As this cavity expands, dirt and potential pathogens, even clothing, are drawn in by the subatmospheric pressure, remaining as contaminants after the passage of the missile and the collapse of the cavity. The result is a major wound associated with tissue contamination and damage often at a considerable distance from the actual wound track.

What the bullet hits will obviously be important in determining its effect. Even a low-energy transfer wound to the heart is likely to be fatal, whereas a high-energy transfer wound to the leg is entirely survivable with good medical care. Similarly, ballistic injuries to other essential organs such as the brain and liver have a very poor prognosis. Because the amount of tissue damage is related to the slowing of the bullet, it is also apparent that denser tissues will sustain more significant injuries than less dense ones. When a bullet strikes bone, it may fragment and will dump its energy almost instantaneously, producing a fracture with multiple bone fragments.

Bullets may also be designed or modified to increase the tissue damage they cause. A sharp-nosed bullet will have a smaller presenting area compared to a snub (flat)-nosed bullet and will be more inclined to tumble, depositing damaging energy. Military bullets have a metal casing around a lead core (a '*full metal jacket*') in order to reduce the chance of them breaking up; other bullets are *designed* to break up on impact, dramatically increasing the energy transfer. A similar effect will be achieved by including a soft or hollow tip which expands on impact. The most notorious of these was the '*Dum Dum*' bullet. Military use of these bullets is banned under international law although they are used by the police to maximize the chance of killing a criminal whilst minimizing the chance of collateral injury due to a bullet passing through its intended victim and injuring someone else and ensuring that the criminal does not have further time to take lethal actions before being incapacitated.

During flight, bullets undergo a series of movements of which the most significant is oscillation of the bullet about its long axis: *yaw*. Depending on the position at the time of impact, the bullet may strike tissue travelling forwards or side on, increasing its cross-sectional area and the energy loss on impact. Once the bullet enters tissue, the greater density of the medium through which it is travelling causes it to become completely unstable and its yaw becomes *tumbling* as it rotates through 360° about its long axis. As a result of this tumbling, its rate of slowing is enormously increased and the potential tissue damage magnified. Tumbling may put sufficient strain on the bullet to cause it to fragment, further increasing the tissue damage. It is because of tumbling that, where complete penetration occurs, the exit wound tends to be larger than the entrance wound.

Types of weapon

Handguns

Handguns generally fire a bullet with a diameter of 9mm and a muzzle velocity of around 1000 feet per second. As such, they are low-energy weapons producing only a small temporary cavity, injury being essentially confined to the bullet track. However, handguns that fire high-energy bullets are also available.

Shotguns

Shotguns fire cartridges containing many small lead pellets rather than a single ball. The diameter of these pellets ranges from 1 to 10mm. Once fired, the pellets disperse in a cone-shaped pattern. The degree and rapidity of dispersion is proportional to the size and number of pellets as well as the diameter of the shotgun barrel at the muzzle. Due to their aerodynamics, the velocity of individual pellets will attenuate over short distances, even in air. Furthermore, the conical dispersion leads to a rapid decline in the number of pellets which will hit a particular target as range increases. As a result, at close range, the pellets act together much like a single projectile but beyond 30–50m spread increases and kinetic energy drops as the pellets slow. At close range, a shotgun can create very severe patterns of injury but it is likely to be virtually ineffective at ranges over 50m. Sawn-off shotguns will have a much greater spread of shot as a result of their shorter barrel.

Shotgun bore is a measure of the number of lead balls a gun could fire which would make up a total weight of 1lb. A twelve-bore shotgun has the same bore (inner diameter) as a 1.33oz lead ball (12 × 1.33oz = 16oz or 1lb), an eight-bore shotgun has the inner diameter of a 2oz lead ball (8 × 2oz = 16oz or 1lb). In practice, shotguns fire cartridges containing variable numbers of smaller pellets, from several hundred to fewer than ten ('buckshot').

Military assault weapons

The commonest assault rifle worldwide is the AK47 (an estimated 125 million such rifles are in circulation), with a bullet of 7.62mm diameter and 39mm in length which leaves the weapon at a speed of around 900m/s (3000 feet/s). The British military assault weapon (referred to as a long-barrelled weapon) is the modified SA80 (A2) which fires a 5.56mm round. In weapons of this kind, rifling of the barrel sets the bullet spinning, which, combined with the increased velocity, leads to greater accuracy at long range. Weapons of this kind (or effective copies) are in widespread use among terrorist organizations. The very much greater kinetic energy of these bullets leads to a much bigger temporary cavity and hence greater damage than is seen in lower-energy weapons.

Bombs and blast injury

Injury as a result of an explosion is referred to as *blast injury*. However, it is important to remember that such injuries may result from a wide range of incidents as well as bombs. For simplicity, we will consider what happens when an explosive detonates, although similar results occur during a chemical explosion or the sudden uncontrolled release of material at high pressure. Explosives are usefully divided into *low explosives*, such as gunpowder burn if ignited and only explode if confined, and *high explosives*, such as Semtex® which do not burn and require an initiating detonation to explode but do not require confinement.

Injury due to blast

When a detonation occurs, a blast wave spreads out from the point of detonation like the ripples on a pond. This blast wave travels faster than the speed of sound in air, compressing the air in front of it and producing an almost instantaneous rise in pressure lasting a fraction of a millisecond before falling away to a negative pressure. Atmospheric pressure is then restored as the blast wave passes. The blast wave is responsible for *primary blast injuries*. When the blast wave impacts upon a surface, it is reflected (again like ripples on water), increasing the blast pressure at reflection.

In addition to the blast wave, the detonation of an explosive also produces a fireball of hot gases and products of combustion (the blast wind) which passes through the air behind and slower than the blast wave. As the blast wind passes, inevitably objects and people in its path will be injured or damaged. Not only will bodies very close to the detonation be torn apart but the resulting fragments together with environmental debris will be energized, forming fragments capable of causing devastating injury. Victims who are not immediately killed may sustain further injuries when thrown against walls or other environmental objects. Injuries caused by fragments energized by the blast wind are termed *secondary injuries*. What has become one of the hallmarks of terrorist attack is deliberate inclusion of material for its fragmentation effect. Nuts, nails, and ball bearings are all typical of the readily available arsenal of the bomb-maker and obviously cause a great deal of the secondary injury seen in these attacks. The injury pattern is much less predictable than that seen in conventional munitions which are designed to fragment in a particular way either by including preformed fragments or by breaking up in a particular pattern. Because body parts may act as fragments, there is a significant risk of transmission of infection following an explosion in a busy confined space. In addition, these injuries may not always be immediately apparent and careful assessment by clinicians is essential. Primary fragments are those incorporated within the explosive device itself such as nails or ball bearings, and commercial explosive devices such as grenades or shells are expressly designed to disintegrate into effective fragments. In terrorist explosions, three types of fragment may be found, with injuries resulting from nails (a crude form of primary fragment), shattered furniture (secondary fragments), and parts of victims. Large fragments have considerable wounding potential but a small range; small fragments have reduced wounding potential but considerably greater range.

Primary blast injury

Injury caused by the blast wave itself is referred to as primary blast injury and is a significant cause of illness and death. It affects the lungs, gastrointestinal system, and less importantly, the ears (presenting as pain and deafness—*all* blast victims *must* undergo ENT assessment). From the perspective of incident management, the important feature of *blast lung injury* (BLI), which presents with shortness of breath, pulmonary haemorrhage (coughing blood), and respiratory failure, is that since artificial ventilation is the key treatment strategy, there is likely to be a need for large numbers of intensive care beds. This capability will probably require distribution of patients around a number of major centres.

It is also important to note that primary blast injury may not be immediately apparent as it can develop over several hours. As a result, triage methods must be capable of identifying those at risk due to their proximity to the detonation and ensuring appropriate medical surveillance and care. Symptoms and signs of blast injury to the abdomen include shock, abdominal pain, abdominal tenderness and swelling, nausea and vomiting, testicular pain, bleeding from the anus, and rarely vomiting blood. The treatment is essentially surgical, adding to the significant operating load produced by the management of fragment injuries and amputations.

All forms of primary blast injury are commoner when the explosion has occurred in a confined space. It is important to remember that in the early stages blast injury can present with little more than anxiety, agitation, and tachypnoea. These features may suggest a diagnosis of anxiety. Such a misdiagnosis may have fatal consequences and such patients must be treated seriously and admitted for observation.

Classification of blast injuries
- *Primary injuries*: due to the blast wave
- *Secondary injuries*: due to fragments
- *Tertiary injuries*: amputation, fragmentation, and translocation
- *Other (quaternary) injuries*: burns, inhalation injury, and psychological trauma.

In view of the fact that highly energized body fragments from victims may cause significant injury to others, the response to any blast incident must include plans for the management of potential inoculation from transmissible infections such as hepatitis and HIV. This is likely to take the form of immunization programmes and treatment with immunoglobulin as well as routine post-exposure prophylaxis for commensals or environmental contamination.

Traumatic amputation and body fragmentation are referred to as *tertiary injuries*. Experience from recent military conflicts has demonstrated that relatively simple measures such as *tourniquets* and *haemostatic dressings* have a key role in preventing death from amputations and both must be available to the emergency services in sufficient quantities. However, the injuries which are likely to follow an explosion will result in many hours of operating time and will have a corresponding impact on health continuity which planners must allow for. In less confined bombings, victims may be thrown significant distances, again sustaining critical injuries. Traumatic amputation is rare in survivors but much more common in those who die early (approximately 20% of victims). The presence of blast amputation is indicative of severe blast effect.

Because these amputations are avulsive rather than 'guillotine like', tissue damage occurs proximal to the level of amputation as blood vessels, nerves, and tendons are torn from the limb. Re-implantation is therefore rarely, if ever, possible and precious surgical time should not be wasted in attempting it. Wherever possible, expert advice in the management of such injuries should be sought, as counterintuitively, different protocols to normal civilian practice may be required.

Burns, inhalational injury, and psychological problems are collected together as *other injuries*, sometimes termed *quaternary injuries*. In the early stages of the incident, psychological trauma is largely a matter of ensuring that all patients from the scene are logged to allow follow-up in due course via their primary care provider.

It has been estimated that on average up to 50% of survivors will require hospitalization.

Sources of expert advice

Inevitably, the *Defence Medical Services* (DMS) have accumulated a great deal of experience in the complex and multidisciplinary management of blast (and gunshot) injury. Particular expertise in the continued management of these patients has been gained by the Royal Centre for Defence Medicine in Birmingham and those responsible for planning and providing the response to such an incident should consider contacting the DMS who are happy to provide expert advice.

Suicide bombers

The first commonly recognized suicide bombing was the assassination of Tsar Alexander II in 1881. Relatively uncommon until the 1990s, such devices have become powerful terrorist weapons in the hands of extremists, especially those of a religious motivation where there is a perceived additional benefit for the bomber of eternal bliss. Beginning most notably in the Lebanon, such attacks became common in Israel and then Iraq and Afghanistan; increasingly frequent use in Western democracies seems inevitable.

Suicide bombing has much to offer the terrorist. Very confined spaces and high-density targets can be attacked and the technology is simple as it does not require remote detonation. Teams can be kept very small for launching the attacks as there is no exfiltration or rescue required. For the same reason, there is no perpetrator to be questioned and to risk the security of operational units.

The majority of attacks conform to the model of an explosive package worn as a belt or waistcoat, commonly with fragmentation weapons incorporated in the design (often just bags of nails, screws, or nuts). Introduced into a confined space, due to blast wave reflection the victims are likely to be struck multiple times by the blast wave, and the injuries will be devastating.

Shrapnel, as originally designed by the eponymous Colonel Henry Shrapnel, consisted of preformed spherical fragments (like ball bearings) contained within artillery shell cases, typical *primary* fragments. The term should not strictly be used generically of secondary fragments.

Managing the scene of a shooting

The UK has, for a variety of reasons, avoided significant numbers of multiple shootings such as are all too distressingly common in the USA. The Dunblane incident of 1996 in which Thomas Hamilton killed sixteen pupils and one teacher and the Whitehaven tragedy of 2011 in which Derrick Bird killed twelve and injured eleven are notable exceptions. The majority of shootings, therefore, which are relatively common, will not reach the status of a major incident. What they will require is medical care when it can be provided safely and security cordoning of the area until the risk is eliminated.

Factors which turn a shooting into a major incident include difficulty in locating and eliminating the perpetrator, as was the case in Cumbria, large numbers of living, or *possibly* living casualties, and major disruption to infrastructure.

It is important to remember that the scene of a shooting has the capacity to turn into a hostage situation which will require careful management. Such situations are beyond the scope of this book.

Zones at a shooting incident

The zones at a shooting incident will be determined and enforced by the police.

Non-permissive zone

Militarily, this is referred to as care under fire (*hot zone*). Under no circumstances should non-specialist medical staff enter this area. The aim is to extract patients from the non-permissive area for treatment and clinical protocols may need to be amended to reflect this. Police firearms teams receive standard, national advanced first aid training relevant to non-permissive environments.

Semi-permissive zone

This is often referred to as the *warm zone* in that risk persists but the direct threat is absent. Minimal care necessary to save life should be provided, under instruction from the relevant commander and ideally by specially trained personnel only. This area is within the police cordon and when treatment is necessary, an escort should be provided. *Hazardous area response teams* are trained to work in environments such as this.

Permissive zone

This is also referred to as the *cold zone*, allowing routine and advanced pre-hospital care to occur with minimal risk to responder and casualty.

Police post-shooting procedures

Whenever the police discharge a firearm causing injury or death there will be an official investigation into the incident. Officers will be immediately removed from the scene and a situation report will be provided to the tactical firearms commander. The investigation will involve the *post incident manager* (PIM) appointed by the police force, a *Police Federation* representative, and representatives of the force's *professional standards department*. Further reports will then be prepared including from police witnesses at the scene. Officers involved have access to legal representation and to their families and will be assessed by a doctor to exclude injury. A senior investigating officer will be appointed to oversee the next stage of the procedure which includes personal statements from the officers involved and from witnesses. Finally, reports will be prepared detailing all the facts of the incident including the justification for the use of force. These accounts will be submitted to the Independent Police Complaints Commission (IPCC) within 7 days of the incident. The officers involved in a shooting will not return to work until they are authorized to do so by senior officers.

Discharged weapons will be forensically examined and clothing may be required for testing in some instances. In the event of a fatality, a coroner's inquest will inevitably follow.

Managing the scene of an explosion

To some extent, the management of the scene of an incident will vary according to the cause of the blast. The key features which will guide such a response include:
- protection of the public, victims, and rescuers from:
  - the possibility of a secondary device
  - building collapse, fire, or further explosion
  - toxic hazards (e.g. products of combustion)
  - associated CBRN risk (rare)
- extrication and treatment of victims
- location and identification of the dead
- location, identification, and custody of surviving perpetrators, if any
- preservation of evidence.

The scene of an incident must therefore be considered to be a non-permissive environment until the nominated person in charge of scene security informs responders to the contrary. Everyone attending an incident must be conscious of the risk of admitting an unidentified perpetrator into the casualty chain. Quite apart from any further deliberate acts, a live perpetrator may suggest incomplete or failed detonation of the device and hence substantial risk to emergency responders.

The decision regarding the placement of cordons at the scene of an explosion will be taken by the senior police officer at the scene, with the advice of ordnance disposal experts. The outer cordon, manned by police officers to prevent unauthorized entry, will be placed to allow an appropriate safe working area for the emergency services outside the inner cordon. In addition to those managing the scene, the police will appoint a *senior investigating officer* who will commence the criminal investigation into the incident and in so far as it is safe to do so, and it does not compromise the treatment and extraction of victims, the forensic investigation of the scene will commence. Exhibits officers and police photographers will play a key role in this process. When it is safe to do so, the area within the inner cordon will be divided into zones for search purposes.

Triage following an explosion

It is in the nature of an explosion, especially one in a confined space designed to cause terrible injuries, that there is likely to be a large number of casualties, many with severe and complex injuries. It will, therefore, be down to effective major incident management to limit the impact as much as possible, and a good triage system will be the mainstay of this. Conventional systems can be used, but the possibility of blast injury developing later must be taken into account as must the position of the casualty at the time of the explosion. Essentially any victim, even if apparently uninjured, who is at risk of having sustained a significant blast effect *must* be formally assessed in hospital and may require a period of observation.

Psychological effects of explosions

As the archetypal terrorist weapon, bombs will be associated with a significant incidence of psychological problems in both survivors and rescuers. Similar injuries are, of course, also seen in non-terrorist explosions, although the numbers are usually smaller.

Blast injuries are devastating and mutilating. Both in civilian (terrorist) and military contexts, victims are likely to be known personally to the survivors and possibly to the rescuers. This can only heighten the horror of the situation. Medical professionals likely to be called upon to deal with such situations may benefit from prior education including exposure to illustrations of injuries resulting from blast. Fragmented, burned, and mutilated bodies, widely scattered body parts, and diffuse projection of blood, brain, and other body tissue over victims and survivors may be expected. Active management of the mental health of both victims and rescuers is essential.

Documentation

Clinical documentation must be thorough. Accurate descriptions, together with detailed measured diagrams, are of immense value to the forensic services. Where possible, photographs should be taken. Wounds should be carefully described. There must be no speculation regarding the nature of entry and exit wounds. It is imperative wherever possible that these descriptions are completed before appearances are altered by surgical intervention. Clear labelling of incisions caused during treatment (iatrogenic wounds) such as thoracostomies or escharotomies is also essential. It is important to resist the common temptation to try to appear an expert on wound ballistics.

Preservation of evidence

There will inevitably be an enquiry after every explosion or major shooting incident, whether a criminal enquiry, or one led by relevant regulatory and safety bodies. In either case, prosecution for negligence or a criminal act may follow. All such scenes must therefore be considered scenes of crime and preservation of evidence is essential unless such preservation would cause risk or injury to victims or rescuers. There are a number of basic principles: if clothing has to be removed, holes made by projectiles must be preserved and not cut through; gunshot residue, carbon, metal fragments, and components of rounds and any fragments should be identified and preserved.

Given that there are likely to be multiple victims, it is vital that clothing and other material is not mixed up but kept scrupulously separate. Wherever possible, any material of potential forensic interest should be handed directly to a police officer. Where this is not possible, it should be bagged and labelled and given into the care of a clearly identified named person. Evidential material must not be left where subsequent allegations of tampering might be made. A chain of custody must be demonstrable at all times.

Bodies and body parts

Bodies or body parts found within the inner cordon should be left *in situ* for later recovery by forensic teams. If these can be seen by the public (remembering the lenses of the media), they should be covered, otherwise they should be left 'as found'. It will be necessary for a medical practitioner to declare life extinct even in obvious cases, and although removal of bodies to a temporary or designated mortuary should take place as quickly as possible to reduce the distress of relatives, the coroner may wish to see bodies *in situ* and this should be discussed with their officer. Bodies that need to be removed for their own preservation or to gain access to the living will be removed to a *body holding area*. Before forensic removal, bodies and body parts will be photographed *in situ* initially with coverings in place if this has occurred. Further photographs will be taken as the cover is removed (and bagged and sealed for future evidential analysis) and as any debris is removed from the body. Following assessment by an exhibits officer, the body will then be wrapped in a plastic sheet, bagged, and removed, with a designated accompanying police officer, to the mortuary facility. A similar procedure is followed for body parts.

After arrival at the designated mortuary facility, each body will be X-rayed to look for bomb and other fragments and the officer accompanying it will identify it to the pathologist. The chain of evidence must be maintained at all times.

Forensic aspects of the bomb scene

The zones of the inner cordon will initially be *walked through* by the forensic recovery team looking for obvious elements of the device which will then be recovered. A more detailed examination including the meticulous searching of debris will then follow. A detailed map of the area showing evidential finds will be compiled by the police. A significant area may need to be swept for debris energized by the blast and thrown considerable distances. The area of the detonation itself will also require swabbing and analysis for the type of explosive and measurement of the crater to assist in estimation of device size. Vehicles near the scene will be lifted onto tarpaulin, covered in a further tarpaulin, wrapped, and removed for forensic analysis. Every item removed from the scene will be bagged and numbered and the process logged, every effort being made to avoid contamination. An air exclusion zone may be requested to prevent damage or movement or evidence due to helicopter downdraft.

The Hospital Response

Introduction

The hospital response is a key component of major incident planning where large numbers of casualties are likely to require onward treatment, specialist services, follow-up and reha-bilitation. A major incident will typically require the support of at least one acute hospital and larger-scale incidents may require a coordinated response involving several hospitals in one region or even over two or more regions, especially where an incident occurs on an administrative boundary.

The hospital response usually applies to acute hospitals where there is an emergency (A&E) department providing 24-hour emergency services. However, the general principles and approach could also reasonably apply to any acute care provider institution such as 'walk-in' centres, urgent care centres or minor injury units. The management of casualties from a major incident will often consist of a coordinated response involving all such facilities. Casualties may well be streamed to different locations depending upon their injury severity, for example, all P1/P2 casualties would generally be transported to acute hospitals whereas many P3 casualties could be managed appropriately and swiftly by a local minor injury or walk-in centre. The key to such an approach is to ensure informed decision-making and effective casualty tracking, coordination and communication.

Planning

Ensuring that every hospital has an effective, well-rehearsed major incident plan is complex although intensive preparation can mitigate the risks and reduces the likelihood of failure. It is the duty of the chief executive of each acute hospital trust to ensure that an effective major incident (MAJAX) plan is in place.

Key components of the hospital response to a major incident include:
- fulfilling responsibilities under Part 1 of the Civil Contingencies Act 2004
- following national guidance
- regular training and exercises
- ensuring that plans are in place to safely reduce or suspend routine/elective work in response to a major incident when required
- effective planning in conjunction with other healthcare providers (walk-in centres, general practices, private sector bodies, and out-of-hours providers), the emergency services, local and regional organizations, and other important responders
- full involvement in planning work in conjunction with sub-region/area teams
- provision of a Medical Emergency Response Incident Team (MERIT) if required (and may be in addition to that already provided by ambulance services)
- an effective hospital command and control structure
- plans for managing vulnerable groups such as children
- contingency plans for a prolonged incident or an incident which compromises the function of the hospital.

A senior manager will usually be designated to lead an implementation and planning team for managing major incidents. This should include a senior clinician such as a consultant in emergency medicine and a senior nurse or departmental clinical manager. The team must be adequately resourced to remain responsive to changing circumstances. Ideally, the function of the planning team should mirror that of a Local Resilience Forum. Sub-working groups will undertake supportive roles such as training and education, CBRN responses and so on.

Government guidance places responsibilities for a major incident response on an acute hospital trust as shown in Box 12.1.

Box 12.1 Hospital responsibilities in the event of a major incident

- Provision of a safe and secure environment for patients and staff
- Provision of initial resuscitation and specialist care to victims
- Liaison with the ambulance service(s), sub-region/area teams, Clinical Commissioning Groups, and other relevant responders
- Support to medical care at the scene (if not otherwise provided) without denuding hospital personnel or resources
- Review and maintenance of essential hospital functions for the duration of the incident
- Provision of support to other hospitals involved in the response
- Provision of limited decontamination facilities for casualties who self-present to hospital (coordinated with the ambulance and/or fire and rescue services depending on local arrangements)
- Procedures for handling the bodies of patients who die at hospital
- Communication with relatives and friends of patients (including those not involved in the incident)
- Communication with the casualty bureau, local media, local community, and VIPs.

The structured approach to the hospital response and surge management

For planning purposes, an acute receiving hospital should maintain the capability to manage up to 40 casualties from a major incident within its locality. It is possible, however, that some hospitals as a result of their remote location will have to manage *all* the casualties from an incident. This possibility must be reflected in the hospital's major incident plan which should include, for example, mechanisms to ensure that those with minor injuries are treated elsewhere. In addition, if the hospital is very close to the incident site, there is the real possibility that facilities may be at least temporarily overwhelmed by patients who make their own way to hospital or are brought by other members of the public. In these circumstances, the best protection is rigorous implementation of an effective well-practised system. For incidents involving mass gathering or stadium events, acute hospitals may be required to manage up to 100 significant casualties across the system. Optimal receiving capacity per hospital should be based upon up to five seriously injured or ill casualties at any one time.

The structured approach to the hospital response is based upon HMIMMS principles (see 'Further Reading', Appendix A) which are essentially the same as those guiding the response at the scene (Box 12.2). Hospital plans should be fully integrated with local pre-hospital plans and be functionally effective across local and regional boundaries and between all services. There must also be a resilient capability to communicate and share information at a regional and national level if this is required.

The four phases to the hospital response may be described as:
- pre-hospital
- reception
- definitive care
- recovery.

Box 12.2 CSCATTT principles (from the Major Incident Medical Management and Support (MIMMS) system)

Management and support principles
Command
Safety
Communication
Assessment
Triage
Treatment
Transport.

Planning and preparation

Key areas

A number of key clinical and administrative areas in the hospital must be prepared early following the activation of a major incident response. These are summarized in Table 12.1. Priority areas will include patient reception areas, particularly the emergency department, and other areas where urgent clinical activity will be taking place such as theatres, critical care units, and nominated acute receiving wards. Once these areas are established, other areas can develop as staff arrive.

Essential administrative areas include the hospital *coordination* and *information centres* as well as those which will facilitate safe discharge of existing ward patients (in order to clear space on the wards) and a press area—ideally placed away from acute receiving locations.

From a hospital perspective, preparation for major incidents requires an up-to-date major incident plan that is practically achievable and well rehearsed. Familiarity with the plan is a vital component for all personnel who may be involved, especially (but not exclusively) in the key clinical and administrative areas as listed. It is clearly too late to read and understand a major incident plan once the response has already commenced. At this stage, the plan should be used as a reference guide and the relevant action cards followed. Major incident response plan briefings and individual and team training should also form part of staff induction programmes with annual refresher sessions.

Other areas that must be identified as part of the major incident planning process include a reporting point for staff where individualized action cards may be collected where appropriate and a discharge waiting area for patients discharged to provide surge capacity as well as those affected by the incident (and where reunions with family can take place). The availability of crèche facilities will significantly enhance the ability of staff to respond to the incident at short notice. A major incident will obviously result in additional demand for portering, catering, cleaning, linen services, and central sterile supplies and all of these areas must have plans in place to enable them to cope.

Table 12.1 Key clinical and administrative areas requiring identification and early preparation

Clinical	Administrative
Reception area (emergency department)	Hospital coordination centre
Staff reporting area	Hospital information centre
Theatres	Discharge/reunion area
ITU	Press area
Wards	
Body holding area	

Priorities

When preparing a hospital major incident plan, the plan must be intelligible and understandable, ensuring that each responder receives only the information they need to respond effectively. Effective training processes must be established. The process of triage and its location, as well as who will carry it out must be clearly established. Sensible estimates of achievable major incident capacity must be made and effective patient tracking systems must be established which are as far as possible compatible with normal operating systems. Procedures for 'locking down' the building and maintaining a limited number of access routes must be clear and effective.

When there is the possibility that CBRN casualties might be received, arrangements for casualty decontamination (in conjunction with the ambulance service) must be developed together with humane but effective methods of preventing access until this process is complete. In addition, it may be necessary to isolate or lock down the emergency department, including shutting off the air conditioning. The processes, technical means, and decision-making process by which this will be achieved must be established in advance. The emergency plan must also establish the ability to 'quarantine' certain groups of patients including provision of a separate reception or holding area away from the main emergency department

Essential principles

The hospital response should be developed and maintained through regular training and exercises at every level, and conceptually can be divided into 'generic' and 'specific role'-related approaches. The generic approach will guide individuals, teams, and departments in how to prepare for, organize, and undertake the response through the hospital-based phases of a major incident. This will be built around the guiding CSCATT principles (see Box 12.2, p. 348) with consideration of local resources and trauma systems.

Specific roles must be well defined and appropriately prioritized. The concept can be referred to as the 'right person, right place, right time, and supported to perform the correct job'. The structure of a hospital major incident response can be developed under the headings shown in Box 12.3. Planning guidance is available centrally from the *Department of Health*, although this is generic and does not address specific roles within the hospital response.

Box 12.3 The structure of a hospital major incident response

- Command and control
- Communications
- Key staff selection
- Key staff tasking
- Team definition
- Key area selection
- Infrastructure.

Writing a major incident plan

This section describes the process of writing a major incident plan. The key to a successful response is a robust plan which limits the need for improvisation and provides clear instructions and areas of responsibility for decision makers at every level. An effective plan cannot be successfully improvised 'on the day' but must be flexible to any potential situation. Everyone involved will *do their best* but this simply won't be good enough without a robust effective framework. Also, plans which rely purely on statements of intent rather than specific actions and requirements are unlikely to be effective during the response. Writing an effective major incident plan is a significant and time-consuming task requiring considerable attention to detail, collaboration, and diplomacy. Plans should always be exercised to ensure that any lessons are learnt in order to further refine the plan over time, particularly when services are changing or potential new threats are identified. The main components of an effective major incident plan are listed in Box 12.4 and discussed below.

The layout

The major incident plan must clearly identify the location of the following areas of the response:
- P1 and P2 areas (invariably in the emergency department)
- P3 area which may use the out-patients department or another suitable large area
- Hospital incident control room and appropriate communication hub
- Triage point (and single point of entry for patients)
- Police casualty bureau
- Point of entry for staff.

Patient flows

The areas and routes to be used in the transfer of patients during the incident must be clearly defined. Such arrangements must avoid bottlenecks and over-reliance on single points of access to departments and lifts. Clearly defined routes and well-demarcated areas are particularly important in the event of a potential CBRN incident. An area in which patients may wait for discharge must be identified, not only for those patients from the incident who are fit for discharge but for those sent home to provide capacity during the incident such as patients whose operations have been cancelled. Routes of access to key areas such as ITU should be established, bearing in mind that access to individual buildings will be restricted to the minimum number of points during the incident. Ambulance loading and unloading points should be identified and processes established to allow all key components of circulation routes for staff and vehicles to be clearly marked and supervised. Pre-determined signage should be stored ready for use and staff allocated to its placement via action cards (usually portering services staff).

Effective staff utilization

It is all too easy in planning a response to a major incident to concentrate on the clinical areas. It should not be forgotten that a wide range of support services will also be required including, for example, catering (for patients and staff working long hours), chaplaincy services,

---

Box 12.4 The components of an effective major incident plan
- Hospital Co-ordination Team and hierarchy
- An effective major incident response framework
- Simple and effective patient flows
- An effective staff utilization programme
- Effective call-in procedures/cascade
- The emergency department response
- Effective record-keeping and patient tracking
- Effective communications
- Appropriate and resilient equipment scalings
- Action cards (see p. 358) and SOPs
- Discharge processes
- Media liaison and family information centre
- Regular maintenance, review, and exercising.

linen and sterile supplies, blood component supply, laboratory and mortuary services, clerical support, pharmacy services, and patient transport. All of these must be included in the plan with those being responsible for their provision clearly identified and tasks for the individual responders allocated to action cards. Given that the hospital response to a major incident is likely to be prolonged, an important component of staff utilization is to ensure that an effective response can be maintained rather than calling in too many staff too soon, resulting in exhaustion and problems maintaining the appropriate level of service: this may mean allocating delayed times for certain staff members to attend the hospital.

Effective call-in procedures
There is a real risk that inadequate call-in procedures could overwhelm the hospital switchboard causing delays in mounting an effective response to an incident if the call-in procedure is left entirely to the duty operators. In addition, call-in information held centrally is often out of date. As a consequence, a cascade system is recommended (see p. 364).

The emergency department response
The response within the emergency department is key to the efficiency of the whole hospital response. It is essential, therefore, that processes within the emergency department are effective, efficient, and rapidly established.

Effective record-keeping and patient tracking
Effective record-keeping and patient tracking during an incident is essential and will result in a considerable clerical burden which is best managed during the incident by those familiar with such systems. Pre-prepared major incident documentation packs should be used (see p. 356).

Effective communications
When a major incident is declared, it is too late to start improvising effective communications. These *must* be in place beforehand. In arranging communications, the volume of material which must be handled and the number of people requiring access to communications must not be under-estimated (see p. 357).

Action cards
(See pp. 358–9.)
   Individual action cards which are role and not person based are the best way of ensuring an effective plan, eliminating uncertainty, and allowing an appropriately staged response.

Discharge processes
Processes must be in place to ensure an effective and efficient process for discharging or transferring in-patients to create capacity during the incident and for those involved in it who have been discharged after assessment.

Media liaison
Effective media liaison is vital and facilities must be provided; constructive engagement with the media can be used to positive effect when managing an incident.

Regular maintenance, review, and exercising
Receiving hospitals are required to regularly practise and update their major incident plan, which must remain fit for use. Changes in building use, areas of clinical responsibility, contact details, contractual suppliers of non-clinical services, and many other components of an effective plan will require regular updating. Major incident practices must ensure that every member of staff is aware of the main components of the plan and their part in it: this latter component is most easily achieved simply by ensuring that every member of staff knows where to report when called in and where to collect their own action card. Unsurprisingly, the greater the level of authority and responsibility borne by an individual during an incident, the more actively they should be involved in planning, practice, and preparation.

   Plans should be regularly exercised in both individual teams and at a multidisciplinary level for assurance purposes and to ensure any organizational lessons can be learnt, and plans adapted accordingly if necessary.

Hospital coordination team

The most senior component of the clinical hierarchy in overall control of the hospital response is known as the *hospital coordination team* (HCT). This must be established as soon as a major incident is declared or standby is announced. The HCT is led by the *medical coordinator*, a senior physician with detailed knowledge of the major incident plan, ideally with knowledge and experience of management structures in the hospital and the wider emergency services community. The remaining roles of the HCT are taken by the senior emergency physician, senior nurse, and senior manager.

All members of this team will have the authority to make decisions without routine recourse to a higher authority. A designated location, the *hospital control room* (HCR), for the team will need to be identified in the major incident plan. All potential members of the team will require regular training for their roles and should be familiar with the response plan.

The senior emergency physician's main responsibility is to organize the reception phase while the senior nurse will coordinate the overall nursing response in the hospital. As such, the senior nurse should be a senior member of the nursing staff from *outside* the emergency department.

Responsibilities of the hospital coordination team

The coordinating team is responsible for ensuring that the following are in place and functioning effectively:
- Hospital command and control
- Communication within the hospital
- Communication with outside agencies
- Assessment of the size of the required response in the light of developing information
- Patient and staff safety procedures
- Triage
- Treatment
- Patient transport
- Liaison with the core business team.

Hospital incident control room

A location for the hospital incident control room must be pre-identified as part of the plan, requirements include:
- accessibility,
- central location
- single point of access
- desk space
- signage
- access to computer terminals, high-speed fax, and telephones
- clerical support
- access to a conference room.

The control room will also hold the designated 'major incident clock' against which all timings will be recorded.

Infrastructure and resource management

This is the primary responsibility of the *senior manager* in coordinating the hospital support services. It is relatively easy to forget support services—in the broadest sense—and the major incident plan should provide action cards for such diverse but essential roles as cleaners, chaplains, mortuary staff, and hospital volunteers.

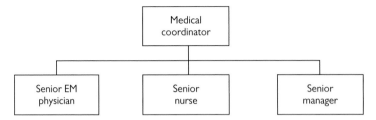

Fig. 12.1 The hospital coordination team (HCT).

Documentation and patient tracking

Where it is planned that written clinical records will be used, a stock of major incident documentation packs should be prepared in advance, complete with all necessary note formats and carrying unique identifiers in order to support rapid management and facilitate casualty tracking. A suggested list of documentation pack contents is shown in Box 12.5. Each component should be clearly pre-marked with the patient's unique identifying number and enclosed in a suitably robust container (e.g. a foolscap wallet), which must also be clearly marked with the identifying number. MAJAX numbered tracking slips forwarded to a central coordination point after completion will allow the tracking of each patient through the system.

Each set of records should have a unique identifying number (e.g.M-000001 to M-000200). These sets of records should be stored in an accessible but locked location near to the designated patient entrance and triage point.

As each casualty arrives, no attempt should be made to collect their personal details. Instead, only the next numerical identifier (M- number) should be assigned to each patient in sequence from the pre-prepared supply. The agreement of all parties to accept such a system must be in place *before* an incident occurs in order to ensure that the laboratories and radiology are prepared to carry out blood tests, cross-matching, and imaging using the unique identifier and that a routine hospital number will not be demanded or samples rejected.

As more staff become available it will be possible to collect further information about each of the patients. The plan should assign sufficient clerical staff to ensure than this can be achieved, and a central location should be identified for the collation of this data and maintenance of a detailed patient database. This area should have easy access to the police cell, or ideally be co-located with it, so that patient information can be easily shared with the casualty bureau. Each note set should include a series of patient tracking slips which can be passed to this central point once a decision has been made regarding the next destination of the patient. Using these slips, the patient can be tracked from the emergency department to operating theatre, from the operating theatre to the ward or intensive care unit. Action cards must task a member of the clerical or support staff, or a volunteer, with the collection and collation of these slips.

Box 12.5 Suggested contents of a major incident documentation pack

- Patient identification device (wrist/ankle bands)
- Admission 'front' sheet/clinical record template
- Continuation sheets
- Drug chart/'kardex'
- Intravenous prescription and fluid balance chart
- Nursing care record
- Patient movement tracking slips
- Laboratory forms for biochemistry/haematology and blood product requests*
- Imaging request forms (computed tomography and plain X-ray).*

* Unless using appropriate electronic alternative system. If so, consideration should be given to printing out 'hard' copies to be kept with written notes for archiving purposes and to act as a permanent contemporaneous record for the post-incident debrief or any future inquest.

Communications

In general, the hospital response should use means of communication which are already in place and with which staff are familiar. Elaborate systems with which staff are unfamiliar are likely to result in ineffective communications. However, certain key personnel will require use of a resilient communication system, such as a digital cordless telephone (e.g. DECT), or radio or cellular communication system so that they remain contactable as they move around the hospital. These individuals will include the medical coordinator, members of the HCT, and others as appropriate (Box 12.6). Training for these individuals is essential and the equipment must be easily obtainable and charged for use. In most cases, equipment will be stored in the emergency department or switchboard but its location must be specified on the action cards of all those who will use it.

Rooms designated as administrative hubs (the control centre, patient data collation point, and police locations) must be provided with appropriate equipment including telephones, faxes, and computers with Internet and email access. Extra activated computer points should be available for this purpose. High-speed fax machines will be required in the hospital control room, police locations, and patient data collation area. Ideally, this equipment should be pre-placed in major incident equipment storage cupboards in the appropriate locations. Keys for such stores can be attached to appropriate action cards for collection and use when an incident is declared, or stored centrally.

In circumstances where heavy telephone usage is expected to occur, extra telephone lines should be installed, ideally colour-coded differently to those in routine use. Additional telephone points may also have to be installed in places such as radiology, laboratories, the resuscitation room, and other main treatment areas where heavy usage is predicted.

Communications resilience is essential and back-up capability must be built into the plan in case of power failure or other forms of communications black-out. This may include the use of runners with memo sheets or radios (while battery power lasts).

Box 12.6 Key personnel requiring access to special incident mobile communications medical coordinator

- Senior emergency physician
- Senior nurse
- Senior manager
- Police casualty documentation team (liaison officer)
- Ambulance liaison officer
- Hospital enquiry point.

Action cards

Plans work more effectively if responders have a written list of specific tasks on an action card. In addition, the majority of individuals only need to be trained regarding where to collect the card and how they will be called in. Everything else should be on the card! Each card should clearly indicate the location to which the individual must report after collecting the card, to whom they are responsible, and for whom they have responsibility. Contact details should be given and should be up to date. Actions should be precisely defined and not vague aspirations but may be divided into primary and secondary tasks.

Writing action cards

Each card within a particular group should be numbered from one (the first card to be collected—e.g. PORTER 1, ANAESTHETIST 1). The number of cards should be based on the best estimate of the likely number of staff who will be available. This can only be determined by detailed consultation with key staff and heads of department. The lowest numbered cards (and therefore those with the most important immediate tasks) should be allocated to those who will already be on site when the incident is called.

These tasks should where necessary be time dependent (e.g. *during normal working hours, bleep the medical consultant, out of working hours, ring the medical consultant at home, ...*) and any necessary contact details must be included with the card and regularly updated.

Every action card must allocate:
- a working location or point of contact (*Go to ...*)
- a responsible senior (*You report to ...*)
- a secondary tasking (*If you are not required for your primary task, you are to ...*).

Each card must also include where relevant a further call-out list of staff from home. This should occur on low-numbered cards to ensure that staff *are* called and no single card should give too many people to call. A specific form of words to be quoted when calling in staff should be given with instructions to adhere to it closely. This will include details of where to park and where to report on arrival which should be confirmed with the staff being called in. A delay to the arrivals of later call-in to ensure sustained staffing in the event of a prolonged response should be built into the cascade system.

Where appropriate (key roles only), an instruction to collect an identifying tabard, radio, keys, signage, or other equipment such as a signing in book for the staff reception area, should be included. A plan showing the main areas of the response including points of access and patient routes on the back of the card is useful. An instruction to return the card at the end of the incident should also be included. (See Box 12.7 for a sample action card.)

Box 12.7 A sample action card

CONSULTANT GENERAL SURGEON 3

Collect: RADIO No 5 from switchboard

Responsibilities:
- You report to the medical coordinator.
- You are in charge of the preoperative surgical teams.
- Your role is to ensure prioritization and preparation of patients for emergency surgery.

Immediate action:
- On being informed of a major incident, proceed to main theatre reception.
- Using the major incident file in theatre reception, call in:
  - two consultant general surgeons*
  - two consultant orthopaedic surgeons.*
- Liaise with senior sister theatres (bleep 4001) to ensure that:
  - support staff are present or have been called
  - you know which theatres are to be used.
- Liaise with senior anaesthetist theatres to ensure that:
  - surgical teams are matched with anaesthetic capability in order of priority.
- As staff become available, allocate teams of consultant surgeon/surgeon in training/ anaesthetist to each patient as they arrive.
- Liaise with senior sister theatres to allocate a theatre to each patient.
- Ensure that all requests for equipment are fulfilled.
- Continually liaise with following key personnel.
  - Medical coordinator (*RADIO 1*)
  - Senior consultant emergency department (*RADIO 4*)
  - Senior consultant intensive care unit (ext. 54201 or 54202).
- Call in extra staff as required, consider delayed call-in to maintain service, consider re-deployment of staff to emergency department.
- Ensure business continuity for urgent non-MAJAX patients.

* You are to say: 'A major incident has been declared, please report to the west entrance to collect and sign for your action card. Please use your normal parking area.'

Equipment

Tabards and identification badges or lanyards as appropriate should be available for key personnel including those who will have to deal with members of the public. Emergency department staff must also be easily identifiable to supporting personnel from other departments. Leaders and members of treatment teams should be clearly identified, as should those with an administrative role. Within each treatment team the use of an armband or tabard is ideal. Administration and non-clinical personnel should remain in their regular clothing or uniform.

A white board with markers is a very straightforward way of managing casualty tracking, at least in the early stages and is a familiar and practical solution for most staff. This allows rapid and reasonably robust recording of identification and information management at the reception and triage areas. It can also operate as a back-up option if electronic systems are usually used, but become unavailable due to power or IT system failure.

It is essential that sufficient stores of appropriate PPE are held and that staff are trained to use it. Supplies should include plastic gowns, gloves, masks, eye protection, and enhanced protective equipment for special circumstances such as CBRN incidents. Some special equipment may have a fairly short shelf-life or be unfamiliar to some personnel. Stores of this equipment must be maintained and training should include familiarization for staff, especially new starters at induction. Clear plans must be in place for resupply in the event of stocks becoming exhausted.

Training

Written plans should be made readily available to all members of hospital staff with an up-to-date version held centrally on hospital information systems. Ideally, a printed copy should not be kept (other than action cards) in order to ensure the version is the most recent one and avoid conflicting direction. Using an action card system means that most responders only need to know the basic structure of the plan, locations of key components, and where to collect their own action card: any required detail can be included on the action card.

Training should be designed to ensure that individuals and teams have an understanding of their likely allocated roles and responsibilities. Collective training is also required to ensure plans remain feasible and effective against any given scenario. Those aspects of a major incident response which most require training are command, control, communication, and triage. This can be carried out in a variety of ways. Individual and team training can take the form of skill and knowledge development (role dependent) and triage exercises (paper based or dynamic as individuals or in groups). Larger-scale training will include communication cascade exercises, multidisciplinary tabletop exercises (walkthroughs or practical exercises without casualties (PEWC)) and multiagency training (e.g. large external exercises at locations such as airports which involve simulated casualties).

Operational exercises should take place as follows:
- A live exercise at least every 3 years
- A tabletop exercise at least every year
- A communications cascade test every 6 months.

The Hospital Major Incident Medical Management and Support: the practical approach in the hospital (HMIMMS) course devised by the Advanced Life Support group and prehospital Medical Management and Support: the practical approach at the scene (MIMMS) courses offer basic training in major incident planning and response. Training in media handling, communication, and leadership skills may be appropriate for some key personnel, particularly those who will be required to offer briefings, work with the public, and interact with the uniformed services.

Hierarchy

Adaptable and collapsible frameworks

The hierarchy of the hospital response must be configured in such a way that it is adaptable and collapsible. This will ensure that the plan is effective during any scale of incident while remaining sustainable and offering the most efficient use of the available resources.

The framework will be made up of core roles, responsibilities, and capabilities. For example, one of the main priorities will be to ensure there are sufficient personnel to provide treatment teams for the resuscitation of P1 casualties. The size of the hospital will also be important and scaling should be a consideration. For example, smaller hospitals will commence the response with a small team initially until it is reinforced. Certain tasks will be prioritized and this may require delegation or amalgamation. Until subordinates become available, the responsibility for certain tasks will go up a level to the next most senior individual. Similarly, there may be a need for 'acting up' from lower level until staff become available.

The key to success is that the hierarchy refers to tasks or roles rather than specific personalities. In HMIMMS terms, essential roles must be filled from the start then the additional roles (which are important but lower priority). The next priority will be services or roles which provide integral support

Medical hierarchy

The following roles make up the medical hierarchy. There are five roles that must be filled at the earliest opportunity:
• Medical coordinator (HCT)
• Senior emergency physician (HCT)
• Senior medical laboratory services officer (MLSO)
• Senior surgeon
• Senior physician.

Action cards will also be needed for radiographers and radiologists, laboratory services officers and consultants in laboratory specialties (biochemistry, transfusion, haematology), pharmacists, anaesthetists and intensive care consultants, surgeons tasked with preoperative assessment and selection, surgeons tasked with postoperative care, operative surgeons (a surgeon will also be tasked to coordinate each of these groups), surgical and medical staff for the minor injuries area, and paediatric specialist teams under an identified paediatric lead. The emergency department will need treatment teams and transfer teams, usually made up of anaesthetists, will also be required. Consultant physicians will oversee capacity creation by reviewing the bed state. In most cases, the emergency department action cards will be held in the department which will initiate its own call in cascade on declaration of a major incident.

Nursing hierarchy

There are six essential roles in the nursing hierarchy that must be filled:
• Senior nurse (HCT)
• Senior nurse emergency department
• Senior nurse wards
• Senior nurse ITU
• Senior nurse theatres
• Team coordinator emergency department.

Nurses will also need to be allocated to the triage area, priority 1 (resuscitation) and priority 2 areas in the emergency department and the priority 3 (minor injuries) area. In practice, this staffing will build on the staff available at the time of the declaration. Action cards must also allocate nursing staff to preoperative and postoperative areas and to the operating theatres and must ensure that appropriately skilled nurse are deployed to the right areas.

Other nursing roles include management and operation of discharge areas and admission wards, intensive care, paediatric services, and emergency department treatment teams. In some cases, roles may be allocated to operating department practitioners rather than nurses depending on local practice. To ensure appropriate prioritization, roles should be allocated to individual specialist groups numerically. Thus, for example, ACTION CARD THEATRE NURSE 1 will have essential immediate tasks and the importance of the tasks will reduce towards ACTION CARD THEATRE NURSE 16. Only tasks which are non-essential should be allocated to cards with a high number in the call-in sequence.

Management and support hierarchy

There are three essential roles that must be filled:
- Senior manager
- Senior porter
- Senior telephonist/communications.

Action cards will also be needed for press liaison staff, staff to handle enquiries, the volunteer coordinator and their staff, security, portering, catering, and transport services and supplies (including sterile supplies and linen). Engineering services will also be needed.

Personnel will also be required (and must therefore have action cards) to run the crèche, care for relatives, and provide pastoral and spiritual support. Others who will require action cards include medical photography, hospital radio (accurate and up-to-date information is important), and mortuary staff.

Declaration and activation

Standardized major incident messages are used to prepare and activate hospital responses. These are shown in Table 12.2. If an incident occurs on a scale requiring a hospital response, the decision to activate one or more hospitals will be made by the senior incident commander and passed onto designated healthcare responders. Messages will subsequently be delivered to the main hospital switchboard from emergency services control before cascading to the main HCT and then further cascaded according to the hospital plan.

Cascade

A cascade process will be initiated from switchboard to key individuals during which information will be passed on including the *incident location, type, time, and estimated number and severity of casualties*. The duty telephonists should begin by notifying key staff on site using pagers or mobile phones whilst informing pre-determined key individuals who are likely to be off-site. These individuals can then be tasked by their appropriate action cards to call in particular groups within their own areas of responsibility. Individuals who are off-site will generally activate their component of the cascade on arrival at hospital, but may be required to keep a copy of their action card at home and commence the cascade process before leaving for the hospital. In the majority of cases (e.g. the emergency department or laboratory facilities), as soon as the initial call has been received, the first action will be to summon assistance as indicated on the relevant action card. Ensuring that the cascade functions within pre-established areas of responsibility ensures that staff are familiar with those being called in and increases the likelihood of up-to-date information being available. Departments will be activated in order of priority with key receiving areas being informed first.

An effective cascade system relies on accurate personnel lists with regular testing of the system. The cascade system will usually involve landline or mobile telephone communications, but other less formal methods may include local media such as radio, television, or social media which may avoid overloading routine communication networks.

Called-in personnel should report to a pre-defined central major incident reporting area which should not be, or be close to, the emergency department. This area should have sufficient space to accommodate arriving personnel and be secure with access strictly limited to those holding hospital identification. The area must hold copies of all action cards in a way which allows staff to take either their specific card, or the next card in sequence for their operational group. In some cases, the plan may identify arrangements for certain groups of cards to be held in alternative locations (e.g. holding the emergency department cards in the emergency department), but this should be the exception rather than the rule to facilitate monitoring of the level of response at any given time. All arriving personnel should be signed in on reception, ID badges checked or temporary ID provided if necessary, and then released to attend their relevant departments.

Updates

As the at-scene response matures, further information will be provided to enable refinement of the hospital response and inform resource management. This may utilize direct communication with hospital emergency departments and/or control centres on a dedicated landline or via the *Airwave* network. A liaison function will be maintained between incident commanders and regional medical advisors, usually via ambulance services and MERIT practitioners.

Table 12.2 Standardized major incident messages

Major incident—standby	This alerts the hospital that a major incident is possibly imminent. A limited number staff needed to be informed
Major incident declared— activate plan	In this case the incident has occurred and the major incident plan must be activated
Major incident cancelled	This is used to cancel a standby call

Reception

The reception phase includes the initial triage of all arriving casualties, their assessment, and emergency treatment. Hospital areas involved in the reception phase must be prepared to manage the arriving casualty load for up to several hours in smaller incidents, up to several days in the most severe scenarios. To maximize use of space in the emergency department, the plan may allocate patient categorized as priority 3 to an alternative location with sufficient space such as the physiotherapy department or outpatients. In this case, stores of equipment for use in this area must be available and in date.

Following activation of the major incident plan, reception areas should be cleared of the existing (non-incident) patient load as much as it is possible and appropriate and safe to do so. Minor ailments and injuries could be redirected to primary care facilities or follow-up arranged in a relevant clinic. Patients with more serious conditions should be moved to a ward that is not designated to be involved in the response. Brief documentation should accompany such patients where possible.

The emergency department is the priority area to prepare for the arrival of the more seriously injured or unwell patients, with expansion into adjacent areas if needed. It is unlikely that most departments will have sufficient dedicated resuscitation room space in which to manage all the priority 1 casualties and plans should therefore consider reallocating the departmental *majors (medical) area* for the sickest patients.

The next highest priority areas include theatres and critical care areas. These should also assess current workload, capacity, and capability as a matter of urgency. The number of available ward beds must be determined and communicated to the hospital coordination cell. Systems for rapid and safe discharge with appropriate paperwork and medication must be in place.

The role of the triage officer is to ensure appropriate dispersal of the arriving patient load to the correct prepared area—the process of triage performed rapidly on arrival and the patient appropriately labelled and logged. Use of pre-determined major incident patient identification numbers is essential. Liaison with the hospital information centre is vital, as well as with the police-coordinated casualty bureau. Some new patient records may well require merging with their existing documentation later, therefore it is vital that patient details are carefully collected and recorded on arrival.

Emergency department staff will coordinate the formation of a number of treatment teams. Each one will include at least one doctor and one emergency nurse allocated by senior personnel. Care will then be provided to the highest priority cases first, based upon initial triage. One team will be required per P1 casualty, although one or two teams will usually be able to manage all P3 (minor) cases.

Mass casualty capacity planning

Acute providers will need to meet the following agreed requirements:
1. All hospitals should be able to enact rapid discharge processes to free up 20% of their total bed base over a period of up to 12 hours and ideally 10% within the first 4 hours.
2. Intensive Care Units should prepare to surge to double their normal Level 3 ventilated bed capacity, and maintain this for a minimum period of 96 hours.
3. Trauma Units should be ready to manage patients that they would usually treat and transfer, potentially for extended periods, along with preparing to receive additional repatriations from Trauma Centres, potentially across a wide geographical area.

Triage

The principles of triage are covered in detail in Chapter 5 on pp. 148–52.

Expectant category

Department of Health guidance states: 'in the event of demand for healthcare exceeding or overwhelming supply, the underlying principle is to achieve the best health outcomes based on the ability to achieve health benefits'. In other words, if it is not possible to treat everyone, treatment must be directed to those who are most likely to benefit from it. By extension, there will be some patients whose injuries or condition are so serious that it would be inappropriate to waste resources (both in terms of people and materiel) on them when such resources could be used to better effect elsewhere. These patients will receive expectant treatment. Protocols should be in place for co-locating these patients, keeping them comfortable and pain free, and ensuring their dignity. Ideally they should be managed by a senior clinician who fully understands the implications of the expectant category. There are likely to be significant psychological issues amongst both carers and relatives of patients.

Triage may use either the triage sieve or the triage sort. The triage sieve is more appropriate for the rapid assessment of patients on arrival in hospital, although the judgement of a senior experienced clinician is also of great value. Once the triage process has been completed, the patient should be labelled. A number of methods are available, but the most appropriate and most widely used is the cruciform triage card. The triage criteria may need to be adapted in special incidents such as those involving radiation (see pp. 302–3).

Resuscitation

The most critically ill or injured patients will require immediate life-saving intervention in the emergency department. Those who are less severely ill or injured will still require treatment and investigation, the components of which can be delayed until after admission to a ward. The majority of patients will require investigations including X-rays and scans and a significant proportion will require surgery. An essential component of this early phase of the response therefore is the relative prioritization of patients for investigation and surgery. This is especially important in the early stages of an incident when it is likely that theatre and imaging capacity will be limited pending the arrival of more staff. This is particularly likely to be the case *out of hours*. Decisions regarding priorities must be made by senior staff with the experience to estimate how long particular interventions are likely to take, the probability of them achieving the desired aim, and the necessity for any particular intervention at any given time. These decisions are best made in discussion between the senior emergency department clinician and the surgeon tasked with patient selection and preparation for theatre. Factors which will influence the order of surgical intervention include the number and severity of patients, the operative time for each procedure, and the availability of theatres, theatre staff (operating department practitioners, surgeons, anaesthetists, specialist surgeons, and nurses), sterile supplies, and specialist equipment. Intensive care capacity after surgery is completed must also be considered.

Surgical care

Once patients requiring immediate life-saving surgery and critical care have been identified, they can be relocated to the appropriate area. Those requiring surgery at a later date will be admitted to a designated major incident surgical admissions ward. The admissions ward will have been cleared first, if necessary by immediate movement of patients to beds elsewhere. The overall control of the surgical process requires effective management by a senior surgeon and effective liaison with surgeons and teams in the pre-op and theatre areas as well as intensive care and designated postoperative wards.

Theatre availability must be assessed by a senior surgeon and the senior nurse for theatres and must include existing and planned surgical care which may need to be abandoned or cancelled. Surgical teams should be formed with surgical and anaesthetic staff of the highest training grade available.

In the longer term, planning will be needed to incorporate the ongoing surgical workload arising from the incident into normal business with the minimum disruption. This may be a role for the hospital trauma coordinator.

Non-surgical (medical) care

A similar approach is required in prioritizing patients for higher-level care (intensive care or high-dependency care) and general ward care. Not all casualties involved in a major incident will arrive with conditions directly attributable to the incident—some may have conditions precipitated or exacerbated by their circumstances. Some of those presenting to the emergency department may also be uninvolved in the incident itself. Plans should take into account the management of such patients and they should receive the same documentation and follow the same casualty flow as those directly involved.

Actual and potential bed availability will need to be assessed; this will usually be the responsibility of the senior coordinator working with the senior physician. A rapid bed-state assessment will be included as a priority tasking on a senior nurse manager's action card. Assessing critical care bed availability will be the responsibility of the senior intensivist and senior nurse on ITU. The majority of hospitals will be unable to accommodate all patients requiring critical care beds and early consideration must therefore be given to the possible transfer of some patients to other units. Selection of patients for limited critical care beds will also require liaison with the senior surgeon and theatre teams. Clinical and non-clinical support services will also be vital components of the in-patient phase of the plan and have appropriate action cards which reflect this.

Forensic considerations

It is possible in the event of a terrorist incident that the perpetrators will be brought to hospital having been injured, and possibly masquerading as innocent victims. They may as a result present a security risk to staff and other patients and security advice from the police should be carefully followed. Similarly, suspicious behaviour by any victim should be immediately reported. Criminal or civil legal proceedings are likely after any major incident and whilst forensic considerations must never hamper the treatment of patients, neither should thoughtless actions by clinicians threaten successful completion of the legal process. All health service staff should follow instructions given to them by police officers, especially following the preservation of evidence, and wherever possible discarded clothing and other items should not be mixed up with those from other patients, but bagged, labelled, and where possible handed to a police officer. Similarly, extrinsic material may be removed at operation and must also be appropriately labelled and saved for forensic purposes. The chain of evidence must be maintained and appropriate documentation completed (see Chapter 8, p. 244).

Recovery/business continuity

From the hospital perspective, there are three elements to the recovery phase of a major incident:
- *resolution* (restoration of normal activity)
- *reflection* (including debriefing)
- *lessons* learnt (audit).

Business continuity is the process by which the normal day-to-day activity of the hospital is carried on after the incident with minimal disruption due to a wide range of factors (see Box 12.8). Some of these factors can be reduced by careful planning before and during the incident itself.

Some, but not all, of these factors can be ameliorated by ensuring that plans are in place for the recovery period of an incident before the incident occurs. Most post-incident problems, although not necessarily their magnitude, can be predicted.

Business continuity

In very large incidents, incidents which are prolonged, or incidents with long-term effects on the ongoing activity of the trust, a *business continuity control team* may be established. Consisting, like the HCT, of senior managers, clinicians, and nurses, the business continuity control team is charged with managing the transition from the emergency period to the full return to normal functions.

Key tasks will include:
- management of the return to normal elective activity
- assessment of the impact of the incident on central performance targets
- communication with patients affected by the incident, for example, by having elective procedures cancelled
- maintaining adequate staffing levels in the transitional period
- quantifying the ongoing surgical and ITU load arising from the incident
- monitoring the impact of major incident patients on the bed state
- ensuring staff welfare
- maintaining adequate supplies of equipment and consumables
- auditing and reporting the incident
- cooperating with and assisting any post-incident reviews or enquiries.

Box 12.8 Potential factors affecting business continuity

- Bed occupancy by incident victims
- Non-availability of operating theatres due to incident-related workload
- Non-availability of ITU beds
- Retrieval of patients transferred to other hospitals
- Out-patient review and management of incident victims
- Shortage of blood products
- Shortage of specialist surgical and other equipment
- Management of large amounts of incident-related patient data
- Centrally imposed performance targets
- Non-availability of staff recovering after prolonged working periods
- Psychological effects on staff
- Decontamination (CBRN incidents)
- Screening of staff (CBRN incidents).

Post-incident recovery

The key feature of recovery is that relevant issues must be considered from the beginning of the response and be part of a proactive agenda, along with all components of business continuity in general.

There are three main stages to the recovery phase: resolution, reflection, and audit.

Resolution

During the resolution phase, restoration of normal services occurs. The management group set up to direct this phase of the response to an incident must ensure that appropriate priorities are followed when returning services to normal (e.g. cancer surgery) and must ensure that those affected are kept informed. A *template* for the recovery period should be in place before an incident occurs and forms an important part of the major incident plan. Like the remainder of the plan it should be regularly reviewed and updated. Essential aspects of recovery include post-incident staffing levels, need for further surgical procedures, general and critical care bed occupancy by major incident patients, and equipment resupply.

Reflection

The reflection phase will involve staff operational debriefs which should not be confused with post-incident support for casualties and relatives. The effectiveness of the site plan, conduct of operative and critical care interventions, and medical care provided will need to be audited and any lessons learnt. The indiscriminate use of *trained counsellors* is as likely to cause harm as benefit. Such interventions are important but need to be focused appropriately and delivered by skilled and experienced practitioners. In practice, visible support and thanks from managers and leaders at all levels and informal *talking* in a social environment with colleagues who trust each other are powerful ways of reducing the mental health effects of a major incident.

Staff require immediate formal operational debrief by heads of department—individual or group as appropriate are important before lessons are forgotten. These are not counselling sessions, nor are they for apportioning blame or responsibility. All who have managerial responsibility for others should remain vigilant for signs of stress and difficulty coping following an incident and should make it absolutely transparent that no blame attaches to such individuals who should be encouraged to come forward.

A number of individuals and groups will be able to offer support to patients. These include social workers, chaplains and faith groups, psychologists and liaison psychiatry services, and members of charitable support groups established by patients. Support from other patients with similar experiences should be facilitated and encouraged and may lead to long-term engagement through survivor or victim groups. Such groups may also act as a focus for appropriate claims for compensation. Patients who are discharged should be followed up and counselling offered. Leaflets should be handed out to provide appropriate advice and post-incident support, including relevant contact telephone numbers. Social workers will usually coordinate out-of-hospital support services.

Audit

A robust post-incident audit process is essential as an opportunity to assess the management of the incident and improve future practice. Elements of this include thorough debrief as part of the reflection of the hospital's ability to cope with the incident. It should be noted that no response can ever be perfect and that recognizing where improvements could be made should be expected and taken as constructive and positive learning. The review should not concentrate on clinical care alone and must include all those involved in the incident response (see Figure 12.2).

Ideally, the audit process should take place within 1 month of the incident occurring. Each department should be required to produce a post-incident report. Liaison with other relevant agencies and responder organizations is essential in order to share learning points. The key tenets of the audit approach are independence, openness, and an explicitly *blame-free* culture of shared learning.

As a fortunately rare event, the results of the reflection and audit following major incidents should offer an opportunity to disseminate learning points at a national level. However, care should be taken not to make significant material changes to existing plans to cope with specific peculiarities of the last incident as the next incident is likely to be very different. Changes should therefore be more generic—concentrating on the common aspects of communication, organization, and hierarchy structure maintaining an all-hazard approach.

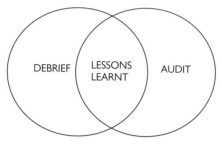

Fig. 12.2 The components of reflection.

Special incidents

Hazardous materials (CBRN)

A full description of the response to CBRN incidents is given in Chapters 8–10. Incidents arising from the irradiation of victims offer few serious organizational challenges. Chemical incidents are effectively managed and controlled by implementation of decontamination processes and restriction of access to healthcare areas until decontamination is complete. More complex measures will be required for those who have been contaminated by radioactive material, but it should be remembered that simple procedures, if followed correctly, will contain and minimize the risks to staff and patients alike. Processes for the disposal of waste must be in place and the responsibility for carrying out such disposal clearly established. By their very nature, biological incidents are unlikely to present in the manner of a conventional major incident, and will usually take the form of gradually increasing numbers of patients presenting with a familiar or unfamiliar set of symptoms. Management of these incidents is based on disease control and expert assistance in order to support victims and protect staff. Relationships with organizations such as PHE must be in place and functional. Staff should work in teams and leadership should be clear and confident. Hospitals must ensure that all equipment (including PPE and radiation monitoring) is functioning and in known locations and staff know how to use it.

The initial response at hospital to an incident involving contamination

All acute hospitals should have plans in place to manage potentially contaminated casualties. Advance warning of an incident may be available from the emergency services or may be given by the appearance of a chemical plume, depending on how close the incident is and its nature. Alternatively, casualties may start to present without warning individually or in small groups. Once it is decided that an incident involving contamination is or might be in progress, the following actions should be taken:

- Contaminated casualties who have entered the waiting room should be removed to outside the hospital.
- Contaminated casualties who present should be refused admission to the building and the doors closed to all but emergent cases.
- Contaminated casualties should be directed outside the building to decontamination facilities or instructed to wait until such facilities are available.
- A safe location should be identified for the initial minimal treatment of casualties during decontamination.
- Non-urgent patients should be asked to leave the department via an alternative route.
- Potentially contaminated casualties already in the department and who cannot be removed safely should be decontaminated and the time spent with them by individual staff limited on a rotating basis.
- The hospital plan should be activated.
- Appropriate protective clothing should be donned.
- Expert advice should be sought from the appropriate authorities.

The normal paradigm of triage, treatment, and transport remains extant. The main differences lie with the addition of a decontamination step during triage; this may include use of a self-decontamination area for walking (P3) cases at, or after, leaving the scene. The rinse–wipe–rinse procedure is the key method for casualty decontamination involving cutting off or removal of clothing. Further information regarding decontamination is given in Chapter 5 (pp. 156–9).

During decontamination, the only potentially life-saving interventions that can be offered are catastrophic haemorrhage control, airway opening manoeuvres, C-spine immobilization, and hand BVM ventilation. Advanced care will need to wait until after decontamination once in the semi-permissive ('warm') zone. Specific therapeutic interventions such as chemical antidotes will rely upon identification of the agent, or agents, involved. The use of toxidromes may help to guide treatment depending on symptoms and clinical signs.

Transport of CBRN casualties represents a significant challenge and a risk to staff that must be mitigated as much as possible. Appropriate respiratory protection and separation between patient and driver and responder compartments are essential. Ambulances leaving the scene of an incident may themselves become contaminated and therefore necessitate the use of both clean and dirty circuits at the receiving hospital site. Staff working at the clean–dirty line must be adequately protected.

The post-incident debrief process will need to take into account any perceived or real long-term post-exposure risks to staff and the local population and may involve specific counselling and physical follow-up. Written information can be particularly helpful. The lead agency for this will usually be the local occupational health department for staff, and PHE for patients.

Multiple burns casualties

Major incidents involving large numbers of burns may rapidly overwhelm available services resulting in a state of decompensation. The UK NHS capability to manage burns is divided into three tiers:

- *Burn facilities* provide acute care for people with less complex burns and are a component of a broader plastic surgery service. More complex patients are referred to burn units and centres. Burn facilities will be involved in the rehabilitation of patients with more complex burns from their catchment area.
- *Burn units* provide care for patients with moderate burns. These services can treat a broader range of more serious burns than *burns facilities* and can provide critical care for burns patients.
- *Burn centres* provide care for patients with the most severe or complex injuries and for those requiring the highest level of specialist critical care.

The majority of ITU capacity inevitably consists of general ITU beds co-located within a burns unit or centre. As ITU bed occupancy is routinely high, there is often little spare capacity to cope with a large-scale incident. The establishment of major trauma centres means that severe burns casualties are likely to go directly to such hospitals.

The Bradford stadium fire, 1985: an example of a major incident involving multiple burns

The Bradford City stadium fire on 11 May 1985 was the worst fire disaster in the history of English football. The fire resulted in the death of 56 fans with injuries occurring in over 250 more.

Legacy

The Bradford Burns Unit was set up by Professor David Sharpe after he received many of the victims following the fire. During the initial hospital response they were reportedly able to gain the assistance of around 10% of the UK's plastic surgeons. Treatment was required for the injuries of over 200 individuals, with many experimental treatments being used. On the 25th anniversary of the fire, the University of Bradford established the UK's largest academic research centre in skin sciences as an extension to its plastic surgery and burns research unit.

The complexity of care for burns requires careful coordination and cooperation between multiple specialities and support services. Preparation for such incidents is essential. Amongst the factors which planners should consider when planning the response to a major incident involving burns include:

- up-to-date knowledge of the location and capacity of nearby burns facilities
- details of mechanisms for identifying the location of available capacity
- the need for a robust activation process which identifies and mobilizes all those with specialist expertise
- local burns incident notification procedures.

Assessment of burn size or complexity is best undertaken by those with appropriate training and experience, such as plastic surgeons or senior emergency department staff; however, there are several validated methods of estimating burn surface area available such as Lund and Browder charts, rule-of-nines, or hand count.

Systems should also be in place for the formation of burns transfer teams in the event of transfer to higher and often distant echelons of care being needed. Specialist equipment needed for the initial management of burns casualties will include cooling dressings, cling film, burns area calculators, and fluid calculators. Additional specific training for severe burns management should be undertaken by emergency department staff wherever possible. Burns-specific triage should also be incorporated into generic skills as well as pre-hospital staff training. Specific action cards should be produced to guide the process.

Planning

Emergency planning should take into account direct transfer algorithms which should be implemented where possible. The receiving unit must always be contacted before secondary transfer is considered and the duration of the transfer must be taken into account, especially in the critically ill. In addition, each transfer is likely to occupy staff and vehicles for a prolonged period. Reception of burns patients should be controlled locally by the senior emergency physician and also coordinated at a regional level by the burns coordinator at the burns centre (this may be co-located with the receiving hospital). Ideally, staff experienced in burns triage or with burns experience should be utilized to assess patients on arrival and make important early decisions such as identification of patients for whom there is no chance of survival. In extreme cases, the receiving hospital (if not a burns unit or centre) may be supported by a visiting *burns assessment team* (BAT). Secondary transfer is likely from non-specialist to specialist units for onward burns care and rehabilitation in the longer term. Close liaison will be required between units, ideally coordinated by the BAT.

More than one tertiary unit is likely to be required to manage a significant incident involving serious burns. Specialist units should be prepared to expand facilities via local measures to manage the expected or predicted patient load. A high level of coordination will be required to ensure that effective mutual support can be provided through complementary arrangements. Burns incidents can have significant long-term consequences including increased requirements for operative time, rehabilitation, and psychological support services as well as limiting the already limited specialist burns capacity.

Multiple paediatric casualties

The prospect of dealing with a major incident which results in large numbers of seriously injured children is daunting and offers particular emotional challenges. Such events do occur rather more frequently than might be thought, often in the context of travel or education. There are clearly practical and humanitarian reasons to remove children from the scene at as early a stage as possible; however, in incidents involving a large number of children, the at-scene response is likely to suffer from a degree of over-triage leading to a failure of effective prioritization.

Particular challenges of a paediatric incident include effective triage, since the normal values have to be altered and maintaining perspective can be difficult when dealing with distressed children. In addition, it may be difficult to mobilize sufficient staff who are experienced in, and comfortable with, managing children. Although emergency department staff are usually familiar with the management of young patients, this is unlikely to be the case with the majority of medical and surgical specialities. It is common practice in many centres to refer all children requiring surgery to a specialist centre, but this luxury may not be available during a major incident. In many areas, paediatric capability is not co-located with general accident and emergency facilities. In addition, the availability of paediatric intensive care beds is likely to be limited and hospitals must also ensure that they have sufficient supplies of paediatric equipment to be able to cope in the event of an incident involving large numbers of children. Inevitably in these incidents, hospitals will have to manage the needs of distressed relatives and the media interest will be magnified.

The considerations discussed above mean that inevitably any incident involving a large number of children is likely to require a regional or multiregional response. Effective mechanisms must therefore be in place in order to pre-alert both general and specialist centres to initiate an effective response. This will require close liaison between pre-hospital, primary receiving hospitals, and specialist children's facilities. This will ideally be coordinated by a strategic-level medical incident advisor ensuring regular communication with the medical advisor at tactical (silver) command level. When a major incident is declared involving children, it is essential that the HCT makes an early and thorough assessment of the capacity to deal with the expected number of paediatric casualties. The appointment of a senior paediatrician can help ensure that the response is appropriately configured. The senior paediatrician will be tasked by a specific action card.

Where on-site or local paediatric support is limited, the mobilization of a *paediatric assessment team* (PAT) from a specialist centre may be considered to support the receiving hospital in the initial triage, treatment, and prioritization for transfer of casualties. Membership of the PAT is usually based around the typical PICU retrieval team. A significant level of coordination is likely to be required to ensure the most appropriate use of limited critical care resources, utilization of specialist care beds, and paediatric surgical expertise. Action cards should be produced for all members of the PAT as well as for specialist paediatric staff within the hospital, allowing them to offer support to those with less experience.

Post-Incident Recovery and Business Continuity

Introduction

The most obvious effects of a major incident are those which arise directly from it, most obviously the casualties. However, depending on the nature and magnitude of the incident, the effects are almost certainly going to be far greater and more prolonged than the initial response might suggest. In some cases, the medium- and short-term effects may be widespread across areas from healthcare, through destruction of buildings to transport disruption, in others, the problems may be restricted to a single agency, small geographic area, or relatively small aspect of life. Whatever the case, the recovery period must be managed to deal with the effects and aftermath of an incident as efficiently and quickly as possible whilst maintaining normal activities, rebuilding infrastructure, and minimizing disruption to individuals and organizations. Needless to say, such aims cannot be achieved by improvisation after the event. In addition, an important component of any recovery process will be a detailed, structured review of the incident and the response to it in order to improve responses in the future.

A major incident will affect those directly involved, emergency responders individually and as organizations, witnesses, the community, businesses, physical and organizational infrastructure (including travel and the health services), and the environment. An effective plan will recognize the involvement of all these individuals and groups and address their needs in an appropriate manner. Some of the bodies involved in an effective recovery plan are likely to be quite surprising, including such organizations as tourist boards, heritage bodies, highly specialist technical companies, and insurance providers.

Recovery is defined in UK Emergency Response and Recovery (EPRR) guidance as:

> 'the process of rebuilding, restoring and rehabilitating the community following an emergency'.

The recovery process

The recovery process following a major incident will be complex and usually prolonged, and importantly will take place observed by the media and the general public. As a result, there is considerable potential for criticism by experts (of varying degrees of insight), politicians, and, later, public and judicial enquiries. In addition, historically, allocation of responsibilities during the recovery period has been less clearly understood than during the initial response phase. These factors, combined with the disruptive effects of a major incident, mean that considerable attention *must* be paid to the recovery process by planners and responders before an incident occurs.

The recovery of a community will occur across four domains:
- humanitarian and health
- the economy
- infrastructure
- the environment.

Examples of problems in these domains are given in Box 13.1, p. 379. In addition some issues may involve more than one domain.

In order to achieve effective recovery, the community affected must be involved and active engagement will be required not only from government (local and national) and the emergency services and statutory bodies, but from charities, community groups, and the private sector. Like every other aspect of major incident management, recovery must be practised. Like justice, the recovery process must not only be done, but be seen to be done.

The recovery process must begin as soon as the emergency begins with the formation of a *Recovery Coordinating Group* (RCG) working alongside the SCG (see p. 382–3).

General aspects of effective recovery

In addition to humanitarian, environmental, infrastructure, and economic issues, there are a number of less specific issues which are nevertheless essential components of an effective recovery process and which must be included in the planning process. These include multiagency collaboration, working with the media (including the social media), ensuring community engagement and cooperation, managing the impact on established performance targets, and preparing for future coroner's enquiries, criminal proceedings, and official enquiries. Attention must also be paid to identifying and learning lessons for the future which can then be incorporated into the planning process.

Box 13.1 Aspects of community recovery: the following issues will require a prompt effective and sensitive response

Humanitarian and health issues
- Physical injury and death
- Psychological effects
- Social needs (shelter, food, financial support, access to services)
- Evacuation from harm and return.

Economic issues
- Physical damage to business premises
- Disruption of essential supporting infrastructure
- Disruption of labour provision or changes in behaviour.

Infrastructure
- Disruption to travel systems, financial systems, communications
- Damage to buildings—stations, schools, hospitals, etc.
- Relocation of workforce
- Damage or interruption to utilities or services
- Breakdown of law and order.

Environment
- Pollution and decontamination (environmental and water supplies)
- Disposal of waste
- Exclusion zones (e.g. following a CBRN incident)
- Damage to natural habitats and agriculture.

Organization of the recovery process

The recovery component of major incident planning is managed, like other components, through the LRF and the local authority is the responsible agency, just as it is for managing the response phase once an incident has occurred. Planning must include all the necessary agencies and is likely to be complex, requiring effective interagency cooperation.

The local authority will chair and provide the secretariat for the RCG. When an incident crosses local authority boundaries, but remains within the area of one LRF, consideration may be given to establishing more than one RCG (in each authority), although this is not ideal and a single RCG is preferred, planning having previously identified the lead local authority were such an incident to occur. In the event of an incident crossing LRF boundaries, establishment of a multi-LRF RCG should be considered. The lead government department (LGD) will be determined by the Civil Contingencies Secretariat at the Cabinet Office based on the nature of the incident and the Department for Communities and Local Government Resilience and Emergencies Division (DCLG RED) will coordinate communication between central and local governments. Like the SCG, the RCG will have access to the Scientific and Technical Advice Cell (STAC). The effectiveness of the recovery process will be greatly enhanced if the affected community is actively involved and consideration should be given to formation of a *Community Recovery Committee* (CRC).

Community recovery committees

A community recovery committee (CRC) may be established to assist in reflecting the views and priorities of the community and keeping it informed of progress in dealing with the emergency. By involving the community in the recovery process, individuals are empowered and hopefully feel less that they are the passive victims of what has happened. The CRC also allows passage of concerns to agencies and organizations involved in recovery and may allow plans to reflect community wishes regarding post-incident regeneration and mitigation of possible future problems.

Membership of the CRC will include representatives of local government (structures will vary with location), residents or tenants associations, schools, businesses, community groups (including faith communities), and of the RCG.

In some circumstances, a charitable *disaster fund* may be established, in which case the fund manager may sit on the CRC. This appeal may be coordinated by the local authority or through an established charity.

Structure and function of the Recovery Coordinating Group

The Recovery Coordinating Group (RCG), as well as having access to the STAC and SCG will have a number of working groups. These are likely to include communications and media, environment, infrastructure, economic and business, health and welfare, and community recovery. Finance and legal aspects will also need attention (see p. 383).

The recovery plan following any incident will begin with an assessment of the impact of what has occurred, often in conjunction with the SCG and a priority profile for restoration of normal function. The utilities and transport are likely to be most important in terms of community recovery. Targets times or dates for specific aspects of recovery should be agreed between agencies. In some cases, the opportunities offered by the recovery process may facilitate previous plans for regeneration and redevelopment and the appropriate authorities and groups will need to be involved in the process. An agreed *end state* for the recovery process should also be agreed. Similarly, as in the case of post-flood recovery, for example, measures are likely to be included which will reduce vulnerability and increase resilience in the event of further similar incidents in at-risk areas. Recovery is an expense process and careful financial planning and budgeting will be required.

Suggested membership of a Recovery Coordinating Group

Representatives from:
- local government
- chairs of RCG subcommittees
- chair of STAC
- chair of CRC (if established)
- health sector
- Environment Agency
- social services
- Public Health England (or equivalent)
- utility and transport companies and providers
- emergency services
- voluntary organizations
- Health and Safety Executive.

This list is not exhaustive: other members might include, as appropriate, representatives of the Ministry of Defence, Animal Health Agencies, Maritime and Coast Guard Agency, Natural England, Government Decontamination Service, and tourist boards.

Where possible, the RCG should be co-located with the SCG, at least in the early stages, as this will facilitate passage of information and coordinated decision-making. As the recovery progresses, organizations and individuals will usually work from their normal locations, meeting to coordinate activity. If the strategic coordination centre becomes unavailable, local authority accommodation is usually found for the RCG. Coordination meetings will become less frequent with time, but initially are likely to occur several times a day.

Recovery Coordinating Group subgroups

The subgroups of the RCG will depend to some extent on the nature of the incident. However, the following groups will usually be established.

Health and welfare

Chaired by the director of public health or local authority head of adult social care, this subgroup is responsible for all aspects of health and welfare including public health, health provision continuity, health data collection, resource allocation (and requests for assistance), provision of shelter and care for evacuees, education, social benefits, and mental health issues. Membership consists of the appropriate health sector and public and private social care and charitable bodies.

Business and economy

The business and economy subgroup supports the local business community and is responsible for devising a recovery plan which minimizes adverse economic effects as well as working towards long-term strategic and regeneration objectives. The chair is usually an appropriate senior civil servant from local government. Areas of responsibility for this group include impacts on employment, industry, retail and tourism, grant support, rate and rent rebates, compensation, and infrastructure including utilities and transport. Suggested membership is given in Box 13.2.

Environment and infrastructure

This subgroup is responsible for setting targets for decontaminating or restoring the built or natural environment. The chair is provided by the local authority and members will include representatives from public health, environmental, heritage and tourist bodies, utility and transport providers, for both humans and animals.

Communications

Arrangements for ensuring effective and consistent communications will have been established early in the response to a major incident, and the same group may continue responsibility, possibly in a modified form, throughout the recovery process. The *communications subgroup* must ensure that messages are clear and consistent and that the public is fully and appropriately informed. A clear communications strategy must be determined and this subgroup will oversee the communications outputs of the other subgroups, each of which should appoint a communications lead. The chair will be a senior civil servant with a background in public relations and communications.

Finance and legal

The finance and legal subgroup must assess the financial and legal consequences of the incident, monitoring expenditure and informing the RCG. It should also identify potential sources of funding as well as maintaining an overview of any likely legal, public, or criminal enquiries or prosecutions and providing expert legal advice to the RCG. Possible financial issues include loss of income from rates or council tax, costs of social services provision or shelter, loss of income from disrupted businesses, uninsured losses, compensation, and legal fees.

Box 13.2 Membership of business and economic recovery subgroup

- Health services representatives
- The emergency services
- The Government Decontamination Service and other agencies will attend as appropriate
- Local government
- National government (if required)
- Business community (including chambers of commerce, trade bodies, and local and national government agencies dealing with business and development)
- Trade associations
- Trades unions
- Employment bodies
- Tourist boards and heritage agencies
- Representatives of the insurance industry (Association of British Insurers (ABI)).

Agency roles

The roles of the major bodies and agencies in recovery from a major incident are listed in Table 13.1 p. 385.

The role of the local authority

The local authority plays the lead role in coordinating the recovery from a major incident and will be responsible for delivering significant areas of the recovery process. In addition, it will provide the chairs and secretariat for the RCG and the majority of subgroups. It will also act as the link between agencies involved in the response and the affected communities, working closely with community, charitable, and other groups to promote recovery and ensure that the public remains informed. Other tasks will include managing disruption to education and other social services, environmental health advice (including waste management), providing humanitarian assistance and shelter if necessary, working to promote restoration of utilities and other services, as well as arranging VIP visits. If VIP visits occur, individuals concerned who might wish to make a statement must be briefed in detail to avoid error.

Table 13.1 Organizations and their role in recovery

Organization, provider, or public body	Role(s) in the recovery process
Fire and rescue	Search and rescue (inland) Access to hazardous areas Provision of equipment and manpower Advice
Police	Ensure RCG is convened (as lead for immediate response) Investigate criminal activity Maintain law and order (prevent looting) Control access Coordinate procedures for dealing with fatalities
NHS	Provide and coordinate primary and secondary care (including maintenance of business continuity) Care for victims, relatives, and the displaced Provision of countermeasures such as vaccines or antidotes Ensure long-term screening where appropriate
Public Health England	Health protection Management of infectious disease and CBRN contamination incidents Provision of expert advice
Health and Safety Executive	Assurance of safety in the workplace and investigation of suspected reaches of guidance or legislation
Animal health agencies (see pp. 166–9)	Prevention management and investigation of animal disease outbreaks Safeguarding public from animal-borne disease Ensuring food production standards (dairy and eggs)
Defra	Safeguard animal welfare Minimize effects on food production and farming
Environment Agency	Lead agency for pollution of the environment Investigation of offences connected to the environment Hazardous waste disposal (including CBRN removal and decontamination)
Food Standards Agency (FSA)	Ensuring food safety Disposal of food unfit to eat
Met Office	Weather forecasts and warnings
Business organizations	Employment, health and safety, grants, IT, tax, sales and marketing, and HR advice Insurance and legal advice Business helplines
Insurance industry	Advice regarding insurance cover Cooperation with the emergency services
Charities	Advice on financial, legal, and social problems (Citizens' Advice Bureau and others) Transport Communications (RAYNET and others) Medical and first aid provision (voluntary aid societies and others)
Faith groups	Provision of spiritual and social support Assistance to the bereaved Hospital chaplaincy

Handover from response to recovery

The handover from the *response phase* to the *recovery phase* of a major incident is an important milestone and a formal process should be followed once set criteria agreed by the SCG and RCG are achieved. At this point, overall control passes from the SCG which is usually chaired by the police to the RCG which is usually chaired by the local authority who will appoint a *senior recovery officer* to manage the recovery process.

End of recovery process

The chair of the RCG will decide when there is no longer any requirement for interagency cooperation and coordination and remaining issues can be managed by individual agencies. This decision will be made in consultation with the all RCG members. This decision will be communicated to other agencies by the RCG chair or secretariat. In some cases, long-term issues such as environmental contamination or health effects will continue to be monitored by individual agencies.

Funding the recovery process

The majority of costs of recovery will fall on local government, individual agencies, and services and commercial providers such as utility companies. The *Bellwin Scheme* (see pp. 94–5) provides financial support to local authorities and other agencies to assist with costs as a result of *immediate actions* to save life and property or to prevent suffering or severe inconvenience, and is not therefore available for assistance with funding the recovery process. Nevertheless, central government funding may be available to assist agencies with the costs of the recovery process. If the incident is of sufficient magnitude to warrant central funding support, this will be provided by the government department responsible for the sector in which the expenditure falls (*Department for Transport* for roads, *Department of the Environment* for contamination) and not with the LGD. Government departments will not pay for costs which are insurable and funding is at ministerial discretion. Decisions regarding granting of central funding will be taken on the basis of an impact assessment across the domains of health, social-economic, and environmental impacts.

European Union Solidarity Fund

The European Union Solidarity Fund (EUSF) offers financial assistance following major disasters where no other funding is available and can be used to support restoration of infrastructure (including utilities and transport, although costs will usually fall on commercial providers), accommodation for the displaced or homeless, rescue, maintenance of infrastructure designed to mitigate effects, protecting buildings and artefacts of cultural importance, and immediate clear up following the incident. To be eligible for assistance under EUSF, the total cost of the damage must exceed 3.2 billion euros or 0.6% of the applying country's gross national income. If the threshold is exceeded, payment is triggered at 6% of the cost over the threshold and 2.5% of the cost under the threshold.

Identifying lessons from a major incident

The term debriefing has, unfortunately, become associated with psychological debriefing, and as a consequence it is better, for the avoidance of confusion, to refer to identifying lessons learnt from all stages of a major incident and its response. In order to learn the most from an incident, it is essential that representatives from affected communities and groups are involved in the process.

The process of learning lessons does not start once the incident is over, although for obvious reasons, more time and resources will be available at this stage. Lessons should be learnt (and recorded) as the response proceeds and this element should be built into plans. Each organization will be responsible for lessons within its own operational area, but forums for interagency review must be established. Lessons of national significance can be circulated via DCLG RED or the LGD to the Cabinet Secretariat who will ensure transmission to appropriate agencies and departments. More locally, the LRF is responsible for ensuring that lessons learnt are incorporated into future policies and practice. Educational case studies can be submitted for wider dissemination through the UK Government resilience website.

Business continuity

Business continuity means that normal services and structures continue to function with as little interruption as possible over as short a period as possible after a major incident. Business continuity is therefore a key component of recovery which runs through the activities of all the groups discussed in this chapter. All public bodies and businesses must have a continuity plan in place should an incident occur and the CCA requires Category 1 responders to maintain plans to ensure that they can continue to exercise their functions in the event of an emergency. Such plans should focus on maintaining the core (essential) functions of the organization, detailing timelines for the recovery of these functions and the equipment, manpower, and arrangements necessary to restore them. The potential impact of disruptions to core functions should also be assessed and plans put in place for mitigation. The location of an incident response control room should be identified and those who will man it identified and trained.

Like all aspects of major incident response, *business continuity planning* (BCP) requires regular practice. Local authorities are required under the CCA to provide advice and assistance to the business community and charities in their areas in relation to *business continuity management* (BCM) during an emergency, and must therefore be actively engaged in planning such continuity before an incident occurs; however, they may seek to recover costs for providing this service. In some areas, a *business continuity forum* may be established which will improve links between the LRF and the commercial sector. Each of the emergency services will provide advice to the commercial sector within its own area of responsibility, for example the police for crime prevention, the fire service for fire safety. Organizations such as the *Confederation of British Industry* (CBI), the *British Chambers of Commerce,* the *Confederation of Small Businesses* and the *Councils for Voluntary Service* (CVS) should all be actively engaged in promoting BCM.

The stages of a business continuity management strategy

Active engagement in the process at senior level
- Leadership—appoint a BCM lead.

Understanding the organization's key outputs (products and services) essential activities, statutory duties, and essential resources
- What are the consequences of failure in these areas over set timescales?
- In each area, how long can failure be accepted?
- Perform a *business impact analysis* (BIA)

Determining a BCM strategy based on an understanding of the organization
- What do we want to achieve?
- Areas to be considered include personnel, premises, technology including IT, information supplies, and stakeholders.

Developing a BCM plan
- How do we achieve it?
- May include details of staff responsibilities, rotas and tasking, prioritization of functions, required external services (including contractors), recovery timetables, public information, and media handling

Exercise, maintain, and review plans
- Tabletop exercises, discussions, and formal exercises.

Ensure that BCM plans are embedded at all levels of the organization:
- Training, information, and implementing change.

Disaster Action

Disaster Action is a registered charity, founded in 1991 by survivors and the bereaved from a number of incidents, which offers support to those affected by disasters, raises awareness of the needs of victims, and promotes measures designed to reduce the likelihood of further incidents. It provides a useful source of advice to agencies involved in disaster planning and response and further information is available at the http://www.disasteraction.org.uk website.

Humanitarian consequences of a major incident

A key component of effective recovery is providing appropriate support to victims and their relatives whilst normality is re-established. This may require the provision of first shelter, then emergency housing for prolonged periods, but also includes medical and psychological support and social support. Financial and legal help may be required, the latter particularly during any coronial or legal process. Advice regarding sources of help and assistance will also be required. Members of affected communities must be kept informed at all times, especially regarding the progress of the recovery effort and facilities should be made available for community members to meet and exchange experiences and offers of assistance. Local authorities are required to assess individuals and arrange care services for those entitled to them. Establishing a public telephone helpline and use of social media and the Internet all have a role to play in supporting the community.

The provision of accommodation in the longer term for those made homeless by a major incident is a statutory responsibility of the local authority, under the *Housing Act 1966*, although many people will prefer to seek shelter with friends or family, or accommodation funded through insurance. In the short term, after the closure of any temporary onsite facility, use is made, where necessary, of bed and breakfast and hotel accommodation. Arrangements for providing support to the friends and family of the deceased are the responsibility of the police through family liaison officers, although charities, faith groups, and other bodies may also be involved.

Consideration should be given to the establishment of a *humanitarian assistance centre* (HAC) as a focal point for provision of assistance, support, and information to survivors, relatives, and community members alike. The HAC may also facilitate the gathering of forensic samples and information from those involved in the incident. The local authority will lead in the establishment of an HAC in conjunction with the police, and is specifically responsible for identifying suitable premises. A *community assistance centre* (CAC) may also be established as a focal point for community engagement and support. The decision to set up an HAC is usually made by the SCG. Once the SCG has been stood down, an *HAC management group* (HACMG) usually chaired by the local authority director of adult or children's social services will normally take over. When the RWG decides to close the HAC, the local authority and other bodies must have alternative arrangements in place.

The number of organizations which might be represented at the HAC is considerable: examples include the *Foreign and Commonwealth Office* (if foreign nationals are involved), victim support services and the *Criminal Injuries Compensation Authority* (CICA), transport carriers, customer care teams, and legal advisors. Staff at the HAC will work closely with the police *forces liaison officers* (FLO). Further detailed guidance is available at the https://www.gov.uk/government/publications/humanitarian-assistance-in-emergencies website.

The HAC and similar components of the response and recovery phases offer convenient opportunities to gather data which will be useful for ensuring comprehensive medical, psychological and social care. Although legislation under the CCA allows data sharing, such data must be handled appropriately under current data legislation. It is recommended that the SCG appoint an *information coordinator* to oversee the management of patient and other data throughout the response and recovery process, and that all involved organizations identify an *information controller*.

Planning assumptions for post-incident shelter/temporary housing

As an estimate, it may be assumed that:
- 60% of affected people leave the area and stay with friends or relatives
- 30% use hotels or similar accommodation away from the affected area
- 10% will need assistance with temporary shelter.

In the case of severe flooding:
- 50% of displaced victims will require accommodation for up to 3 months, 30% for up to 6 months, and 20% for up to a year (these periods may, however, be significantly longer in severe or more extensive flooding).

In the longer term, those involved in an incident will have changing needs. The requirement for information about the incident itself will become a need for information regarding the process of investigation and identification of responsibility; the medical and psychological challenges will change and require the intervention of different groups; and the financial and social issues will become those of community reconstruction, establishment of normal function, compensation, and longer-term accommodation.

Services provided by the humanitarian assistance centre (HAC)

- Registration and data recording—establishing lists of those involved
- Shelter (including feeding and sanitary facilities)
- A quiet area for reflection and confidential interviews
- Opportunities for communication and exchange of views, information, and experience
- Landline and mobile phone access
- Crèche facilities
- First aid provision
- Information about the incident as it develops
- Interpreters (if required)
- Emotional support
- Financial, accommodation, travel, and legal advice
- Advice regarding 'next steps' for those involved in the incident
- A focal point of longer-term contact and support
- Links to police and other investigations.

Planning the humanitarian aspects of major incident response usually lies with a multiagency *humanitarian assistance working group* (HAWG) as part of the resilience process (national guidance is available via the http://www.gov.uk website) which must ensure that sources of such assistance and the capability to provide it are identified and available based on a detailed assessment of community needs. Like all aspects of resilience, regular practice and updating is essential. The HAWG should establish timelines for the provision of humanitarian services following an incident.

Resistance and resilience

Those who are minimally distressed or not distressed as a result of their involvement in a major incident are sometimes referred to as *resistant people*.

Those who show mild temporary distress but continue to function normally, and those who are more distressed but function reasonably at least in the short and medium term may be referred to as *resilient*.

Some of those involved will either suffer sustained distress from which they recover slowly or permanent distress, or may be in the course of developing a defined mental disorder.

Foreign nationals

Foreign nationals involved in a major incident in the UK will receive immediate medical treatment for significant injury under the NHS. For other assistance they should approach their embassy or high commission (Commonwealth countries). The relevant embassy or high commission will automatically be notified in the event of the arrest of a foreign national on charges connected with the incident. Death of foreign nationals in a UK incident would be investigated in exactly the same manner as for a UK citizen. Contact will be made with the relevant consular officials, and at the end of the process, the coroner will issue authority for the body to leave the UK. Central government mechanisms are in place for the immediate notification of the diplomatic community of a UK major incident.

Memorials and commemorations

Those involved in recovery following a major incident in which there have been fatalities should work carefully with community representatives and others (e.g. faith groups) to ensure that memorials and commemorations are culturally and religiously appropriate, sensitive, and inclusive (see Appendix C). Attention should be paid to avoiding dates with other cultural significance. Invitations to ceremonies is a potential area for embarrassment and should be handled carefully. There will almost inevitably be issues with security, access, and media engagement. Councils and other organizations should consider opening a book or books of remembrance or establishing a condolence website.

Shelter

Apart from providing people with medium- or long-term accommodation, temporary shelter (*rest centres*) may be required until more appropriate arrangements can be established. Plans should identify potential accommodation for such temporary shelters in the event of an incident. Such facilities will need heating, light, communications, and toilet facilities, and catering will need to be available. Given appropriate access to communications, many people will be able to arrange their own accommodation. When only small numbers of people are involved, it may be more appropriate and cost-effective to use nearby commercial accommodation such as hotels and guest houses. Local councils should be able to make immediately available interim supplies of items such as bedding and clothes whilst larger-scale arrangements are put in place. Plans should also have identified who will staff shelter facilities and how medical care will be provided.

Rest centres may not be suitable for those with additional needs and alternatives such as hotels and care homes should be considered if support from family members is not available. All those accommodated at rest centres will be anxious, either about what has happened, or potential future events, or both. Welfare facilities including support and advice (financial, social, and legal), as well as adequate information, should be made available. Separate arrangements should be made for pets which will not generally be accommodated at rest centres, but at local commercial facilities. Following evacuation, it is important that those involved feel that their vacated property is as safe as possible and steps should be taken to demonstrate and confirm that an appropriate crime prevention strategy is being implemented.

Return

Return to an area affected by a major incident is likely to be phased, with those involved in key services or assisting with the recovery effort returning first. The return of evacuated members of the public may also be phased, although such plans may be difficult to enforce. The decision to return will be taken by the SCG and may require temporary facilities such as water bowsers or temporary shopping facilities. Early return of children to school will facilitate the return of their parents to work.

Investigations and enquiries

There will inevitably be some form of investigation or enquiry following a major incident. Options include:
- criminal investigation
- statutory enquiry
- public enquiry
- coroner's inquest.

In significant incidents which have resulted in deaths, there may be all four types of enquiry and the duration of this phase of the recovery process will be prolonged.

Criminal investigation

The scene of a major incident will be treated as crime scene and investigated as such until the police confirm that no crime has taken place. The police will appoint a *senior investigating officer* who will determine whether there is sufficient evidence to justify criminal proceedings. Such evidence will then be passed to the *Crown Prosecution Service*.

Statutory enquiries

A number of bodies including the Air, Marine, and Rail Accident Investigation Branches, the Ministry of Defence, and Health and Safety Executive will be required to carry out technical enquiries following certain types of incident.

Public enquiries

Following all major incidents there is likely to be a public enquiry, usually chaired by a judge or senior Queen's Counsel. Such an enquiry will review the causes of the incident and the response to it. This enquiry can take months or even years to complete and will result in the preparation of a comprehensive report detailing what happed and why, and importantly making recommendations for future planning and response to a similar incident. Failings commonly identified by public enquiries are listed in Box 13.3. Public enquiries are not trials, but unlike coroner's inquests, they may apportion blame.

Box 13.3 Issues commonly identified by public enquiries
- Failure of integrated planning, absence of planning
- Inadequate training
- Lack of attention to safety procedures and equipment before the incident
- Failure to carry out appropriate risk assessments
- Organizational management failings and unclear lines or responsibility
- Organization culture inhibiting disclosure of information or decision-making
- Lack of a coordinated emergency response
- Poor communications
- Command and control failures
- Inadequate management of large crowds or events
- Inadequate legislation (such as to prevent long working hours, firearms licensing)
- Poor handling of relatives and victims.

Coroner's inquests

In the event of an incident involving fatalities, HM Coroner is responsible for establishing cause and circumstances of death and for identification of remains. A coroner's officer will act as coroner's representative and liaison between the coroner and hospitals, the incident scene, and mortuaries. The coroner will request a forensic post-mortem examination of all the deceased following a major incident. Following this, the coroner will hold an inquest. Once this inquest is complete, the coroner will assign the cause of death to one of a number of categories only some of which are relevant to a major incident (Box 13.4). Alternatively, a narrative verdict (describing what happened) or an open verdict (when there is insufficient evidence for any other outcome) can be issued. The coroner is not responsible for any form of criminal investigation into the deaths, but may pass on information to the police. If criminal charges have been brought, the coroner will adjourn the inquest until the criminal trial is over.

Box 13.4 The potential causes of death following a coroner's inquest

- Accident or misadventure
- Lawful killing
- Unlawful killing
- Industrial diseases
- Alcohol or drug related
- Natural causes
- Road traffic collision
- Stillbirth
- Suicide
- Open verdict
- Narrative verdict.

Victim identification

The relatives of victims will inevitably be distressed and anxious whilst human remains are unidentified since absolute confirmation of loss of a loved one is unavailable and the normal procedures of mourning cannot be carried out. It is essential therefore that the identification process is carried out as quickly as possible and in a respectful and sympathetic way which avoids error and keeps relatives informed at all stages.

Therefore *disaster victim identification* is a key component of the recovery process following any incident involving fatalities, although the nature of the incident will clearly determine how challenging this process is likely to be. Each police region has an identified lead for *disaster victim identification* (DVI). These individuals are trained in the identification, labelling, recovery, and mortuary management of bodies and body parts. Final identification will be by a variety of methods including location of body parts, DNA analysis, dental and medical records, documentation, visual identification, and reconstruction.

UK disaster victim identification

There is a national police *disaster victim identification* (DVI) cadre of individuals coordinated by ACPO and trained to work in this area. The UK DVI coordinator is located at the *Police National Information Coordination Centre* (PNICC). UK DVI includes specially trained police officers, victim recovery officers, police mortuary officers, forensic specialists (pathologists, odontologists, podiatrists, imaging specialists, biologists, and photographers), forensic support staff, and others. There is a national DVI management team under the ACPO lead. International DVI arrangements are coordinated by INTERPOL and UK DVI personnel may be deployed abroad.

Family liaison officers

Family liaison officers assist the SIM and SIO by collecting evidence, gathering ante-mortem data, and assisting with patient identification. They also provide information to the family about police and coronial investigations and procedures, providing support and a link to other statutory and voluntary agencies. In addition, FLOs will assist families in dealing with the media, facilitate visits to the incident scene, and ensure personal property is returned. Although they should be supportive and sympathetic, they do not offer any form of counselling. A *family liaison coordinator* will coordinate and facilitate the FLOs.

Coroner's officers

Coroner's officers are usually civilians (although often ex-police officers). Their responsibilities include arranging the transfer of bodies from the scene to a mortuary, liaising with victim recovery teams, liaising with pathologists about samples and the extent of permitted examinations, acting as a link between hospitals and the coroner, and assisting with the establishment of mortuary facilities and membership of the mortuary management team. The coroner will also assist the bereaved in conjunction with the families' liaison officers.

Methods for identification of the dead are given in Box 13.5 p. 395. The process by which ante-mortem data is analysed and compared with post-mortem samples for identification purposes is known as *reconciliation*. In the event of a mass fatality incident, an *identification commission* may be established to oversee the identification process. Members will include the coroner (as chair), SIM, SIO, family liaison coordinator, ante- and post-mortem data coordinators, and forensic experts.

Box 13.5 Methods of identifying the dead

Primary identifiers
- Fingerprints
- DNA
- Dental records.

Secondary identifiers
- Serial numbers on implanted medical prostheses
- Scars and tattoos
- Blood groups
- Previously recorded medical conditions and medical records
- X-ray examination
- Jewellery and personal effects
- Distinctive clothing.

Assistance
- Location of remains
- Visual identification (requires corroboration)
- Photographs.

Psychological Aspects of Major Incidents

Introduction

Human beings are not only physically vulnerable to adverse events, but psychologically vulnerable too. Every major incident will have mental health consequences for some of those involved. Lives will be disrupted to a greater or lesser extent, for short periods or permanently. People will be killed or injured. Victims will be left to recover, survivors to mourn. It has been estimated that up to 80% of those affected by a major incident or disaster will have short-term mild distress, 20–40% a psychological disorder in the medium term, and up to 5% may be left with a long-term problem. Fortunately, the majority of those affected will recover without professional intervention.

In addition, although psychological effects will occur as a natural *consequence* of a major incident which is a consequence of human error or natural forces, in the case of terrorist incidents, it is the precise *aim* of the perpetrators to inflict psychological damage. Not only will the mechanism be chosen to inflict wounds associated with maximum horror or to cause anxiety and panic, but an element of deliberate malice is introduced which in itself is likely to increase the adverse psychological consequences. Actions designed to minimize psychological consequences both in rescuers and victims, as well as to identify such problems when they do occur and treat them promptly, are thus a key component of the response to any incident. In addition, means must be in place after any traumatic incident to establish a follow-up registry so that victims with mental health issues can be identified and offered assistance. Conversely, it must not be forgotten that for some, their role in a major incident may actually be life-enhancing, perhaps because the feelings of others towards them became clear, perhaps because they found and demonstrated new strengths or new or previously unknown abilities to cope and to assist others.

It is essential that expert mental health advice and mental health services engagement occur at all stages of planning, response, and recovery.

Prompt and regular release of accurate, credible information by individuals with appropriate expertise and authority can significantly reduce the risk of post-incident psychological problems.

Psychological aspects of a major incident

As stated in the previous section, the psychological effects of an incident are likely to be more severe and more widespread if there was an element of malice in its causation. This is exactly and deliberately the case with a terrorist incident, which by its nature is designed to cause mass anxiety, fear, or panic. In the early stages following an incident such as a bombing, and more chronically if a series of incidents occurs, helplessness or hopelessness may follow with questions being raised over the competence of the authorities. Such pressures, from terrorist and victim or potential victim alike, may cause those authorities to make mistakes or act precipitously, perhaps under political pressure. All of these effects may reduce or destroy a sense of security and safety, exacerbated by the destruction of civilian infrastructure.

Fortunately, the available evidence suggests that panic is rare and incidents have repeatedly demonstrated that altruistic behaviour, often at some risk to the individuals concerned, is more common. When panic does occur, those who demonstrate it are likely to be trapped and unable to help themselves, afraid that the situation is out of control and there is no leadership, or wish to ensure that they receive help which they fear may be on a first come, first served basis with some victims being left without assistance.

Although experience may suggest that the occurrence of adverse psychological symptoms following a traumatic incident is universal, it is nevertheless true that the majority of people emerge unscathed from traumatic events, although there may be a prolonged period before normality is re-established. Those who enjoy warm interpersonal relationships, are able to control their emotions, have a positive self-image, and are able to apply themselves to practical and positive tasks in a sustained way are more likely to cope effectively. Thus there is a lot to be said for adopting an encouraging approach and emphasizing the positive consequences of involvement wherever possible. Constructive participation, the feeling of having made a positive contribution, of having been part of an effective team, is a powerful protective mechanism. Strong, effective, confident leadership is essential. There may also be positive effects as a result of a major incident not just at an individual level but also for society as a whole. Individuals may discover previously unknown strengths and societies may be drawn closer together and be strengthened, typified in Britain by the 'Blitz mentality'.

Individual risk factors for an adverse psychological reaction

Given sufficient provocation, everyone has the potential to develop mental health symptoms after a significantly stressful event. However, there are certain factors which increase the risk that an individual will develop problems of this kind. These can be divided into factors preceding the event, features of the traumatic event itself, and factors which apply to the circumstances following the incident. Children are at a particular risk of developing problems following a distressing and traumatic event, and women are also at greater risk than men.

Pre-traumatic factors

Pre-traumatic factors include a previous psychiatric history or history of unresolved loss or trauma and a history of childhood sexual abuse. Social or economic disadvantage, poor education, and drug abuse are also risk factors. Perhaps not surprisingly, those with other simultaneous life stresses are more likely to react adversely to a major traumatic event as are the young compared to the old.

Peri-traumatic factors

Features of the event itself which predispose to an adverse psychological reaction include a threat to life, whether genuine or perceived, exposure to terrible injuries or sensory experiences, and a sudden and unexpected rather than gradual and predicted onset of the event. Incidents that result from the deliberate malevolent acts of other people as well as those that result in considerable personal loss to the individual are also associated with an increased incidence of psychological problems. In addition, those closer to the event and exposed to it for longer are more likely to have problems.

Post-traumatic factors

Lack of support and adverse reactions from others as well as a feeling of guilt are all associated with an increased incidence of mental health problems as is perceived loss of societal structure or norms and previous social certainties.

Adverse psychological effects

Psychological features of *post-traumatic stress reactions* may be emotional, cognitive, or behavioural, or may affect the victim's personality. Alternatively, physical symptoms such as insomnia may predominate. These include an increased heart rate (tachycardia), shaking, nausea, sweating, tiredness, headache, non-specific aches and pains, sleep problems, and hyperventilation syndrome (commonly referred to as panic attacks). These issues collectively may be referred to as *distress*; when they become persistent or debilitating they can be referred to as *disorder*. Whatever the level of problem, it is essential that plans ensure that those at risk are identified and offered the assistance they need.

Victims and rescuers are more likely to suffer an acute stress reaction than debilitating long-term problems. Stress symptoms usually occur within a few minutes of the precipitating event and disappear within a few days. When these symptoms do persist for more than a few weeks, a diagnosis of *post-traumatic stress disorder* (PTSD) should be considered. Features of acute transient reactions include numbness, feeling dazed, insomnia, impaired concentration, restlessness, and autonomic arousal. Avoidance behaviours can also occur as may maladaptive coping mechanisms such as substance or alcohol misuse. Transient 'flashbacks' are common, but in most cases will stop relatively quickly. Individuals may be divided into those who are resistant and do not demonstrate (or show only minimal) transient distress, the resilient who show transient or longer-term distress but with normal function, and those who develop persistent debilitating distress, some of whom will go on to develop an established psychiatric diagnosis.

A list of emotional, cognitive, behavioural, and personality problems is given in Box 14.1.

Box 14.1 Common mental health problems following a traumatic event

Emotional problems
- Fear
- Anger
- Edginess and irritability
- Blame (self and others)
- Sadness
- Depression
- Emotional numbness
- Inability to cope.

Cognitive problems
- Poor concentration
- Poor memory
- Difficulty in making decisions
- Loss of faith
- Increased alertness and disorientation
- Intrusive and unwanted memories ('*flashbacks*')
- Reduced self-esteem/confidence
- Denial.

Behavioural and personality problems
- Emotional outbursts
- Anger and argumentativeness
- Inability to settle.
- Sleep problems
- Withdrawal
- Loss of the desire to communicate with others
- Reduction/loss of appetite (or may be increased as a coping mechanism)
- Reduced or lost libido
- Increased use of tobacco, drugs, and/or alcohol
- Increased risk-taking behaviours.

Post-traumatic stress disorder

PTSD is estimated to affect about 1 in every 3 people who have a traumatic experience. It is characterized by:
• a delayed or prolonged reaction
• re-experiencing the event in flashbacks, dreams, nightmares, and unbidden memories.

In addition, there is usually a background of numbness, detachment, and emotional blunting. Hyperarousal with hypervigilance and fear and avoidance behaviour may also occur, along with anxiety, depression and suicidal thoughts.

The diagnosis of PTSD cannot be made in the immediate aftermath of a traumatic event (diagnostic criteria ICD-10). Although it is one of the most severe reactions following a traumatic event, it is not the most common long-term mental health issue. Depression, anxiety, increased alcohol or tobacco use, family conflict, or unexplained somatic symptoms are all more common.

Inevitably victims of PTSD are less able to carry out the activities of their daily lives (impairment). Substance abuse, risk-taking behavior, and deliberate self-harm are all more common in victims of PTSD. The severity of the precipitating trauma is a good predictor of persistent PTSD. The key to management of PTSD is anticipation. There is no convincing evidence that 'psychological debriefing' prevents PTSD.

Re-experiencing
This may take the form of nightmares, disturbing dreams, unpleasant thoughts, emotions, or disturbing reactions to events which remind the victim of the original event. Flashbacks are common and can take the form of smells, sights, or sounds associated with the original event.

Avoidance
The individual may change their behaviour to avoid people, places, or activities associated with the event. Enjoyment of activities which were previously pleasurable is reduced.

Hyperarousal/hypervigilance
Features of hyperarousal include loss of concentration, difficulty in sleeping, an enhanced startle response, and problems with controlling anger.

Psychological 'first aid'

Psychological first aid (PFA) is a technique designed to be used in the early stages of the response to a traumatic event. Access to shelter, food, sanitary provision, and facilities for a physical recovery will promote the return to mental health. Giving victims something constructive to do is also a powerful force in recovery. Beginning to re-establish order by the return of simple elements of everyday life is an important aim. Accurate and authoritative information should be provided at the earliest opportunity and links with family, friends, and loved ones should be facilitated in order to reduce stress in survivors. Acute significant mental health problems are not the norm, but all those involved in responding to an incident should be alert to the signs and prepared to direct individuals to appropriate assistance. Psychological first aid is summarized in Box 14.2.

Box 14.2 Psychological first aid

- Comfort and console
- Protect from further harm
- Provide immediate physical care
- Engage purposefully and encourage a sense of being in control
- Provide accurate information
- Re-establish order
- Facilitate links with loved ones
- Provide psychological triage.

Management of mental health issues resulting from major incidents

Wherever appropriate, plans for the identification, surveillance, and management of medium- and long-term psychiatric and psychosocial problems must be included in major incident plans. An effective response will result from integrated cooperative working and ready access to specialist advice. Central planning guidance describes a stepped model of care as illustrated in Figure 14.1 below p. 404. Such plans will include schools and communities, employers, therapists, the NHS, community services, primary healthcare staff, and mental health professionals. Conventional planning structures (see Chapters 2 and 3) must ensure integrated working in this as in other areas.

The NHS has a key role in coordinating and ensuring appropriate planning but will also provide expert advice to commanders during and after an incident as well as offering appropriate training for those likely to be responsible for managing psychosocial issues. Crucially, the NHS must ensure that adequate mental health resources will be available following an incident and that such staff are aware of, and trained for, their role. Establishment of regional teams of healthcare professionals and managers is recommended, the members of which will be involved in both planning and care provision following an incident, as well as providing specialist advice to responding agencies and training staff.

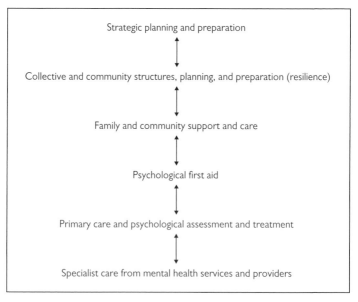

Fig. 14.1 A structure for managing the mental health consequences of a major incident.

Components of an effective response

Immediately following an incident, as well as the practical support of psychological first aid, written information should be available detailing where further help may be obtained. These materials must be appropriate for the communities and individuals concerned. A telephone helpline number should also be made available offering access to appropriately trained advisors. Information may also be made available through websites and from *information and advice shops* (if the incident is of a sufficient size). A mental health presence at the survivor reception centre or humanitarian assistance centre is also advised. Particular emphasis should be placed on the normality and transience of most psychological symptoms whilst facilitating access to help for those who may need it. With time, mental health services should identify all those in need of professional intervention (including emotional, physical, welfare, and social needs) and ensure that appropriate relationships are established, often through primary care services. Interventions may include trauma focused *cognitive behavioural therapy* (CBT) and stress management teaching. In the medium term, interventions are likely to be provided by mental health professionals who will also manage those with long-term problems.

Dealing with psychological problems in emergency personnel

It is perhaps inevitable, depending on the nature of the incident, that there will be individual responders who will develop psychological problems following a major incident; however, there is much that can be done to reduce the incidence of such problems. The key is an appropriate occupational climate and the responsibility for this lies not only with leaders and managers but with all members of the team. There are a number of important features of organizations which are tuned to deal effectively with these issues:

Strong, but sensitive leadership

Feeling part of a well-motivated and well-led professional group with a strong group dynamic protects against later mental health issues.

Trust

When individuals know that there is nothing to fear or be ashamed of in disclosing that they are suffering psychological problems following an incident, they will be more willing to be open about them and they will be more effectively dealt with. It must be made clear that genuine psychological issues will not be a bar to career progression, seen as a sign of weakness, or a cause of breaches of personal confidentiality.

Responsibility

Individuals should know that the culture will identify legitimate responsibility but not search for scapegoats.

Caring

Individuals should consider themselves to have a responsibility to each other regarding the recognition of psychological problems; in addition, organizations should be well prepared for possible problems, free from stigma, and have a well-established process for seeking help. At its simplest level, professionals who are well rested, well fed, and feel valued are less likely to develop psychological problems.

Openness

Responders must be encouraged to, and feel able to, share their experiences informally with each other.

Assistance

Personnel must be aware of sources of help should they require it.

Recognition

It is vital that personnel are made to feel aware that they are performing an important public service which is recognized and valued.

It might be argued that, in an attempt to reduce the stigma of mental health issues, the consensus has been allowed to swing too far. Psychological problems are not 'normal' in any conventional sense and most responders will not suffer them. This is not an indication of an absence of empathy or compassion as it has been recognized since the First World War that everyone has a threshold of exposure beyond which they are more likely to have problems. Fortunately, most never reach this threshold and will retain an ability to function normally. Most will suffer transient distress, equilibrate with it, and move on. No one called to deal with the aftermath of, for example, a terrorist atrocity will be unaffected and all will in some way be changed by the experience. However, it must also be emphasized that there is absolutely no shame to be attached to those who do develop psychological problems as a result of their experiences.

Counselling

The observation that personnel should be encouraged to share their experience in an open way should not be seen as an endorsement of so-called counselling or more formally *critical incident stress debriefing* (CISD) which, if delivered at the wrong time or by inadequately trained personnel (or worse still untrained personnel), *may* be positively harmful in formalizing and 'medicalizing' problems and re-traumatizing the individuals concerned. This is particularly the case with single-session interventions focused on the individual or group's emotional reactions. Conversely, informal 'conversational' discussion among normal support groups (including family and work colleagues) is likely be helpful.

Responders requiring further professional help

It may, as time passes following an incident, become clear that an individual requires help from a mental health professional, such as a psychologist or psychiatrist. Potential indicators of this are:

- the inability to carry out the activities of daily living or normal working life
- personal neglect (no longer eating, sleeping, or washing)
- substance misuse (usually, but not always, alcohol)
- relationship difficulties and breakdown, sometimes violence to family members
- sustained post-traumatic symptoms (see p. 401)
- exacerbation or re-occurrence of previous mental health problems.

Mass sociogenic illness

Following specific incidents where there is the risk of widespread exposure to a potentially noxious agent, *mass sociogenic illness* (or *multiple unexplained symptoms*) may occur. As a result, large numbers of people may report to healthcare professionals complaining of symptoms or supposed symptoms of exposure to an agent in the absence of any evidence of such exposure. This situation perhaps most commonly occurs therefore when there is a deliberate or accidental release of chemicals or a biological agent. It relies on the presence of uncertainty regarding the possibility of exposure. In essence, it is not possible to be concerned that one might have been shot, it is possible to worry that one might have been exposed to anthrax or pesticides. Similarly, fewer people will be concerned that they might have been harmed by an explosion than will be concerned that they have been affected by unseen radiation. Mass sociogenic illness occurs in normal people without a history of psychiatric illness. Episodes of mass sociogenic illness are usually short lived but may recur if the precipitating event reoccurs.

Mass sociogenic illness is not the same as panic, and experience clearly demonstrates that victims are more likely to help each other than run for safety leaving the injured in their wake. Mass sociogenic illnesses have a number of characteristic features (Box 14.3) and symptoms (Box 14.4).

Management

Prompt reassurance is essential in limiting the effects of outbreaks, but genuine causes for the symptoms must not be missed. Mass sociogenic illness is therefore a diagnosis by exclusion and managers and clinicians must ensure that means are in place for dealing with it when it happens. People with mass sociogenic illness must be rapidly separated from those who are well, otherwise further spread will occur. Removal from the environment associated with the outbreak is key to effective management. Reassurance should be offered once genuine physical illness can be excluded.

Individuals should be given something to do and encouraged to eat, sleep, and drink normally. Prompt reunion with family is important. Open scepticism among health professionals must be avoided.

Examples of mass sociogenic illness

In October 1965, at a girls' school in Blackburn, several girls complained of dizziness and fainting Within a few hours, 85 girls from the school had been taken by ambulance to the nearby hospital suffering from fainting, moaning, chattering of teeth, hyperventilation, and muscle spasms.

After a radioactive contamination incident in Brazil in 1987 which eventually resulted in the deaths of four people, 125,000 people presented to healthcare professionals for examination. Of the first 80,000, 8% had somatic symptoms including rash, vomiting, and diarrhoea. Not a single one of the 125,000 had any evidence of exposure.

In the period immediately after the 1995 sarin attack on the Tokyo subways, 4000 people who had no history or evidence of exposure presented to the healthcare services.

Box 14.3 Features of mass sociogenic illness
- May have a trigger such as an index case, a smell (actual or imagined), or a rumour
- Is more common in closed groups such as schools or the workplace
- Is more frequent in groups under physical or emotional stress
- Reflects the prevailing beliefs or concerns of the group or society in which they occur
- More common in females
- Spreads from high-status to low-status individuals within communities.

Box 14.4 Characteristic clinical picture of mass sociogenic illness
- Associated with anxiety
- Is of rapid onset and 'spread' from case to case
- Mimics victims' beliefs about the symptoms of the presumed cause: 'they get what they think they should get'
- Symptoms also include non-specific complaints such as headache, nausea, and pain
- Is associated with transient and benign symptoms which have a rapid onset and recovery
- Symptoms are often made worse by media and emergency services attention.

Behavioural changes following an incident.

It is worth noting that there are likely to be changes in behaviour following an incident which do not suggest psychological harm, but rather rational (or perceived to be rational) attempts to reduce risk. These might include changes in travel patterns (for instance, to avoid tube journeys or particular journey times), changes in dress (to reduce identification with a particular group), or more broadly, changes in attitudes towards groups perceived to be supportive of extremist minorities which may in turn lead to further incidents.

Psychological problems in children following a major incident

The psychological effects of an incident on children will be affected by many of the same factors which affect adults; however, their age, developmental stage, and the reactions of their parents, especially if they were involved in the incident, will also be important. Death or critical injury of a parent may also remove a vital layer of support. Children may demonstrate behavioural or emotional regression following an incident but this usually resolves with support from family, school, and health professionals if necessary. Adolescents may show increased levels of substance abuse following involvement in an incident. Access to care from an expert in the management of children with psychological and psychosocial problems is essential.

Dealing with the Media

Introduction

The media in all their forms are often seen as an irritation, an added complication in the already stressful and complicated process of managing a major incident. There is no doubt that less scrupulous journalists from all media, and some media organizations have motivations which are incompatible with the ideals of the emergency, charitable, and public services and could well be done without. However, the vast majority of those in the media are simply motivated by the need to inform (and entertain, although not in this context) and used appropriately offer powerful tools in incident response. The two main roles of the media in such a situation might be summarized as dissemination of information about the incident itself (cause, casualties, and response: news) and dissemination of useful information to the public designed to reduce the impact of an incident and prevent it escalating. It is essential in any emergency situation to be able to disseminate information to the public which is accurate, clear, and timely and to ensure that they have all the advice they need. Accurate information reduces anxiety and panic and prevents overuse of stretched resources. Radio, television, and the print media are thus key components of any effective response.

The first briefing

It is essential to ensure not only that information is provided in good time, but that its content is appropriate for the audience. Highly technical language should therefore be avoided for public information releases and it may on occasion be necessary to sacrifice some information to ensure that the key elements are available when they are needed and intelligible to those who need the information. The likely impact of the information on those who receive it should always be considered before it is released and responding agencies should also ensure that information released through the media is clearly labelled as, and identifiable as, official information. Responding organizations must, in addition, ensure that their own staff remain fully and appropriately informed at all times.

The first media briefing after an incident has occurred should include:

• the time and location of incident
• a brief description of the scene
• a brief description of what has happened without speculation regarding cause or blame
• a brief description of the response to date with reassurance that everything necessary is being done or is imminent
• whether or not there are casualties (without details of numbers of fatalities) and whether anyone is trapped
• which hospitals are responding
• any immediate actions for members of the public (not normally needed)
• the contact details of the casualty bureau
• information for the public regarding (as appropriate) access restrictions, transport disruption, and weather conditions
• time of next briefing.

Warning and informing the public

The Civil Contingencies Act 2004 (CCA), COMAH, and REPPIR regulations all mandate a duty to provide timely and accurate advice to members of the public. The CCA mandates that all *Category 1 responders* inform the public regarding the risks of emergencies affecting a local area and how they should respond if such an incident does occur. They are also required to inform the public if an incident has occurred, or is likely to occur. Naturally, the public will also want to know what is being done to protect them. Both REPPIR and COMAH require operators to provide information to members of the public who are at risk of being affected by an incident at their establishment. The local authority has a supervisory role in ensuring that this requirement is complied with. It is absolutely vital that during any significant incident contradictory, inaccurate, or incorrect information is not released. Communication with the public is covered in more detail in Chapter 3.

Challenges of working with the media

Working with the media is not always straightforward. The scale of media interest is often underestimated and with modern 24-hour satellite news channels is likely to be continuous and international. The number of media representatives at a significant incident is likely to be in the hundreds and may be considerably larger even than this. It should not be forgotten that these individuals will bring vehicles and technical equipment with them and will require food, water, shelter, and energy whilst present. Thus provision of parking space and a suitable building for representatives of the media are essential components of any response.

The nature of modern media with live streaming from the scene of an incident also means that information will be broadcast ahead of the responders being able to assess, assimilate, and respond to it. Not only does this increase the potential for responders to be 'wrong footed' but footage may be used in any subsequent enquiry. Conversely, the media may be able to provide information which can be used either in the immediate response or as part of any subsequent enquiry or criminal investigation.

Central government media arrangements

In the event of a very significant incident, the *Cabinet Office Communications Group* will establish a *News Coordination Centre* (NCC) in Whitehall to support the lead government department during and after the incident. The NCC will assist in the preparation of briefings, management of requests for interviews (ministers and senior civil servants and advisors), dissemination of information via websites, and ensuring a consistent message. The NCC will also liaise with staff from the *Central Office of Information—News and Public Relations Department*. Ministers may be required to issue statements which should be checked for technical accuracy by the appropriate technical advisor as well as the relevant command structures.

National Resilience Extranet

The National Resilience Extranet is a secure collaborative platform designed to share information and which is available over any broadband connection.

BBC 'Connecting in a Crisis'

The BBC 'Connecting in a Crisis' initiative encourages planners to work closely with BBC local radio to incorporate local stations into their plans as emergency broadcasters of information to the public. The BBC website contains the contact details of all local radio station editors.

Engaging the public

Now that everyone has a camera on their mobile phone, the general public are no longer the passive victims of an incident. They have access to and can communicate all kinds of information which may be of use in response to an incident or during the subsequent investigation. The conventional media can be used to gain access to this information.

New media

Twenty years ago, this section would have been confirmed to radio, television, and the printed media. Now, any effective strategy must include the Internet and social media such as *Twitter* and *Facebook*. Information released through websites must be accurate and therefore regularly updated, and every agency should ensure that the details of its website are issued early during an incident. Prior planning should ensure that these websites have the capacity to cope without crashing with the increased workload which will follow an incident. This may involve reducing the content to an essential minimum whilst the incident is ongoing. Organizations must ensure the availability of technical personnel to manage such media during and after an incident.

Social medial is an equally effective medium for disseminating accurate official information and inaccurate information based on rumour. Therefore incorrect information and rumour should be specifically and rapidly corrected and difficult questions raised through social media specifically answered. Thus information from official bodies must be clearly recognizable as such.

The *Defence Scientific and Technical Laboratories* (Dstl) have produced guidance to assist in the use of social media management during an emergency: 'Using social media in emergencies smart tips'. This is available via the http://www.gov.uk website. Use of social media in an emergency is likely to be most effective for those organizations which have established a following before the event occurs.

Social media may also be used as part of the response. Following the riots and looting of 2011, the social media were used as a means of coordinating community efforts to assist businesses and clear the streets of debris. During the recovery phase, social media can be used to inform the community about the availability (or otherwise) of health, transport, and other disrupted services.

Roles of the media at a major incident

The main role of the media is the dissemination of information, although this may be coloured by reader or local demographics, house style, or political stance. However, during an incident the reputable media accept that their responsibilities are broader and will include:
- dissemination of information regarding the incident (news)
- advice to the public regarding the most appropriate steps to take for their own protection
- advice regarding the availability of emergency call centres, information bureaux, and support lines
- provision of public information such as details of road closures, transport and utility disruption, or extreme weather
- reassurance and prevention of panic through appropriate messages and information
- requesting information or assistance on behalf of responding agencies.

Working with the media

In order to impose some control on the media and to ensure the flow of accurate and timely information, as well as to discourage dangerous and unauthorized access to the site by media representatives, a *media communications cell* (MCC) (or *strategic media advisory cell* (SMAC) in radiation incidents) should be established at strategic (gold) level. This facility will act as the press office for the incident. The MCC reports to the *strategic coordinating group* (SGG), feeding information not only to the media (usually through the *emergency media centre*) but from it to the SCG. Media organizations are not normally granted access to the MCC. The police take the lead in dealing with the media during the incident response phase.

The *emergency media centre* (MC) or *media briefing centre* (MBC) will offer shelter, heating, lighting, sanitary facilities, and communications (Internet and telephone) to the assembled media presence and acts as the single location at scene through which information is disseminated. As the incident develops, a media communications specialist will usually take charge of the media relations strategy, working with a team of media specialists from the responding organizations. In smaller incidents, a *media rendezvous* or *liaison point* (MLP) may be established as a location near the incident at which representatives of the media meet, their good standing can be checked, and they can be briefed.

The media communications specialist

The roles of the media communications specialist in charge of the media response to an incident include:
- maintaining an overview of media coverage, including that of activity remote from the scene
- engaging with the media regarding requests that specific details are not broadcast, or the broadcast is delayed.
- liaison with the *news coordination centre* (NCC)
- provision of media advice to the SCG
- agreeing '*lines to take*' and statements
- overseeing the MLP
- managing the MCC
- management of the MC if established
- arranging media visits to the scene
- ensuring appropriate web coverage
- supporting those who are interviewed and preventing the 'ambush' of those who do not wish to be interviewed.

The media liaison officer

The media communications specialist has an essentially supervisory and managerial role. A *media liaison officer* (MLO) will be appointed as the direct interface between responders and the media. In very large incidents, each responder will have an MLO, although the use of a single individual to represent more than one organization can be considered. It is essential that the MLO has the experience and skills to establish a relationship of trust with the media as this will facilitate such issues as information sharing by the media following access to the site of limited numbers of representatives. Such a relationship will be achieved by regular release of information and an awareness of media working practices including deadlines.

Regular briefings are perhaps the most important component of effective relations with the media. Access to the site should be allowed (in a controlled and safe manner) as well as to senior representatives of responding organizations and services and suitable facilities must be made available for this.

Controlling media access at the scene

Control of access to the scene of an incident is a police responsibility. Inevitably restrictions have to be placed on the media in order to protect the privacy of victims, prevent contamination of crime scenes, and for their own safety and that of others. However, the site chosen for the media must be reasonably close to the scene (safety permitting) and it is desirable to allow controlled and supervised access when this does not distract from more important priorities. The media may attempt to view the scene from aircraft (usually helicopters) although this can be curtailed if there are compelling reasons for doing so. Alternatively, arrangements may be put in place to allow multiple media concerns access to footage taken during a single over-fly. The principle of pooling is useful and can be extended to the establishment of a nominated pool who agree to share their images more widely, for example during a site visit. In some situations, it may be possible to establish a designated *forward media briefing point* from which a good view of the site is available.

Inevitably, there will be focuses of media activity away from scene at the headquarters of involved bodies or national agencies, at the homes of individuals, or at central government departments. The MCC is responsible, as far as is practical, for ensuring that the messages given out at these locations are correct and consistent with the media strategy endorsed by *strategic (gold)*. Similarly, information will be released by the press offices of the responding agencies and this too must be correct, consistent, and appropriate.

Arrangements must be in place for accrediting and registering foreign media organizations and personnel. UK media personnel must be required to show valid identification before access is granted: bona fide representatives will carry a *UK Press Card* recognized by ACPO. Such a card does not carry any rights of access.

Casualty figures and briefings

Special care must be taken when issuing casualty figures or estimates and no information about individual casualties should be issued during the incident response. Names cannot be released until the next of kin and the coroner have been informed and consent is granted. The collection and analysis of this data is usually coordinated by the police through a *casualty bureau* which does not have a responsibility for briefing the media. The role of the casualty bureau should be clearly stated when the contact details are released. Consideration may be given, at least until the situation becomes clearer, to issuing regular briefing statements rather than answering questions, although as the situation develops, interviews with key personnel will be demanded. The ambulance service will usually release information regarding casualty numbers. Details of fatality numbers can only be issued by the police. In some circumstances, consideration may be given to single joint statements on behalf of all the emergency services.

Features of an effective briefing
• Accurate, up-to-date information
• Avoidance of ambiguity or confusion
• Consistency of message
• No personal information or names
• Avoidance of speculation
• Not apportioning blame
• Commitment to provide additional or new information as soon as it becomes available
• Electronic form of briefing made available immediately afterwards
• Time of next briefing given.

VIP visits

Visits by VIPs can be a mixed blessing. However, properly handled, they can bring significant support to, and act as a morale boost for, both victims and responders alike. In addition, ministers may also visit in order to be able to report back to Parliament. Other VIP visitors may include the local MPs, members of the Royal Family, HM Lord Lieutenant or High Sheriff, local council dignitaries, church or military leaders, or representatives of foreign governments in the UK if foreign national have been involved. The various levels or command must be involved in the timing of visits to ensure that rescue and life-saving is not interrupted as well as that the site is safe to visit. Inevitably, VIPs will bring their own security and facilities must be available to accommodate these individuals. VIP visitors will require briefing before or at the start of a visit, although the level of briefing will vary with the purpose of the visit. Ministers will require more information, purely pastoral visits less.

Appendix A

Further Reading

Current texts

Chemical Incident Management Handbook. Medical Toxicology Unit, Guy's and St Thomas' Hospital Trust, 2000.

Major Incident Medical Management and Support: The Practical Approach at the Scene. Advanced Life Support Group, first published 1995.

Major Incident Medical Management and Support: The Practical Approach in the Hospital. Advanced Life Support Group, first published 2005.

Medical Response to Terrorism: Preparedness and Clinical Practice. Daniel C Keyes (Ed), Lippincott Williams & Wilkins, 2005.

Oxford Handbook of Pre-Hospital Care. Ian Greaves and Keith Porter, Oxford University Press, 2007.

Responding to Terrorism: A Medical Handbook. Ian Greaves and Paul Hunt, Churchill Livingstone, 2011.

Ryan's Ballistic Trauma. Adam J Brooks, Jon Clasper, Mark J Midwinter, Timothy J Hodgetts and Peter F Mahoney (Eds), Springer, 2011.

Reports of official enquiries

There is inevitably an independent report after every major incident. Although somewhat dry, there is much to learn from these documents. A representative (but far from complete) selection is given here:

MV Herald of Free Enterprise. Report of Court No 8074 Formal Investigation. HMSO, 1987.

Investigation into the King's Cross Underground Fire. Desmond Fennell, HMSO, 1988.

Investigation into the Clapham Junction Railway Accident. Anthony Hidden, The Stationery Office, 1989.

Report No: 4/1990. Report on the accident to Boeing 737-400, G-OBME, near Kegworth, Leicestershire on 8 January 1989. Air Accidents Investigation Branch, HMSO, 1990.

The Public Enquiry into the Piper Alpha Disaster (2 vols). Lord Cullen, The Stationery Office, 1990.

Report of the Official Account of the Bombings in London on 7th July 2005. The Stationary Office, 2006.

Rail Accident Report: Derailment at Grayrigg 23 February 2007. Rail Accident Investigation Branch, 2008 (also downloadable at https://assets.digital.cabinet-office.gov.uk/media/547c9037ed915d4c0d000199/081023_R202008_Grayrigg_v5.pdf).

Official regulations and guidance

Emergency Planning for Major Accidents COMAH 1999. HSE Books, 1999.

A Guide to the Radiation (Emergency Preparedness and Public Information) Regulations 2001. HSE Books, 2002 (also downloadable at http://www.hse.gov.uk/pubns/books/l126.htm).

Civil Contingencies Act. HMSO, 2004

Guide to Safety at Sports Grounds (Green Guide) (5th Edn). TSO, 2008 (also downloadable at http://www.safetyatsportsgrounds.org.uk/sites/default/files/publications/green-guide.pdf).

A Guide to the Control of Major Accident Hazards Regulations (3rd Edn). HSE Books, 2015 (also downloadable at http://www.hse.gov.uk/pubns/books/l111.htm).

NHS England Emergency Preparedness, Resilience and Response Framework, 2015

Useful Websites

Useful websites

Organization	Website
Air Accident Investigation Branch	www.aaib.dft.gov.uk
Association of Ambulance Chief Executives (AACE)	www.aace.org.uk
Atomic Weapons Establishment	www.awe.co.uk
Bahá'í Faith National Spiritual Assembly of the UK	www.bahai.org.uk
BASICS	www.basics.freeserve.co.uk
Board of Deputies of British Jews	www.bod.org.uk
British Civil Defence	www.britishcivildefence.org/
British National Formulary	www.bnf.org
British Red Cross	www.redcross.org.uk
British Standards Institution	www.bsigroup.com
British Transport Police	www.btp.police.uk
(Network of) Buddhist Organisations (UK)	www.nbo.org
Business Continuity Toolkit.	www.gov.uk/government/uploads/system/uploads/attachment_data/file/137994/Business_Continuity_Managment_Toolkit.pdf
Cabinet Office	www.cabinet-office.gov.uk/
Central Government Emergency Response Training (CGERT)	www.gov.uk/guidance/emergency-planning-and-preparedness-exercises-and-training
Central Office of Information	www.coi.gov.uk
Centre for the Protection of National Infrastructure	www.cpni.gov.uk
Chief Fire Officers Association	www.cfoa.org.uk
Church of England	www.churchofengland.org
Citizen aid	www.citizenaid.org
Civil Aviation Authority	www.caa.co.uk
Church of Jesus Christ of the Latter-day Saints	www.lds.org
Churches Together in Britain and Ireland	www.ctbi.org.uk
Civil Contingencies Secretariat	www.gov.uk/government/policies/emergency-planning
Defence Science and Technology Laboratory (dstl)	www.dstl.gov.uk
Department for Communities And Local Government	www.communities.gov.uk
Department for Environment, Food & Rural Affairs	www.defra.gov.uk
Department for Transport	www.gov.uk/government/organisations/department-for-transport
Department of Health	www.gov.uk/government/organisations/department-of-health

(Continued)

Organization	Website
Department of Health National Poisons Information Service	www.npis.org
Department of International Development	www.gov.uk/government/organisations/department-for-international-development
Disaster Action	www.disasteraction.org
Disaster Information	www.disasterinformation.org
Disaster Research Centre	www.drc.udel.edu/
Emergency Planning College	www.epcresilience.com
Emergency Planning Society	www.the-eps.org
Emergency response and recovery	www.gov.uk/guidance/emergency-response-and-recovery
Environment Agency	www.gov.uk/government/organisations/environment-agency
Fire Service College	www.fireservicecollege.ac.uk
Flood Information Service	www.flood-warning-information.service.gov.uk/
Foreign and Commonwealth Office	www.gov.uk/government/organisations/foreign-commonwealth-office
Free Churches	www.freechurches.org.uk
Government Decontamination Service	www.gov.uk/government/groups/government-decontamination-service
Health and Safety Executive	www.hse.gov.uk
Hindu Council (UK)	www.hinducouncil.org
Home Office	/www.gov.uk/government/organisations/home-office
Home Office (Terrorism)	www.homeoffice.gov.uk/terrorism
HSE Control of Substances Hazardous to Health (COSHH)	www.hse.gov.uk/coshh/index.htm
HSE Hazardous Installations Directorate	www.hse.gov.uk/hid/index.htm
(British) Humanist Association	www.humanism.org
Humanitarian assistance Sharepoint	www.the-eps.org/humanitarian-assistance-sharepoint/
Interfaith Network for the UK	www.interfaith.org.uk
International Air Transport Association	www.iata.org
International Atomic Energy Authority	www.iaea.org
Interpol	www.interpol.int
Jains	www.jaincentre.org.uk
Jehovah's Witnesses	www.watchtower.org
Jewish Emergency Support Service	www.thecst.org.uk
Joint Emergency Services Inter-operability Programme (JESIP)	www.jesip.org.uk

(Continued)

Organization	Website
Joint Services Command and Staff College (JSCSC)	www.da.mod.uk/Colleges-Business-Units/JSCSC
Local Government Association	www.local.gov.uk
London Emergency Services Liaison Panel	www.leslp.gov.uk
London Resilience Forum	www.london.gov.uk/about-us/ organisations-we-work/london-prepared/
Marine Accident Investigation Branch	www.gov.uk/government/organisations/ marine-accident-investigation-branch
Maritime & Coastguard Agency	www.gov.uk/government/organisations/ maritime-and-coastguard-agency
Metropolitan Police, Counter Terrorism Command (Specialist Operations) Centre	content.met.police.uk/Site/specialistoperations
Meteorological Office	www.metoffice.gov.uk/
Ministry of Defence	www.mod.uk
Muslim Council of Britain	www.mcb.org.uk
National Assembly for Wales	www.assembly.wales/
National Health Service (England)	www.england.nhs.uk
National Risk Register for Civil Emergencies (2013 edition)	www.gov.uk/government/publications/national-risk-register-for-civil-emergencies-2013-edition
National Security Strategy (2010)	www.gov.uk/government/uploads/system/uploads/ attachment_data/file/61936/national-security-strategy.pdf
National Statistics	www.ons.gov.uk
National Steering Committee on Warning & Informing the Public	www.gov.uk/government/groups/national-steering-committee-on-warning-informing-the-public
Nuclear Safety Inspectorate	www.onr.org.uk
Office of Rail and Road	www.orr.gov.uk
Pagans	www.paganfed.org
Police	www.police.uk
Public Health England	www.gov.uk/government/organisations/ public-health-england
Public Health Laboratory Service	www.gov.uk/government/collections/ public-health-laboratories
Red Cross	www.redcross.org.uk
Resilience Direct	www.resilience.gov.uk
Roman Catholic Church (England and Wales)	www.catholic-ew.org.uk
Scottish Government's Resilience Division	www.readyscotland.org/ready-government/ resilience-division/
Seventh-day Adventists	www.adventist.org.uk
Shinto	www.shinto.org
(Network of) Sikh Organisations	www.nsouk.co.uk

(Continued)

Organization	Website
St John Ambulance	www.sja.org.uk
Survive: The Business Continuity Group	www.thebci.org/
Toxbase	www.toxbase.org/
UK Parliament, Assemblies & HMSO	www.legislation.gov.uk
United Kingdom Airlines Emergency Planning Group	www.ukaepg.org
Wales Resilience	www.walesresilience.gov.uk/?lang_eng
WRVS	www.wrvs.org.uk
Zoroastrians	www.ztfe.com

Religious and Cultural Issues

Religious and cultural issues

Religion and culture are relevant to a major incident not only because those of all faiths (and none) and backgrounds may be victims of such an incident, but also because terrorists may claim a religious or cultural justification for their actions. Such claims may contribute to an already charged and difficult working environment and require particular sensitivity from the agents and individuals involved. Sensitivity to individuals' religious and cultural (often religious in origin, but without associated beliefs) perspectives is therefore essential. Conversely, misplaced lack of rigour in a desire to avoid offence or complaint must be avoided. Where compromise is necessary, a simple, honest explanation should be offered.

The requirements of different faith groups are likely to relate to the areas of language, dress, diet, religious observance and attitudes, and rituals associated with the sick, dying, and dead. A list of the UK's major faith groups is shown below. Representatives from the faith groups should be actively involved in emergency planning, not only to ensure that responses are appropriately sensitive, but because these groups are active and effective providers of support and assistance within and beyond their own communities, for example, in the provision of large quantities of food acceptable to a broad range of religions. Most areas will have an identified lead for their faith communities. Planning and decisions during the response phase should not be based on ill-founded assumptions which, for example, might conflate different ethnic groups with specific religions. The websites of many of the UKs faiths are given in Appendix B, 'Useful Websites'.

It should be remembered that the requirements of the criminal justice system, statutory enquiries, and the coronial system will if necessary override the religious wishes of the deceased and their families in matters such as post-mortem examination and time of burial. When this is the case, detailed and sensitive explanation is essential.

Major faith groups in the UK

- Christian (multiple denominations)
- Christian Scientist
- The Church of Jesus Christ of the Latter Day Saints (Mormons)
- Seventh-day Adventists
- Jehovah's Witnesses
- Judaism
- Islam
- Buddhism
- Hinduism
- Sikhism
- Jainism
- Zoroastrianism (Parsees)
- Rastafarianism
- Buddhists
- Bahá'í Faith
- Chinese faiths (including Confucianism and Taoists)
- Shinto
- Paganism
- Humanism.

This chapter is intended to provide basic guidance and cannot possibly cover the details of every religious group within the major faiths. Care should therefore be taken before the information in the following sections is applied to any specific group. Most faiths and groups are very happy to explain their own requirements if asked and are similarly keen to increase knowledge of their faith outside their own community.

Christianity

Because the Church of England is the state religion (the Queen being Head of the Church), many people describe themselves as 'C of E' (and other denominations) without implying any deeply held belief, rather expressing the cultural tradition within which they were raised. In such circumstances, religious considerations are likely to be of little relevance. Many individuals, however, profess profound Christian faith which will affect the way they respond to a wide range of situations. Practices will, however, vary widely between different denominations, and at times the differences between the various denominations may appear as important as their shared beliefs.

Language

Many languages depending on the ethnicity of the church, usually English.

Diet

No special dietary requirements, although some Roman Catholics may avoid fish on Fridays.

Dress

No specific requirements except for clergy.

Medical treatment

No specific requirements, transfusion and all other forms of treatment are generally acceptable.

Daily observance

Many Christians will pray daily, otherwise formal observance usually occurs on Sundays and specific church festivals.

Death and dying

Some individuals may seek the presence of a priest to perform 'last rites', communion, or simply to provide comfort. Post-mortems are accepted and Christians may be buried or cremated at a convenient time.

Christian Scientist

The essential tenet of Christian Science is that ill health can be cured by prayer, although this does not prevent adherents from seeking medical aid.

Language

In the UK, usually English.

Diet

There are no specific dietary requirements.

Dress

There are no specific dress requirements.

Medical treatment

Christian Scientists may decline conventional medical treatment, although they will accept treatment designed to protect others. There are no restrictions regarding gender of carers.

Daily observance

There are no prescribed daily religious observances.

Death and dying

There are no specific requirements, but where possible, the body of a female should be prepared for burial by a female. There is no specific religious objection to post-mortem.

The Church of Jesus Christ of the Latter-day Saints (Mormons)

Mormonism was founded by Joseph Smith in the USA in the 1820s. After his death, most of his adherents called themselves *The Church of Jesus Christ of the Latter-day Saints*. The word Mormon is originally derived from the *Book of Mormon*, one of the faith's religious texts: the term *latter-day Saint* is preferred. Latter-day Saints use and believe in the Bible as well the Book of Mormon and other texts. Plural marriage is no longer accepted except amongst some fundamentalist sects. Latter-day Saints believe that the Father, Son, and Holy Ghost of conventional Christian teaching are separate and distinct.

Language
Usually English.

Diet
No specific requirements.

Dress
Endowed members wear a special undergarment ('Temple Garment'). Latter-Day Saints are always soberly dressed.

Medical treatment
There is no objection to any form of medical intervention.

Daily observance
Like other Christian denominations, services occur on Sundays and other holy days. Reading from holy books is important.

Death and dying
A blessing by a priest may be requested. Burial is preferred to creation but not mandatory. There is no objection to post-mortem examination.

Seventh-day Adventists

The Seventh-day Adventist Church is a Protestant Christian church which marks the Sabbath on Saturday. Seventh-day Adventists believe in the imminent second coming of Christ. Much Seventh-day Adventist Church practice and belief corresponds to conventional protestant teachings.

Language

English, unless part of an immigrant Adventist community.

Diet

Practices vary, although all Seventh-day Adventists avoid alcohol, tobacco, and recreational drugs, and some avoid caffeine. Vegetarianism is preferred and is common, and those who eat meat avoid pork, offal, and shellfish.

Dress

Conventional dress.

Medical treatment

There are no specific issues relating to examination or treatment.

Daily observance

Seventh-day Adventists mark the Sabbath from sunset on Friday to sunset on Saturday. During this time, secular work and recreation (e.g. competitive sport) are avoided.

Death and dying

The presence of an Adventist priest is preferred, but if this is not possible, a Christian priest from another denomination is acceptable. Bodies can be cremated or buried. Post-mortem examination is permitted.

Jehovah's Witnesses

Jehovah's Witnesses reject the Holy Trinity, predetermined immortality (believing in true immortality for a limited number), and the existence of Hell as well as festivals which they believe have pagan origins such as Christmas. Social interaction with non-Witnesses is generally limited. There have been a number of so-far unfulfilled predictions of the end of the World and the coming of Christ.

Language
Normally English.

Diet
There are no dietary restrictions other than avoidance of foods containing blood or blood products. Some Jehovah's Witnesses are vegetarian.

Dress
Conventional Western dress.

Medical treatment
Jehovah's Witnesses doctrine objects to allogenic blood transfusion and Jehovah's witnesses may carry an advanced directive that they are not to be given blood or its components—red cells, white cells, platelets, and plasma. However, the refusal of blood products is not universal amongst Jehovah's Witnesses and the beliefs of each individual should be established. Jehovah's Witnesses in the UK have established a series of hospital liaison committees to advise in these circumstances as the doctrinal rules are complex and some products (including factor VIII and globulins) and procedures may be permitted. The decision of parents to refuse transfusion on behalf of a child may in appropriate circumstances be overruled by a court.

Daily observance
Daily Bible reading.

Death and dying
A pastoral visit from a church elder is usually welcomed. Post-mortems are permitted and bodies may be either buried or cremated.

Rastafarianism

The Rastafari movement, like Christianity, Judaism, and Islam, is an Abrahamic religion which began in Jamaica in the 1930s. Rastafarians worship Haile Selassie I, Emperor of Ethiopia from 1930 to 1974. Members are known as Rastas, or the Rastafari, and dislike the term Rastafarianism, although it is widely used. The Rastafari share many Jewish and Christian beliefs and accept the existence of a single God who sent his son to Earth as Jesus and manifested again as Haile Selassie I.

Language
English with Jamaican patois.

Diet
Most Rastafari are vegetarian, some will eat certain types of fish. They avoid alcohol, tea, and coffee.

Dress
Cutting the hair is forbidden and it is worn as dreadlocks. If hair needs to be removed for medical reasons, this should be discussed where possible with patients. Some Rastafari men wear hats, and women headscarves.

Medical treatment
There are no restrictions regarding physical contact or to medical procedures of any kind.

Daily observance
There are no set daily religious rituals.

Death and dying
There are no set rituals associated with death and dying.

Judaism

Language
English with some Hebrew and Yiddish (an essentially German-based language with Hebrew script and the traditional language of Ashkenazi Jews).

Diet
Greater and lesser degrees of observance are found, but Jews do not eat pork or game and shellfish is not permitted. Red meat and poultry must be Kosher. Milk products are not eaten during or immediately after a meal.

Dress
Devout Jews keep their head covered, men with a skull cap (*kippah*) and women with a hat, scarf, or wig. Strictly orthodox men dress in black, often in an old-fashioned manner, and may wear ringlets and beards.

Medical treatment
The very orthodox avoid any contact with the opposite sex outside marriage. Procedures such as blood transfusion are normally accepted, although the very orthodox may object to transplantation.

Daily observance
Prayers are said three times a day.

Death and dying
Someone will normally stay with the individual until death, reading or saying prayers. The individual may also recite prayers and should not be touched or moved as it is believed this may hasten death. After death, the eyes are closed and the jaw tied. Following washing, the body is wrapped in a white sheet and placed feet towards the door, with, in the case of men, a prayer shawl with the corner fringes removed wrapped around the body. Ideally the body should not be left alone. Members of the community will arrange the funeral which should occur if possible before sunset on the day of death. Bodies are not moved on the Sabbath. Orthodox Jews require burial, reform and liberal Jews permit cremation. Orthodox Jews object to post-mortem examination, although this would be overridden if there are legal reasons for such an examination.

Islam

Muslims believe in one God and Islam is an Abrahamic faith based on the *Qur'an*, which is believed by Muslims to be the literal word of God. Muslims believe Muhammad to be the last prophet and thus that Islam is the completed version of a faith that was revealed previously by prophets including Abraham and Jesus. The Qur'an is therefore the final revelation of God. Islamic law affects many aspects of life including finance, family life, and the community. Most Muslims are either Sunni or Shia.

Language
Many languages including Arabic, Turkish, Punjabi, and Urdu.

Diet
Muslims do not eat pork or food that has been prepared with utensils that have touched pork. Muslims may eat fish and poultry, beef, or lamb as long as it is Halal. Alcohol is forbidden.

Dress
Western or traditional dress may be worn, women will usually at least keep their head covered. More orthodox Muslims may wear more complete covering.

Medical treatment
Where possible, patients should be treated by clinicians of the same sex. Blood transfusion is permitted, but some Muslims object on religious grounds to transplantation.

Daily observance
Muslims pray facing Mecca five times each day. Pre-prayer washing facilities (*wudu*) should be available and men and women do not pray together.

Death and dying
A dying Muslim should be turned to face Mecca with their head raised above their body. Males should prepare male bodies and females, female bodies. They may say the testimony of faith. Ideally, after a major incident, Muslim bodies should be kept together and males separate from females. The body is covered with cloth and the head turned to the right shoulder, the face towards Mecca. Bodies are buried, ideally within 24 hours of death. Postmortem examination is forbidden, but may be carried out if the law demands it.

Hinduism

Hinduism is an ancient polytheistic religion from the Indian subcontinent with many different schools or sects. Hindu practices include daily rituals such as *puja* (worship) and recitations, annual festivals, and pilgrimages. The most important scriptures include the *Vedas, Upanishads Mahabharata, Ramayana, Bhagavad Gita,* and *Puranas.*

Language
Guajarati, Tamil, Hindi, Punjabi, and other languages from the Indian subcontinent as well as English.

Diet
Hindus do not eat beef and orthodox Hindus are strictly vegetarian, avoiding fish, eggs, and animal fat for cooking. Very orthodox Hindus may avoid garlic or onions. Many Hindus do not drink alcohol. One-day fasts are common.

Dress
Men normally wear Western dress, but may wear a loose shirt and baggy trousers. Women normally wear a sari or dress and baggy trousers.

Medical treatment
Hindus prefer to be treated by a clinician of the same sex, all treatments are permitted.

Daily observance
Most Hindus will perform an act of devotion each day in their own home.

Death and dying
Prayer with a rosary is helpful, as is the presence of someone of their own sex. Where there is more than one Hindu body, if possible they should be kept together. Post-mortem examination is permitted, although many Hindus dislike the idea. The arms of a body are placed at the side, the legs straightened, and the body washed and covered in white cloth, the head facing north, feet south, eyes closed, face pointing upward. Bereavement rituals last at least 2 weeks following which the body is cremated, unless it is a child who will normally be buried.

Sikhism

Sikhism is a monotheistic religion founded in the 15th century by Guru Nanak and developed by successive Sikh Gurus. The *Guru Granth Sahib* is a collection of the Sikh Gurus' writings.

Language
Mainly Punjabi and English.

Diet
Devout Sikhs are vegetarian (they do not eat eggs) and avoid alcohol (except in medication), tobacco, and recreational drugs. Those who eat meat avoid beef and meat killed according to ritual (Halal and Kosher meat). Some Sikhs avoid pork.

Dress
Male Sikhs wear a turban and five ritual items (the five Ks): *kes* (uncut hair), *kangha* (a small wooden comb), *kara* (a steel bracelet), *kirpan* (a short dagger), and *kachhera* (a special undergarment for the more devout, conventional underwear for the majority in the UK). Women wear the five items and may cover their hair with a scarf.

Medical treatment
Treatment by members of the same sex is preferred. There are no restrictions regarding medical interventions. The kachhera should ideally only be removed by the wearer. All five ritual items should be nearby.

Daily observance
Sikhs must shower or bath daily especially before dawn prayers. Prayers are also said at sunset and when going to bed.

Death and dying
The dying will require access to Sikh scriptures. After death, the five Ks are left on the body which is cleaned and dressed. Contact by a member of the opposite sex should be avoided unless closely related. There is no objection to post-mortem and disposal is by cremation.

Jainism

Jainism is an Indian religion that prescribes a path of non-violence towards all living things. Other key tenets of Jainism include truthfulness, non-materialism, chastity and tolerance. Asceticism is a major focus of the Jains.

Language

Most UK Jains speak English; a minority only understand Gujarati (most common), Hindi, Tamil, Punjabi, or other Indian subcontinent languages.

Diet

Jains are strict vegetarians and do not eat meat, fish, seafood, poultry, or eggs. Most Jains drink milk, but some refuse cheese or butter. Some Jains also avoid root vegetables especially onions and garlic and veganism is common. Most Jains do not drink alcohol and tobacco is forbidden.

Dress

Most male Jains wear Western dress. Women may wear traditional Asian or Western dress.

Medical treatment

Jains prefer to avoid contact with the opposite sex, although this is not mandatory with medical staff. Separate-sex accommodation is preferred. Both blood transfusion and organ transplantation are acceptable.

Daily observance

Jains follow a formal sequence of prayers throughout the day.

Death and dying

Bodies are always cremated (except for infants). Cremation must take place as soon as possible after death, ideally within hours. The family will normally prepare the body.

Zoroastrianism (Parsees)

Zoroastrianism is an ancient monotheistic religion originating in Iran. Zoroastrians believe that there is one god, Ahura Mazda, and participation in good deeds is necessary to ensure happiness.

Language

The majority of UK Zoroastrians (Zarathustrians) speak English. Other languages include Gujarati, Persian, and Farsi.

Diet

There are no specific dietary requirements.

Dress

Zoroastrians wear Western dress with traditional dress for ceremonies. A muslin vest called a *sudra* is worn which should be changed daily and only removed for medical reasons. Zoroastrians also wear a *kusti* (girdle) around the waist.

Medical treatment

There are no issues with any form of medical intervention.

Daily observance

Zoroastrians pray each day, and may cover their head to do so.

Death and dying

Traditionally Zoroastrians followed the practice of ritual exposure, most commonly identified with the so-called *Towers of Silence*. This now only occurs on the Indian subcontinent. In the UK, Zoroastrian communities either cremate or bury the dead in graves that are cased with lime mortar. There is no objection to post-mortem examination.

Buddhism

Buddhism is a non-theistic religion based on teachings attributed to Siddhartha Gautama, the Buddha. The ultimate goal of Buddhism is the attainment of the state of *Nirvana*.

Language
English, Tibetan, Cantonese, Hakka, Japanese, Thai, and Sinhalese.

Diet
Buddhists are often vegetarian, although they will eat eggs or fish. Some refrain from garlic and onions.

Dress
There is no dress requirement for lay Buddhists, although some monks may wear robes and shave their heads.

Medical treatment
There are no issues and all medical practices are accepted. Patients may be touched by medical staff of either sex.

Daily observance
Buddhists meditate rather than pray.

Death and dying
Buddhists may refuse strong analgesia if these impair mental alertness. A monk may be asked to perform some chanting of sacred texts before death. There is no objection to post-mortem examination; relatives may wish to be involved in preparation of the body which is usually cremated either dressed in its own cloths or wrapped in white cloth. There are no restrictions regarding timing of cremation.

Bahá'í Faith

The Bahá'í Faith is a religion with three core principles: that there is only one God, that all major religions have the same spiritual source and originate from the same God, and that all humans have been created equal.

Language
English, although the elderly from the Middle East may speak very little English.

Diet
No special dietary requirements.

Dress
There are no special requirements other than moderation and modesty.

Medical treatment
No special requirements. There is no objection to being touched or treated by members of the opposite sex. Blood transfusion is acceptable. There is no objection to mixed wards, but older Bahá'ís may prefer single-sex wards.

Daily observance
Every Bahá'í aged 15 years and over must recite daily one of three obligatory prayers each day, as well as reading a passage from the Bahá'í scriptures each morning and evening. Prayers are said privately and facing the '*Point of Adoration*' (the Shrine of Bahá'u'lláh, roughly south east from the UK). Before reciting the prayers, Bahá'ís wash their hands and face, but ablutions do not require special facilities.

Death and dying
There are no special religious requirements for Bahá'ís who are dying, but they may wish to have a family member or friend to pray and read the Bahá'í scriptures with them. After death, the body is washed and wrapped in white silk or cotton and a special burial ring may be placed on the finger of a Bahá'í aged 15 or over. Bodies are not cremated or embalmed but buried within an hour's travelling time from the place of death. Prayers for the dead are recited for Bahá'ís aged 15 or over.

Chinese faiths (including Confucianism and Taoism)

Many members of the UK Chinese community do not profess any faith and a significant number are Christian. Taoism is an ancient Chinese philosophy with a unifying impersonal God.

Language
English and Chinese dialects including Cantonese and Mandarin.

Diet
No generally applicable special dietary requirements. Chinese food should be offered where possible and the Chinese community will assist with this. Some Taoists are vegetarian.

Dress
Western dress sometimes including trousers and loose tops.

Medical treatment
Ideally, women will be treated and nursed by females and single-sex wards are preferred.

Daily observance
Regular prayer within the appropriate community.

Death and dying
The family will wish to be present and a priest may be called. Bodies may be buried or cremated, usually within a week of death. There is no objection to post-mortem examination.

Shinto

Shinto, which means 'the way of the gods' is the largest religion in Japan, practised by nearly 80% of the population. It was founded in 660 BC and was originally a diverse collection of local beliefs. Today, Shinto is a term that applies to the religion of public shrines devoted to the worship of many different gods.

Language
Most UK adherents of Shintoism speak both Japanese and English.

Diet
There are no dietary restrictions although the diet is based on rice rather than Western carbohydrates.

Dress
Western dress is worn with occasional traditional Japanese dress for festivals.

Medical treatment
There are no religious objections to any medical interventions including blood transfusion.

Daily observance
Some followers of Shinto will carry out Buddhist meditation.

Death and dying
Dying followers of Shintoism will wish to meditate. Cremation after a Buddhist funeral rite is preferred.

Paganism

There are many pagan religions of which the most significant in the UK are the *modern pagan religions*. Pagans are generally, but not invariably, polytheistic. Broadly, the term pagan simply applies to polytheistic non-Abrahamic religions. Modern paganism, also known as *contemporary paganism* and *neo-paganism*, includes religions which are influenced by, or claim to have origins in, early historical pagan beliefs. The pagan religions cover a very broad range of such beliefs. Common features include polytheism, animism (believing that animals, plants, and objects have a spiritual essence), and pantheism (believing that nature and divinity are the same).

Language
English.

Diet
Many pagans are vegetarian but this is often a feature of their world view rather than religion per se.

Dress
Normally, conventional Western dress. Ceremonial jewellery may be worn when appropriate. Some pagans wear a symbolic ring.

Medical treatment
The are no restraints on physical contact or medical treatment.

Daily observance
Many pagans will have a shrine or other place for religious observance and will pray when they wish to do so. Group celebrations are likely to occur on festival days usually based on the lunar calendar.

Death and dying
Disposal is by burial or cremation. There is no objection to post-mortem.

Humanism

Humanism is not simply the absence of faith, although humanists do not accept the existence of a deity or an afterlife. They believe in moral behaviour arising out of human nature as well as rational analysis and critical thinking.

Language
English.

Diet
No specific dietary requirements.

Dress
No specific dress requirements.

Medical treatment
There are no restrictions on medical treatment or human contact.

Daily observance
None.

Death and dying
Cremation is more common than burial. Post-mortems are permitted. Rites may follow the wishes of the bereaved rather than the deceased and be celebratory rather than commemoratory. Prayers and religious symbols should be avoided.

Index